Immunological Methods

VOLUME II

Immunological Methods

VOLUME II

EDITED BY

IVAN LEFKOVITS

The Basel Institute for Immunology
Basel, Switzerland

BENVENUTO PERNIS

Health Sciences Center
Columbia University
New York, New York

1981

ACADEMIC PRESS
A Subsidiary of Harcourt Brace Jovanovich, Publishers
New York   London   Toronto   Sydney   San Francisco

599.029
I 33
V. 2

ACADEMIC PRESS, INC.
111 Fifth Avenue, New York, New York 10003

United Kingdom Edition published by
ACADEMIC PRESS, INC. (LONDON) LTD.
24/28 Oval Road, London NW1 7DX

Library of Congress Cataloging in Publication Data
Main entry under title:

Immunological methods.

    Includes bibliographies and indexes.
    1. Immunology--Laboratory manuals. 2. Immunology,
Experimental. I. Lefkovits, Ivan. II. Pernis,
Benvenuto. [DNLM: 1. Immunologic technics. QW 525
I324 1979]
QR183.I43   599.02'9'028   78-3342
ISBN 0-12-442702-2 (v. 2)

Contents

1 Determination of Equilibrium Binding Parameters of Monoclonal Antibodies Specific for Cell Surface Antigens

Massimo Trucco and Stefanello de Petris

2 Biochemical Characterization of Cell Surface Antigens Using Monoclonal Antibodies

Béla J. Takács and Theophil Staehelin

17 The Technique of Hybridoma Production

Georges Köhler

18 Enzyme Immunoassay for the Detection of Hybridoma Products

John W. Stocker, Fabio Malavasi, and Massimo Trucco

List of Contributors

Numbers in parentheses indicate the pages on which the authors' contributions begin. Affiliations listed are current. All but the authors whose names are preceded by an asterisk are or were at The Basel Institute for Immunology, Basel, Switzerland, at the time the chapters were written.

Lucien A. Aarden (75), Department of Autoimmune Diseases, Central Laboratory of the Netherlands, Red Cross Blood Transfusion Service, 1006AD Amsterdam, The Netherlands

Vernon L. Alvarez (83), The Basel Institute for Immunology, Basel, Switzerland

Andrei A. Augustin (213), Department of Microbiology, Columbia University, College of Physicians and Surgeons, New York, New York 10032

Robbert Benner (247), Department of Cell Biology and Genetics, Erasmus University, 3000 DR Rotterdam, The Netherlands

Rosa R. Bernabé (187), The Basel Institute for Immunology, Basel, Switzerland

Salvatore Cammisuli (139), Pharmaceutical Division, Preclinical Research, Sandoz Ltd., Basel, Switzerland

António Coutinho (187, 213), Department of Immunology, Umeå University, 90185 Umeå, Sweden

Stefanello de Petris (1), Tumor Immunology Unit, Department of Zoology, University College London, London WC1E 6BT, England

C. Garrison Fathman (277), Mayo Clinic, Department of Immunology, Rochester, Minnesota 55901

Luciana Forni (187), The Basel Institute for Immunology, Basel, Switzerland

Gianni Garotta (163), Cattedra di Immunologia, Università di Milano, Milano, Italy

Donald F. Gerson (105), The Basel Institute for Immunology, Basel, Switzerland

Hans Hengartner (277), Experimentelle Pathologie, Universität Zürich, 8032 Zürich, Switzerland

Ole Henriksen (83), The Basel Institute for Immunology, Basel, Switzerland

* *Dan Holmberg* (187), Department of Immunology, Umeå University, 90185 Umeå, Sweden

Sarah Howie (199), Department of Microbiology, Edinburgh University Medical School, Edinburgh EH8 9AG, Scotland

* *Fredrick Ivars* (187), Department of Immunology, Umeå University, 90185 Umeå, Sweden

* *Guus Koch* (247), Department of Cell Biology and Genetics, Erasmus University, 3000 DR Rotterdam, The Netherlands

Georges Köhler (285), The Basel Institute for Immunology, Basel, Switzerland

Jean Langhorne (221), The Basel Institute for Immunology, Basel, Switzerland

Kirsten Fischer Lindahl (221), The Basel Institute for Immunology, Basel, Switzerland

Alma L. Luzzati (241), Laboratorio di Biologia Cellulare e Immunologia, Istituto Superiore di Sanita, Rome, Italy

* *Fabio Malavasi* (299), Istituto di Genetica Medica, Università di Torino, Torino, Italy

Carlos Martinez-A. (187, 213), The Basel Institute for Immunology, Basel, Switzerland

Tauro M. Neri (163), The Basel Institute for Immunology, Basel, Switzerland

* *Adrianus van Oudenaren* (247), Department of Cell Biology and Genetics, Erasmus University, 3000 DR Rotterdam, The Netherlands

Carolyn A. Roitsch (83), The Basel Institute for Immunology, Basel, Switzerland

Max H. Schreier (263), The Basel Institute for Immunology, Basel, Switzerland

Charles Sidman (57), The Basel Institute for Immunology, Basel, Switzerland

* *Ruud Smeenk* (75), Department of Autoimmune Diseases, Central Laboratory of the Netherlands, Red Cross Blood Transfusion Service, 1006 AD Amsterdam, The Netherlands

Theophil Staehelin (27), Hoffmann-La Roche, Inc., 4002 Basel, Switzerland

John W. Stocker (299), Hoffmann-La Roche, Inc., 4002 Basel, Switzerland

Béla J. Takács (27), Hoffmann-La Roche, Inc., 4002 Basel, Switzerland

Reet Tees (263), The Basel Institute for Immunology, Basel, Switzerland

Massimo Trucco (1, 299), The Wistar Institute, Philadelphia, Pennsylvania 19104

Margaretha Tuneskog (187), Department of Immunology, Umeå University, 90185 Umeå, Sweden

Preface

The development of research methodology suited to its special needs has been a major factor in propelling immunology to its present unique position among the biological sciences. Impressive as is the record of this timely emergence of methodology, ever newer and more innovative research methods continue to evolve.

Dissemination of this newer, changing methodology is at best an uncertain, diffuse affair. Eventually most of it appears in one form or another in the traditional experimental journals, but at the time of their inception the details of individual methods, their potential, and, thus, limitations are to a large extent communicated informally by personal contact. It is in this latter context that investigators at The Basel Institute, operating in the "hot-spots" of immunology, play an important role in that they constitute a lively, critical, interacting environment with associations that favor the verification, refinement, and consolidation of novel experimental procedures. In this respect The Basel Institute has become a kind of proving ground and clearing house for experimental design, probes, and approaches to coping with basic biologic issues. It is our aim to have these volumes, insofar as possible, reflect the methodologic advances that emerge from this informal, spontaneous, sorting-out process.

In the preceding volume a selected group of procedures was assembled with a view toward representation of diverse applications and areas of wide interest for most immunology laboratories. Our original concept, to which we remain committed, was to publish methods that were judged timely, compelling, or especially useful. In this sense, it was intended that volumes subsequent to the first one would *supplement* it rather than *supercede* it. This then is the first of such follow-up volumes, which are intended to provide a timely, fresh, updated assemblage of procedures judged especially appropriate for contemporary studies in immunology. It is not intended to seek a balance in such collections. Rather, it seems more appropriate to have each collection reflect the kind of activities prevailing at the time.

Such an ambitious projection of our intent might seem unduly optimistic were it not for the fact that The Basel Institute for Immunology has functioned so far as an international center for both young and established investigators from all over the world. It has become agreeably evident that visitors and staff as well continue generously to share, via these volumes, their methodologic knowledge and experience with colleagues everywhere.

Ivan Lefkovits
Benvenuto Pernis

Contents of Volume I

Abbreviations List

ACD	acid citrate dextrose
AET	2-aminoethylisothiouronium
ars	arsanilic acid
BBS	borate-buffered saline
BRC	bovine erythrocyte
BSA	bovine serum albumin
BSS	balanced salt solution
CBRC	coupled bovine erythrocytes
CFA	complete Freund's adjuvant
CGG	chicken gamma globulin
C-Ig	cytoplasmic Ig-containing
CMC	critical micelle concentration
CML	cell-mediated lysis
Con A	concanavalin A
CSE	charge shift electrophoresis
CTAB	cetyltrimethyl ammonium bromide
CTL	cytotoxic T lymphocyte
CTL-P	cytotoxic T lymphocyte precursor cell
DBSS	Dulbecco's balanced salt solution
DEAE	diethylaminoethyl
DHB	methyl-3,5-dihydroxybenzimidate
DMEM	Dulbecco's modified Eagle's medium
DMF	dimethyl formamide
DNP	dinitrophenyl
DOC	deoxycholate
EB	Epstein–Barr
EIA	enzyme immunoassay
E-RFC	E-rosette-forming T lymphocytes
EWB	egg white buffer
FA	fluorescent antibody
FBS	fetal bovine serum
FCS	fetal calf serum
FDA	fluorescein diacetate

FITC	fluorescein isothiocyanate
gal	galactoside
glu	*p*-aminophenylglucoside
GPC	gel permeation chromatography
HAT	hypoxanthine-aminopterinthymidine
HB	hepatitis B antigen
HEPES	*N*-2-hydroxyethylpiperazine-*N*¹-2-ethanesulfonic acid
HLB	hydrophile–lipophile balance
HPGPC	high-pressure gel permeation chromatography
HPLC	high-performance liquid chromatography
HRC	horse erythrocyte
HSL	hapten sandwich labeling
HT	hypoxanthine–thymidine
Ia	immune-associated
IEF	isoelectrofocusing
IFT	immunofluorescence technique
Ig	immunoglobulin
IgG	immunoglobulin G
IL–2	interleukin 2
IMDM	Iscove's modified Dulbecco's medium
IMDM–ATL	IMDM supplemented with albumin, transferrin, and lipids
KLH	Keyhole limpet hemocyanin
lac	*p*-aminophenyllactoside
LCH	*Lens culinaris* hemagglutinin
LPS	lipopolysaccharide
LSM	lymphocyte separation medium
MAR	monoclonal antibody-rosetting
ME	2-mercaptoethanol
MEM	minimal essential medium
MHC	major histocompatibility complex
MLC	mixed lymphocyte culture
MLR	mixed lymphocyte reaction
moi	multiplicity of infection
NCI	National Cancer Institute
NEPHGE	nonequilibrium pH gradient electrophoresis
NIH	National Institutes of Health
NP40	Nonidet P–40
N–SRBC	neuraminidase-treated sheep red blood cell
PBL	peripheral blood lymphocyte
PBS	phosphate-buffered saline
PEG	polyethylene glycol

PFC	plaque-forming cell
PFU	plaque-forming unit
PHA–P	phytohemagglutinin P
PMSF	phenylmethyl sulfonyl fluoride
PRS	primed responder cell
P–SRBC	papain-treated sheep red blood cell
RFC	rosette forming cells
RIA	radioimmunoassay
SDS–PAGE	sodium dodecyl sulfate–polyacrylamide gel
SLE	systemic lupus erythematosus/electrophoresis
SmIg	surface membrane immunoglobulin
SP	3-(p-sulfophenyldiazo)-4-hydroxyphenyl
SPA	*Staphylococcus aureus* protein A
SRBC	sheep red blood cells
SRC	sheep erythrocyte
TCA	trichloroacetic acid
TCGF	T cell growth factor
TD	thymus-dependent
TEMED	*N,N,N′,N′*-tetramethylethylenediamine
TNBS	2,4,6-trinitrobenzene sulfonic acid
TNP	trinitrophenyl
TNP–SRBC	trinitrophenyl-conjugated sheep red blood cell
Tris	Tris(hydroxymethyl)aminomethane

1

Determination of Equilibrium Binding Parameters of Monoclonal Antibodies Specific for Cell Surface Antigens

Massimo Trucco and Stefanello de Petris

I. INTRODUCTION

Individuals of a given species respond to the inoculation of a foreign substance by producing several different antibodies able to recognize this "nonself" antigen. Also, in the case of an extremely simple and almost

IMMUNOLOGICAL METHODS, VOL. II

completely homogeneous antigen (e.g., a chemical hapten), at least 5–10 different antibodies carrying the same specificity are found in the serum of the recipient and they are considered a random sample of the total antibody repertoire peculiar to that species (Shulman and Köhler, 1979). The heterogeneity of the antibody population, specific for the same antigenic determinant, is a severe limiting factor in evaluating the affinity of these antibodies for the antigen (see, for example, Fazekas de St. Groth, 1979). Dealing with a heterogeneous antibody population only allows estimation of a mean value for the different antibody affinities; these values are likely to differ in reactions where the same antigen but a different serum is used. These difficulties can be minimized if monoclonal antibodies against a specific antigen are available. Determination of the precise characteristics of binding may be of particular interest when the antibody is directed against a cellular antigen, precisely a surface antigen, as in this case the reaction may have important functional significance. Moreover, the data may provide useful information for understanding the characteristics of chemical reactions at the cell surface.

Köhler and Milstein (1975) obtained the first evidence that the production of monoclonal antibodies with a desired specificity was possible. In our laboratory several monoclonal antibodies against human lymphocyte surface antigens have been prepared (Trucco *et al.*, 1979). By taking advantage of the homogeneous nature of monoclonal antibodies, it is possible to obtain an accurate estimate of several thermodynamic parameters of the antigen–antibody reaction. When the reaction is between monoclonal antibodies and target determinants present on a complex multivalent antigen (e.g., a cell), a quantitative determination of the number of such determinants per single carrying unit is also possible.

We describe here a simple method which allows precise calculation of these quantities. A general treatment of the theoretical and experimental aspects of the determination of the parameters defining antigen–antibody reactions at equilibrium has been presented in the first volume of this series (Fazekas de St. Groth, 1979). The determination of these parameters in the reaction of a monoclonal antibody with a cell surface antigen represents another example of these techniques. The experimental procedure used in the determinations reported here follows that generally used in studying the binding of antibodies, lectins, and other ligands to cell surface components and differs somewhat from the methods previously described. Some of the problems of interpretation of the experimental data, which arise when the antigen is a plasma membrane molecule, are discussed in Section V.

II. THEORETICAL BACKGROUND

The data are analyzed on the assumption that the binding of a bivalent monoclonal antibody to a cell surface antigen can be represented by a single-step bimolecular reaction:

$$[a] + [b] \underset{k_r}{\overset{k_f}{\rightleftharpoons}} [a \cdot b] \tag{1}$$

where k_f and k_r are the forward and reverse reaction rates, respectively.

If $[A]$ is the initial concentration of the antibody, $[B]$ that of the antigen reacting units (one unit being the quantity of antigen capable of binding to one antibody molecule), and $[AB] = [x]$ the concentration of the complex, i.e., the concentration of the bound antibody, at equilibrium we have

$$K = [x]/[A - x][B - x] \tag{2}$$

The equilibrium constant K is formally defined here as the ratio $K = k_f/k_r$ between the forward (k_f) and reverse (k_r) reaction rates in Eq. (1). With this definition, a high affinity of the antibody for the antigen corresponds to a high numerical value of K. If the concentrations of the reacting units are expressed in moles/liter (i.e., as molarity M), K is given in liters/mole (i.e., M^{-1}). If cgs units are used, concentrations are expressed in molecules/cm^3 and K in cm^3/molecule. As 1 mol contains $N = 6.023 \times 10^{23}$ molecules (Avogadro's number), $1 M = 6.023 \times 10^{20}$ molecules/cm^3 and numerically $K_{cgs} = K_M \times (1/6.023) \times 10^{-20}$.

Equation (2) can describe accurately the equilibrium of reactions between monovalent antibody and monovalent antigen (either in solution or cell-bound) or between divalent antibody and monovalent antigen in solution. It is also valid for the reaction of divalent antibody and divalent antigen in solution, provided the concentration of one of the two reagents is in excess (for example, so that the concentration of the complexes formed by antibody and antigen connected only through one of the binding sites can be neglected). The equation is not, in general, suitable for describing the binding of a divalent antibody to monovalent or divalent cell-bound antigens, as K would not be a constant independent of the concentration of the reagents (Section V). Its use in the case we are considering is justified, however, if certain conditions are satisfied. Some of the problems of interpretation which arise in this connection are discussed in Section V.

For practical use it is convenient to transform Eq. (2) into the linear form first used by Scatchard (1949). By multiplying both sides of Eq. (2) by $[B - x]$, we obtain

$$[x]/[A - x] = K[B] - K[x] \tag{3}$$

Provided it is possible to separate experimentally x (the molar concentration of bound antibody at equilibrium) from $A - x$ (the molar concentration of unbound antibody), K and B can be calculated from the parameters of the line obtained by plotting $x/(A - x)$ versus x. K is the slope of the line, while B is the value of the intercept of the line with the x axis. B is an extrapolated value obtained when $x/(A - x) = 0$, namely, when $A \rightarrow \infty$. It corresponds to the maximum amount of antibody which can be bound to the cells in the unit volume under the conditions of the experiment, and therefore to the concentration of the antigenic units. If the concentration $[b]$ of cells/cm^3 is known, the average number n of antigenic units per cell can be obtained from the relationship $[B] = n[b]$. As b is usually given in number of cells/cm^3 (a cell can be considered equivalent to a "molecule" of valency n) B must also be expressed in number of molecules/cm^3.

If both sides of Eq. (3) are divided by $[b]$, we obtain

$$([x]/[A - x])\,(1/[b]) = K([B]/[b]) - K([x]/[b]) \tag{3a}$$

In this equation $[x]/[b]$, a ratio of two concentrations, is a dimensionless number which we indicate by r and which represents the actual number of antibody molecules bound per cell. Equation (3a) becomes

$$r/[A - x] = Kn - Kr \tag{4}$$

where each term has the dimensions of [concentration]$^{-1}$. Thus, if $r/[A - x]$ is expressed in M^{-1}, K will be in the same units, whereas r and n will be numbers. Here n is the value of r at the intercept of the line with the x axis. [Equation (3) is equivalent to Eq. (lla) in the article by Fazekas de St. Groth (1979) in the first volume of this series. Using the notation $x = \alpha B$ (where α is the fraction of antibody A bound to the cells), $B = bn$, and an equilibrium constant defined as $K^* = k_r/k_f = 1/K$, Eq. (3) can in fact be written as $\alpha/(1 - \alpha) = nb/K^* - (A/K^*)\alpha$.

The experimental data can be plotted according to either Eq. (3) or Eq. (4). Although the use of Eq. (3) is more straightforward, for illustrative purposes the representation in Eq. (4) has the advantage that the value of n

can be read directly on the graph of $r/[A - x]$ versus r. In the examples given in this chapter we will use the latter form.

III. TECHNICAL APPROACH

In the following examples we will consider reactions between murine monoclonal antibodies and cell surface antigens of human lymphocytes. The treatment is of more general application, as it has been used by several authors to study the equilibrium binding of antibodies and lectins to cells in suspension.

A. The Antigen

Target cell populations must be as homogeneous as possible, so that in the same population the surface area and the number of determinants per cell, and therefore (as theoretically more important; see Section V) the density of receptors on the cell surface, can be assumed to be constant. Cloning, standardization of culture conditions and harvesting time, and removal of dead cells on a dense layer of Ficoll–Isopaque (density 1.094) are useful in reducing heterogeneity. An accurate enrichment in B or T cells reduces the "natural" heterogeneity of the peripheral blood lymphocytes or of splenocytes or lymph node cells. Thymocytes or erythrocytes form more homogeneous populations. Homogeneity among different cell preparations should be taken into consideration when the results from different experiments are compared.

B. Monoclonal Antibodies

1. Production

Hybridization between myeloma and spleen cells from immunized animals has been shown to be a successful tool in the derivation of cell lines producing antibodies of predefined specificity (Köhler and Milstein, 1975). Soft agar cloning makes it possible to obtain cell cultures secreting a specific and strictly homogeneous population of immunoglobulins (Ig's)—monoclonal antibodies. While the monoclonality is generally supported by isoelectric focusing analysis of L-[^{14}C]leucine biosynthetically labeled products (Cotton *et al.,* 1973), sodium dodecyl sulfate-polyacrylamide gel electrophoresis (SDS–PAGE) (Laemmli, 1970) (Figs. 1 and 2) is the best tool for evaluating the composition of the secreted Ig's.

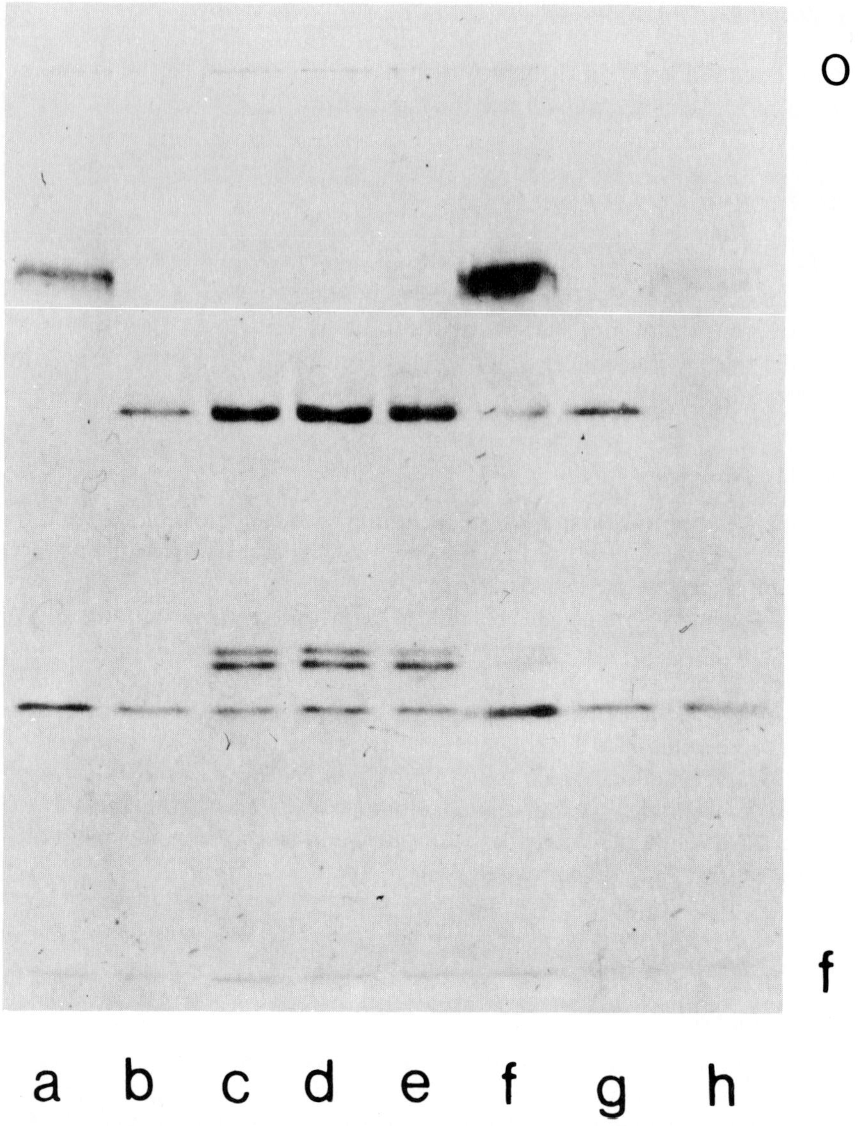

Fig. 1. Sodium dodecyl sulfate polyacrylamide gel electrophoresis (SDS–PAGE) autoradiograph of L-[^{14}C]leucine biosynthetically labeled antibodies from culture supernatants. Slots b and g contain, as a marker, myeloma protein of the P3/X63.Ag8 line (IgG γ_1, $\varkappa$) from which the NS1/1–Ag4–1 mutant used for the fusion was derived. In slot f are proteins produced by a primary culture which contain (from top to bottom) μ and γ heavy chains and two different $\varkappa$ light chains (one of latter is further split into two bands, probably because of different glycosylation). Slots a and h contain proteins produced by two clones derived from the primary culture. They secrete only a μ chain and the light chain from the myeloma used for fusion. Slots c–e contain proteins secreted by three other different clones; they still secrete the myeloma light chain plus the γ_{2a}, $\varkappa$ Ig derived from the spleen. Only supernatants containing the γ_{2a}, $\varkappa$ Ig retained the specific antibody activity of the primary culture against the target. o, origin; f, front.

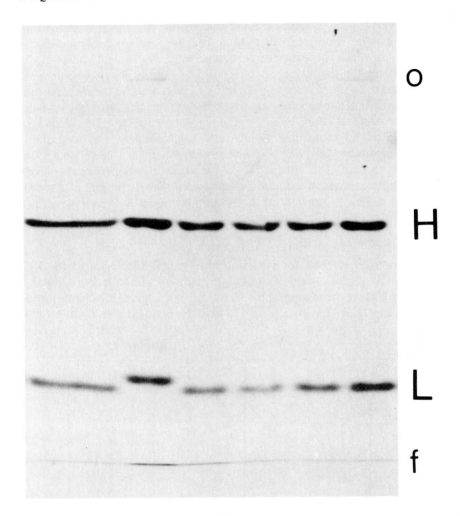

Fig. 2. Autoradiographs of SDS-PAGE representing Ig's in supernatants of repeatedly cloned cultures. Slot X contains as a marker P3/X63.Ag8γ_1, $\varkappa$ Ig, while all the other slots contain IgG's which have lost the myeloma $\varkappa$ light chain. H, heavy chain; L, light chain; o, origin; f, front. (From Trucco *et al.*, 1980.)

IgG's, regardless of subclass, are, in principle, the best reagents for binding experiments (as compared with IgM's), because they are divalent. An important drawback is the incidental presence of heavy or light chains of the myeloma used in the fusion, which drastically reduces the homogeneity of the reagent. Repeated cloning of hybrid cell lines and the use, as a partner in the fusion, of a nonproducing myeloma mutant, are two ways to overcome the problem (Figs. 1 and 2). Fluids from an ascites tumor secondary to hybrid cell lines implanted in mice may be contaminated by natural antibodies and other Ig's, and consequently they might not be suitable as an antibody source for this kind of experiment. Supernatants from monoclonal cultures in medium supplemented with 10% fetal calf serum deprived of Ig's by previous absorption on a protein A–Sepharose gel are the best source of pure antibodies (Fig. 3).

2. Purification

The simplest method for purifying monoclonal antibodies of the IgG class is by *Staphylococcus aureus*-Protein A (Pharmacia, Uppsala, Sweden) affinity chromatography. Practically all mouse IgG's bind to protein A at pH 8 (Ey *et al.*, 1978); acid elution from a 6-ml protein

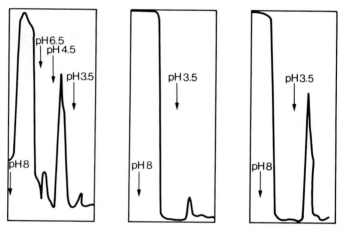

Fig. 3. All mouse IgG's are retained by the protein A-Sepharose 4B column at pH 8. γ_1 is generally eluted at pH 6, γ_{2a} at pH 4.5, and γ_{2b} at pH 3 (Ey *et al.*, 1978). (Left) Elution peaks of the IgG's contained in the fluid from an ascites tumor secondary to hybrid cell lines implanted in mice. (Middle) Elution peak of the IgG's present in 50 ml of fetal calf serum (FCS). 50 ml of FCS is approximately the quantity of FCS used to supplement 300 ml of culture medium. (Right) Elution peak of specific antibody obtained from 300 ml of supernatant fluid supplemented with FCS deprived of bovine IgG's. From 300 ml of supernatant 7–10 mg of pure antibody can generally be obtained.

A–Sepharose 4B column by 0.1 M acetic acid buffer, pH 3.5, allows recovery of about 10–15 mg of a specific Ig from 300 ml of supernatant fluid (see Fig. 3). Before chromatography the column must be cleaned by equilibration and washing with the acid buffer used for elution and re-equilibrated at pH 8.0 with 0.15 M phosphate-buffer at room temperature. The antibody-containing fractions are collected in tubes containing a few drops of 1 M Tris-HCl buffer, pH 8.5, to neutralize the acetic acid buffer instantly. After overnight dialysis against 0.15 M PBS, pH 7.2, the antibody suspension is concentrated to 2–5 mg/ml. The samples are kept in 0.01% NaN$_3$ at 4°C and are active for at least 1 yr. The eluted proteins are quantitated by nitrogen determination following a Lowry modified method (Lowry *et al.*, 1951) (see Appendix A).

3. Radiolabeling

Radioiodination by either the chloramine-T (Greenwood *et al.*, 1963) or the Bolton and Hunter (1972) labeling technique can be used (see Appendixes B and C). With the antibodies used in the present studies only 15–20% of the labeled monoclonal antibodies after chloramine-T iodination were able to bind to the target cells at saturation (Fig. 4). It is possible

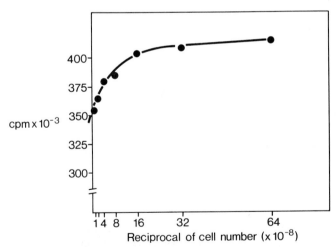

Fig. 4. Curve for the maximum uptake of target cells as determined by incubating a fixed amount of 125I-labeled anti-HLA, A + B + C antibody with increasing concentrations of cells in a 1-ml volume. The value of the maximum uptake after antibody radioiodination by the chloramine-T method (11) was mainly in the range of 15–20% of the input. In this particular example, by subtracting the maximum radioactivity contained in the supernatants after centrifugation of the target cells (350,000 cpm) from the input (441,438 cpm), we obtain a maximum value for the uptake equal to 91,400 cpm, corresponding to 20% of the nominal input.

that by modifying the conjugation conditions better yields could be obtained (Mason and Williams, 1980). Iodine substitution in critical tyrosine residues present at the combining site, or chemical damage due to exposure of the protein to both strong oxidizing or reducing agents during iodination are some of the possible causes of the lower uptake. Sometime loss of antibody efficiency after ^{125}I-labeling may be overcome by using the Bolton and Hunter conjugation method. The uptake of some of the antibodies on target cells reaches a maximum of 65–70% of the nominal input (Fig. 5), while other antibodies fail to work satisfactorily.

In our experience, [^{3}H]leucine biosynthetically labeled antibodies were not satisfactory. The problems due to the preparation of samples in liquid scintillation fluid, mandatory because of the β-ray emission, greatly decreased the reproducibility and precision of the test.

The maximum target uptake, ranging from 15–20% to 65–70% according to the iodination method, should be determined after labeling. These values are taken as 100% actual input for calculation of the binding parameters (Section IV). This assumes that the activity of labeled and unlabeled antibodies is the same after iodination. If this were not the case, some systematic error would be introduced in determination of the binding parameters (the product Kn would remain constant, but the values of n and

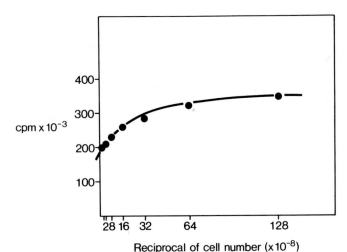

Fig. 5. Curve for the maximum uptake of target cells corresponding to that shown in Fig. 3 using a monoclonal antibody ^{125}I-radioiodinated by the Bolton and Hunter method. The maximum uptake using this method can reach values of about 65–70% of the nominal input. In the example shown the nominal input was 603,021 cpm; the graphically calculated maximum value of radioactivity remaining in the supernatant after centrifugation of target cells was 193,000 cpm. The difference, 410,000 cpm, corresponded to boundable antibody, equal to 68% of the nominal input.

r would be altered by a constant factor). Whenever feasible, the validity of the assumption should be tested by independent experiments.

C. Antigen/Antibody Ratios

An optimal range of concentrations of reactants must be chosen in order to determine the values of K and B (or n) with maximum precision. The criteria for the selection of this range have been discussed by Fazekas de St. Groth (1979). Ideally, the system should be far from saturation, i.e., with only a small fraction (say, not more than 10%) of the antigenic units occupied by the antibody, to avoid interactions between sites. Under the latter conditions, the binding can be generally represented by linear equations of the form of Eq. (3) or (4) (Section V). Moreover, in order to obtain significant differences between the measured quantities, a large fraction of the input should be bound ($[x] \geq 0.5[A]$). To satisfy these criteria, a fixed amount of antibody should be incubated with increasing concentrations of cells. This approach can be applied successfully when working with low antibody concentrations. However, in view of the uncertainties in the interpretation of data for binding antibody to cell membrane components (Section V), it is clearly advisable to perform measurements over a range of antibody concentrations as wide as possible. For intermediate and high antibody concentrations the above approach is not practical, especially when working with nucleated cells (in particular with large culture cells or with human peripheral blood lymphocytes), not only because too large a number of cells would be required for each experiment but also because the increased precision obtainable at higher cell concentrations is offset by increased variation and lower reproducibility. In practice this means that a concentration of 10^7 cells/ml cannot normally be exceeded, and this value is insufficient to satisfy the above criteria if the equilibrium constant is on the order of $10^8 \ M^{-1}$ (or less), as in most of the cases discussed here. [For example, if the bound antibody is to be $\geq 50\%$ of the input, namely, if $[x]/[A - x] \geq 1$, and if $K \simeq 10^8 \ M^{-1}$, we see from Eq. (2) that $[B - x]$ should be $\geq 10^{-8} \ M$ and therefore that $[B]$ should be $> 10^{-8} \ M$, however small the value of $[x]$. A system of 10^7 cells/ml each carrying 5×10^5 antigenic units corresponds to an antigen molarity of $(5 \times 10^5 \times 10^7)/(6.023 \times 10^{20}) = 0.9 \times 10^{-8} \ M$. The ideal cell concentration range for such cells would be 10^7 cells/ml and upward for each experimental point.]

The alternative procedure is to work with a fixed concentration of cells and decreasing concentrations of antibody. This procedure is applicable also with a relatively high antibody concentration and is the one normally followed in this type of measurement. A minor drawback is that generally $[x]$ is $\leq 0.5[A]$ (see Section IV). In principle a more serious disadvantage is the fact that a large fraction of the antigen determinants can be occupied at the highest antibody concentrations, although in the present case this did not affect the linearity of the binding curve (see also Section V). In our measurements cell concentration was typically 1 or 2 × 10^6 cells/ml. Samples containing more than 2–3 × 10^6 cells cannot be used when the separation of cells from the supernatant is carried out using Millipore filtration (Section III, E), as problems of clogging of the filter and incomplete separation can introduce large experimental errors.

The workable range of antibody concentrations, which depends on the value of K, must be determined in preliminary tests.

D. Performance of the Test

A suitable number of target cells is resuspended in McCoy's medium or PBS containing 0.1% bovine serum albumin (BSA) and the chosen antibody concentration. Then 5–20 × 10^5 cells are mixed with the labeled antibody in a final volume of 1 ml (if desired, smaller volumes, even on the order of 50–100 μl, can be used). The reaction is performed in Falcon tubes (No. 2051) which allow free mixing of the cells during the incubation on a shaker and easy handling of the material. The above-mentioned quantity of cells neither blocks the Millipore filter nor (for antibodies with K values on the order of 10^8 M^{-1}) requires a large quantity of iodinated antibody (Section IV). Usually the incubation time necessary to reach equilibrium is relatively short and does not exceed 2 hr even at low temperatures.

Ordinarily measurements at 6–10 different dilutions result in a good K determination. The number of replicates is important and should be three to five. Moreover, parallel experiments with different dilutions of the same cell preparation and with relative amounts of monoclonal ^{125}I-labeled antibodies are suggested as internal controls for reproducibility. The degree of overlapping of the curves is a test of confidence for the assay (Section III, G).

E. Separation of Reactants

Separation of the reactants is carried out by filtration, by vacuum aspiration through a Millipore filter. Filtration gives a better separation of the reactants than centrifugation and generally results in less scatter of the experimental values. Complete separation of the reactants [i.e., of cells with antigen-antibody complexes x from unbound antibody $(A - x)$] is almost instantaneous, and the background is negligible. To decrease the nonspecific uptake by the filter membrane, 5 ml of a mouse myeloma culture supernatant [we have used (P3)X63Ag.8 myeloma] are passed through the filter immediately before use. Without allowing the filter to dry, 0.5 ml is removed with a Gilson syringe from the cell–^{125}I-labeled antibody suspension and filtered, and the membrane with the retained cells is then immediately washed with 5 ml of PBS. The entire procedure takes about 10 sec. The dried filter membranes are directly counted in a gamma counter. An antibody quantity equal to that employed in the first dilution is separately counted to obtain the value of A necessary for calculation of the various inputs. An equal amount without cells is passed through the filter to measure the background of radioactivity nonspecifically retained by the filter. The latter, usually very low or negligible, is subtracted from the experimental cpm.

F. Analysis of the Data

The equilibrium constant K and the maximum number n of antibody molecules which can be bound to a single cell are obtained by graphical extrapolation from Eq. (3) or (4). The points through which the line will be drawn are all derived from the measurements of the first input A_1 and of the different x obtained at different antibody concentrations.

The values of the inputs A_2, A_3,. . . A_{10} are calculated from A_1, knowing the dilutions (direct experimental determination of the actual inputs at the various dilutions was not found to improve significantly the accuracy of measurements). Obviously, all the terms of the equation must be expressed in the same units (Section IV). Thus, if Eq. (4) is used, and K is to be expressed in M^{-1} units, $x/(A - x)$ must be in the same units. This can be obtained by dividing the dimensionless ratio $r/(A - x)$ by the concentration of cells expressed in M units. The latter is equal to the number b of cells/cm^3 divided by the conversion factor 6.023×10^{20} cm$^{-3} M^{-1}$, 6.023×10^{20} being the number of cells ideally contained in 1 cm^3 of a "molar" concentration of cells. The variable r is the dimensionless ratio x/b which can be calculated by converting both x and b into M units, or, alternatively, into number of molecules (cells)/cm^3.

Regression analysis is performed with the aid of a computer. The regression line, drawn through the points of the scatter diagram, is fitted by the minimum square method. The K and n values are calculated together with their standard deviation (SD) (Section IV).

G. Controls

The reliability of the method can be assessed by additional tests or by the intrinsic consistency of the experiments.

A control has already been mentioned and consists in the comparison of results obtained using different quantities of the same cells with the appropriate antibody dilutions. The K and n values should remain constant. This test must be carried out using the same preparation of cells to avoid differences not due to the experimental procedure. In Fig. 6 are reported curves obtained using 0.5, 1, and 2×10^6 cells from the same Epstein–Barr (EB) virus-transformed line against opportune dilutions of the same antibody; the curves are almost completely overlapping. The consistency of the method can also be checked from the experimental data, for example, by comparing results obtained in equivalent experiments performed at different temperatures. The n values should remain constant—at least for the same cell population at a given time—while K values generally decrease with increasing temperature (Trucco *et al.*, 1980).

On the other hand, comparison of the binding of the same antibody to cells from different tissues carrying different amounts of the specific target determinant may give the same K value, while n values are generally different (Fig. 7). In this case the resulting curves are parallel. However, in principle, both K and n could vary (Section V).

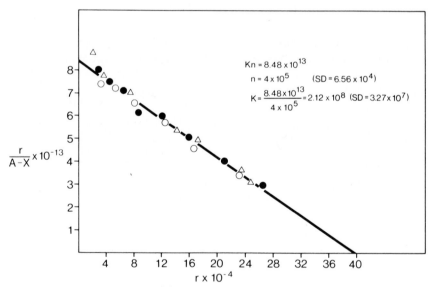

Fig. 6. Linear transform of the law-of-mass-action equation. The binding of the same monoclonal nonpolymorphic anti-HLA DR antibody at different dilutions to samples containing different numbers of cells (triangles, 0.5×10^6; open circles, 1×10^6; solid circles, 2×10^6; cells/cm³) from an EB virus-transformed line is plotted according to Eq. (4). The overlapping of the three curves can be considered good evidence of the reliability of the method.

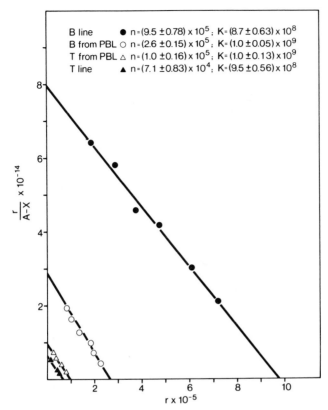

Fig. 7. Comparative binding of ^{125}I-labeled monoclonal anti-HLA, A + B + C antibody to B (WT20) and T (Molt 4) lines and to B- and T-enriched peripheral blood lymphocyte populations. B- and T-enrichment was approximately 87 and 95%, respectively, as checked either by E rosetting or with the aid of specific antisera. Experiments were performed at 0°C. The same starting concentrations and the same dilutions of the anti-HLA antibody were tested against all four different target cells. Because of graphical limits, several experimental points are not reported on the diagram. (From Trucco *et al.,* 1980.)

IV. EXAMPLES

The points discussed above are illustrated by a detailed experimental example.

The experiment involved determination of the equilibrium constant and of the number of HLA, A + B + C determinants on the lymphocyte surface using a nonpolymorphic anti-HLA monoclonal antibody and WT 20, an EB virus-transformed line, as target (Trucco *et al.,* 1980).

In this case anti-HLA antibody had been labeled using a Bolton and Hunter kit. The highest uptake on the target cell was approximately 68% (Fig. 5). The starting (nominal) concentration of monoclonal ^{125}I-labeled antibody dilution was chosen equal to 1 μg on the basis of preliminary experiments.

An antibody concentration of 1 μg corresponds to a molarity of 0.67 × 10^{-8} M (assuming a molecular weight of 1.5 × 10^5 for IgG) or 4 × 10^{12} molecules/cm³. There were 10^6 cells/ml, and 1 μg of antibody had an activity of 124,179 cpm as determined by gamma counting, of which 68% was active antibody capable of binding to the cell (Fig. 5). The actual starting concentration of antibody A_1 was therefore assumed to be 0.68 μg/ml, corresponding to a total activity of 84,441 cpm. For the sake of brevity, in this experiment, only six points were evaluated using dilutions in the ratio 2:3 (2 parts of antibody plus 1 part of medium) in triplicate (if a higher dilution had been employed, a higher cell concentration would have been required to compensate for higher statistical errors). The actual data are reported in Table I and have been plotted in Fig. 8 according to Eq. (4).

The first column (A) gives the inputs A_1 to A_6, in cpm, calculated from

TABLE I

Experimental Data Plotted in Fig. 8 According to Eq. (4)[a]

A	$x/2$	x_a	$x_b \times 10^{-11}$	$r \times 10^{-5}$	$A - x$	$x/A - x$	$(r/A - x) \times 10^{-14}$
84,441	11,016 11,071 11,926	22,142	7.159	7.159	62,299	0.35	2.14
56,223	9,328 9,117 9,474	18,656	6.032	6.032	37,567	0.49	2.98
37,586	7,868 7,673 7.442	15,346	4.961	4.961	22,240	0.69	4.16
25,088	5,497 4,709 5,960	10,994	3.554	3.554	14,094	0.78	4.72
16,717	4,162 4,277 4,200	8,400	2.716	2.716	8,317	1.01	6.11
11,110	2,706 3,004 2,947	5,894	1.905	1.905	5,216	1.13	6.79

[a] 1 μg antibody = 124,179 cpm = 4 × 10^{12} antibody molecules.

A_1, knowing the dilutions. The column $x/2$ gives the triplicate value of the cpm bound to the cells in 0.5 ml of suspension; x_a are their median values, multiplied by 2, which are taken as actual experimental points; x_b are the values of x_a expressed as number of molecules of antibody/cm^3; and r is the number of antibody molecules bound to each cell, which is obtained by dividing x_b by the number of cells/cm^3. In this case, $r = x_b/10^6$. The difference $A - x$ is the free antibody expressed in cpm, and $x/(A - x)$ is the dimensionless ratio obtained by dividing x_a by $A - x$. The last column is the ratio $r/(A - x)$, obtained by dividing the number $x/(A - x)$ by the concentration of cells expressed in moles/liter, which is equal to the number of cells/cm^3 divided by 6.023×10^{20}:

$$\frac{r}{A - x} = \left[\frac{x}{A - x}\right]_{cpm} \times \frac{6 \times 10^{20}}{10^6} M^{-1}$$

A plot of $r/(A - x) \times 10^{-14} M^{-1}$ on the ordinate versus $r \times 10^{-5}$ (dimensionless) on the abscissa gives the line shown in Fig. 8. From the value of

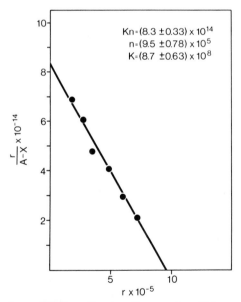

Fig. 8. Linear transform of the law-of-mass-action equation. Data were obtained from the experiment as described in detail in the text (Section IV and Table I). Regression analysis was used to verify whether the regression was significant and then linear. The regression line was drawn through the points on the scatter diagram so as to minimize the sum of squares of the distances of the observed points from the expected ones on the line. The values of the slope and the intercepts of the curve were calculated with their standard deviations. (From Trucco, *et al.,* 1980.)

the intercepts $y_{x=0} = Kn$ and $x_{y=0} = n,$ the value of K in M^{-1} and of n are immediately obtained.

V. CRITICAL APPRAISAL

As observed in Section II, Eqs. (3) and (4) can represent correctly the binding of monovalent antibody to monovalent or multivalent antigen either in solution or bound to the cell surface, or the binding of divalent antibody to monovalent antigen in solution. The reactions between bivalent antibody and divalent or polyvalent antigen in solution, or between divalent antibody with mono- or polyvalent cell surface antigens are not in general single-step reactions. The approximation is valid only under certain limiting conditions.

According to the simplest model (e.g., Bell, 1974; Bell and De Lisi, 1974; Dembo and Goldstein, 1978; Reynolds, 1979; Perelson, 1979) the binding of antibody to cell surface antigens can be described as a two-step reaction (Fig. 9). In the first step the divalent antibody binds to one antigenic determinant at one of its binding sites. In the second step a second bond forms, with another determinant which may be present either on the same dimeric (divalent) antigen molecule (Fig. 9a) or (if the molecules are free to diffuse in the plane of the membrane) on a different antigen molecule (Fig. 9b and c). In the latter case, if the antigen is monovalent (Fig. 9b), only dimeric

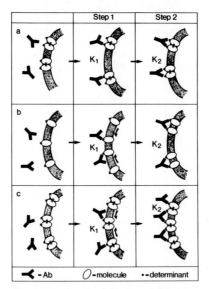

Fig. 9. Schematic diagram illustrating the three binding models discussed in the text (Section V).

complexes can be formed. If the antigen is divalent, linear polymeric complexes can be obtained (Fig. 9c). The latter can have either open or closed ends, corresponding, respectively, to linear or cyclic aggregates (cf. Dembo and Goldstein, 1978). In all cases the first step can be described as a simple bimolecular reaction. Let $c = A - x$ be the concentration at equilibrium of free antibody (expressed in molecules/cm³), S_0 the total concentration of antigenic sites per unit cell surface area, p the surface concentration of singly bound antibody molecules, and P the surface concentration of doubly bound antibody molecules. Then the cell surface concentration of free antigenic determinants is

$$S = S_0 - p - 2P \tag{5}$$

where S_0, S, P, and p are expressed in molecules/cm² and are related to the bulk concentrations per unit volume (in molecules/cm³) used in the previous sections by the relations

$$B = S_0 \sigma b \qquad x = (P + p)\sigma b \qquad B - x = S \sigma b \tag{6}$$

where σ is the (average) cell surface area in cm² and b is the number of cells/cm³.

In all the cases, singly bound antibody complexes (Fig. 9, step 1) will form at a rate proportional to the concentration of free antibody c and of free antigenic sites S according to the reaction

$$[c] + [S] \underset{k_{r1}}{\overset{k_{f1}}{\rightleftharpoons}} [p] \tag{7}$$

where k_f and k_r represent the forward and reverse rates of the reaction, respectively.

The equations describing step 2 are, however, different for the various cases illustrated in Fig. 9. In the following we will discuss these cases briefly.

Case a. This case corresponds to the formation of cyclic intramolecular complexes between divalent antibody and dimeric antigen (Fig. 9a). In this scheme the formation of intermolecular cross-links is neglected. This is correct if the dimeric antigen molecules are immobile and separated by a sufficiently great distance. Even in the case in which molecules are freely mobile, the assumption may be justified, as the divalent binding of an antibody molecule to two determinants on the same antigen molecules (when sterically possible) is in general highly favored in comparison to binding to two independent molecules. This case is formally identical to the reaction between divalent antibody and divalent antigen in solution discussed by several authors under similar assumptions.

The second step (formation of a second bond) is independent of the concentration of free antigen molecules and can be represented by the reaction

$$[p^*] \underset{2k_{r2}}{\overset{k_{f2}}{\rightleftharpoons}} [P] \tag{8}$$

where k_{f2} represents the rate of formation of a second bond and k_{r2} the rate of formation of singly bound antibody complexes by dissociation of a bond of a doubly bound antibody. The statistical factor 2 accounts for the fact that a doubly bound antibody can dissociate in two ways to give a singly bound antibody. The asterisk indicates that, when a large fraction of antigenic sites are occupied, the amount of singly bound antibodies $[p^*]$ which can form a second bond with an adjacent site on the same divalent molecule is less than $[p]$, as part of the adjacent sites are already occupied by another singly bound antibody. It is easy to see that

$$p^* = p \left[1 - \frac{p-1}{S_0 - 2P - 1} \right] \simeq p \left[1 - \frac{p}{S_0 - 2P} \right] \tag{9}$$

At a low-occupancy level (i.e., at $p << S_0 - 2P \simeq S_0$), $p^* \simeq p$. At equilibrium we therefore have from Eqs. (7) and (8)

$$p = K_1 cS \tag{10}$$

$$2P = K_2 p^* \tag{11}$$

where $K_1 = k_{f1}/k_{r1}$ and $K_2 = k_{f2}/k_{r2}$. In this formulation K_1 has dimensions of cm^3 and K_2 of cm^2.

Using the relations (5) and (9), (10) and (11) become

$$p = K_1 c (S_0 - 2P - p) \tag{10a}$$

or

$$p = [K_1 c/(1 + K_1 c)] (S_0 - 2P) \tag{10b}$$

and

$$P = (K_2/2)p[1 - p/(S_0 - 2P)] \tag{11a}$$

Two limiting situations are of practical interest. For $K_1 c << 1$, we have $p << S_0 - 2P$, $p^* \simeq p$, and $P \simeq (K_2/2)p$. Since in general $K_2 >> 1$, in this approximation we have $p << P$, and the total antibody bound P_{total} is equal to the antibody bound bivalently, i.e. $P_{total} \equiv P + p \simeq P$. Equation (11a) becomes

$$P = (K_2/2) \, p \simeq (K_2/2) \, K_1 c \, (S_0 - 2P) \tag{12}$$

or

$$P/c = K_1 K_2 (S_0/2) - K_1 K_2 P \tag{13}$$

The latter equation, except for a constant multiplicative factor σb [or σ, cf. relationships (6)] is identical to Eq. (3) [or, respectively, (4)]. A Scatchard plot would therefore give a line with a slope $K_{exp} = K_1 K_2$. The extrapolated concentration of divalently bound antibody at saturation would be $P_0 = S_0/2$ [or $n = n_0/2$ when using Eq. (4)], as expected.

At the other extreme, i.e., for $K_1 c >> 1$, Eq. (10b) becomes

$$p = [K_1 c/(1 + K_1 c)] (S_0 - 2P) \simeq S_0 - 2P \tag{14}$$

That is, $S \simeq 0$ (saturation limit). Under these conditions [from Eq. (11a)] we have $P \simeq 0$ and $p \simeq S_0$; i.e., all sites tend to be occupied by singly bound antibody.

Since $2P << p$, Eq. (10) tends to the limiting form:

$$p \simeq K_1 c (S_0 - p) \tag{15}$$

or

$$p/c = K_1 S_0 - K_1 p \tag{16}$$

Then, near saturation, the binding plot also approximates a straight line but with slope $K_{exp} \simeq K_1$ (Fig. 10).

Case b. (Fig. 9b). When the antigen is monovalent and mobile in the plane of the membrane, the first step is identical to that of case a. The rate of formation of the second bond (Fig. 9, step 2) will depend on the concentration

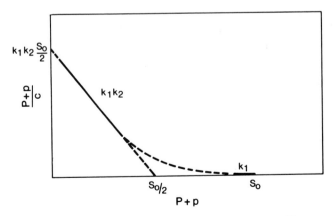

Fig. 10. Theoretical Scatchard plot describing the course of the curve either near saturating conditions ($K_{exp} \cong K_1$) or far from saturation ($K_{exp} \cong K_1 K_2$). See also text.

S of free antigenic sites and of singly bound antibody according to the reaction

$$[p] + [S] \overset{k_{f2}}{\underset{2k_{r2}}{\rightleftharpoons}} [P] \tag{17}$$

At equilibrium (with notation identical to that used above) we have

$$p = K_1 c S \tag{18}$$

$$P = (K_2/2)\, pS \tag{19}$$

namely,

$$p = [Kc_1/(1 + Kc_1)]\, (S_0 - 2P) \tag{18a}$$

$$P = (K_1 K_2/2)\, c\, (S_0 - 2P - p)^2 \tag{19a}$$

A simple relationship between the total bound antibody, $P_{total} = P + p$, and free sites, $S = S_0 - (p + 2P)$ cannot be obtained. Even if p were negligible ($p << P$), Eq. (19a) would become

$$P/c \simeq (K_1 K_2/2)\, (S_0 - 2P)^2 \tag{20}$$

That is, a plot of (P/c) versus P, or of $x/(A - x)$ versus x, would not in general be linear.

Experimental values of the reaction parameters can be obtained, however, as in the previous case, if certain limiting conditions are satisfied. The condition that p is negligible with respect to P is not necessarily satisfied for sufficiently low antibody concentrations c as in case a but, as Eq. (19) indicates, requires that

$$P/p = (K_2 S/2) >> 1 \tag{21}$$

As the second term is maximum for $S = S_0$, a necessary condition for $p << P$ is that $K_2 S_0/2 >> 1$. In physical terms relationship (21) means that the rate of dissociation (k_{r2}) of doubly bound antibodies into singly bound antibodies must be small compared with their rate of formation (k_{f2}) by the collision of singly bound antibodies with free sites. It is clear that these conditions can be satisfied only if the value of $K_2 = k_{f2}/k_{r2}$ and/or the density of free antigenic sites are sufficiently high.

Under conditions in which practically all the bound antibody is attached divalently (i.e., $P_{total} \simeq P$) and for a range of concentrations for which $K_1 c << 1$ the binding can be described by Eq. (20), which can also be written as

$$P/c = K_1 K_2 S_0\, [(S_0/2) - P][1 - (2P/S_0)] \tag{20a}$$

This represents a curve with upward concavity and therefore with variable slope. It is possible, however, to calculate the reaction parameters from the curve, as has been done for case a by noting that the intercept of the curve with the y axis (i.e., for $P = 0$) is equal to

$$[P/c \,]_{P = 0} = K_1 K_2 S_0 [S_0/2] \tag{22}$$

and the slope at the interception is

$$[d(P/c)/dP]_{P_2 = 0} = - 2K_1 K S_0 \tag{23}$$

In terms of the variables r and $c = A - x$, and of the total number of sites n_0, the respective values are

$$[r/c]_{r = 0} = K_1 K_2 S_0 [n_0/2] \tag{22a}$$

$$[d(r/c)/dr]_{r = 0} = - 2K_1 K_2 S_0 \tag{23a}$$

from which experimental values for $K_{exp} \equiv K_1 K_2 S_0$ and n_0 can be derived.

In conclusion, for the model in Fig. 9b, the binding curve should show a more-or-less marked departure from a straight line and a limiting slope for $r = 0$ which depends on the density of the antigenic sites.

Case c. The reaction between divalent antibody and divalent antigen can be described by a model similar to that discussed for case b (see, for example, Dembo and Goldstein, 1978).

If the formation of cyclic *intra*molecular complexes is sterically possible, the relative term in the equilibrium equations is predominant at least for values of c sufficiently small, and the case is essentially equivalent to case a. If intramolecular bonding does not occur, behavior similar to that discussed in case b is expected, with the additional complication that the formation of cyclic oligomeric aggregates is to be taken into consideration. If the latter is neglected, the system can be described (under very general assumptions) by the same equations used for case b. Detailed treatment of this case does not appear to be necessary in the present context.

This brief discussion of binding models illustrates the difficulty of interpreting unambiguously antibody binding data in terms of molecular quantities when the antigen is membrane-bound, even when linear relationships of the form of Eqs. (3) and (4) are obtained. Comparing binding data relative to different cells and carrying out measurements over a wide range of concentrations should help to discriminate among the possible alternatives.

When linear plots are obtained, as in the examples illustrated in this chapter, theoretical considerations suggest that bound antibody corresponds essentially to divalently bound molecules (P), with a negligible contribution from singly bound molecules (p). It should be noted that, when the filtration method is used to separate cells from unbound antibody, such a situation can also arise artifactually if during the brief washing most of the singly bound molecules have time to dissociate. This can occur, however, only if the dissociation rate of the singly bound antibody is on the order of 10^{-1}/sec or higher, which would probably correspond to an equilibrium constant K_1 for monovalent binding of less than 10^7 M^{-1}. As suggested by independent kinetic experiments, this does not seem to be the case for the antibodies we have studied.

In case of uncertainty, kinetic studies or comparisons of binding measurements carried out in parallel by filtration and by centrifugation methods should be able to clarify the point. When the cells are separated by centrifugation (i.e., by pelleting without washing, see Fazekas de St. Groth, 1979), the measured amount of cell-bound antibody should always correspond to the sum $(P + p)$ of singly and doubly bound molecules.

In the case illustrated above the binding seems to follow a linear relationship as expressed by Eq. (3) or (4) for a remarkably wide range of concentrations. In the example described, if the binding is divalent, using the parameters obtained experimentally, a linear approximation appears to apply at least until up to 70% of the total binding sites are occupied.

This result suggests the simple model described in case a as the most suitable for describing the system. This conclusion is also in agreement with the fact that the experimental values of K determined for different cells (Fig. 7) are very similar. According to model b in Fig. 9, K_{exp} should be proportional to the concentration S_0 of antigenic determinants on the cell surface, whereas according to model a in Fig. 9 it should be independent of the latter. Although the measurements provide values for the total number n of antigenic sites per cell but not for their surface density S_0, appreciable differences in the latter would be expected to exist between some of the cells described in Fig. 7.

Although further studies are required before a definite conclusion is reached in this particular case, the example illustrates the potential value of studies on equilibrium binding of monoclonal antibodies to membrane antigens in testing the validity of different molecular models and in examining the physical characteristics and behavior of the surface antigens.

VI. APPENDIX

A. Lowry Modified Method

Solutions
  A: 2% Na_2CO_3 in 0.1 N NaOH
  B: 1% $CuSO_4$
  C: 2% sodium potassium tartrate

Procedure

a. Prepare solution I: 10 ml A + 0.1 ml B + 0.1 ml C.

b. Add 10–100 μl of sample solution to 2 ml of solution I; mix well and leave for 10 min at room temperature in the dark.

c. Add 0.2 ml Folin phenol reagent 1:1 in H_2O; mix well and leave for 30 min at room temperature in the dark.

d. Read the OD at 700 nm.

B. Chloramine-T Protein Labeling

Reagents

Protein: 5–40 μg/10–20 μl of PBS in a collodium bag (SM 132 00, Sartorius GmbH, Göttingen, West Germany) at room temperature

$Na^{125}I$ (100 mCi/ml) about 500 μCi (5 μl)

Chloramine-T: (Fluka, No. 23270), 1 mg/ml in phosphate buffer, 0.3 M, pH 7.3 (10μl)

Procedure

a. Shake gently, close the bag with a rubber stopper, and leave for 2–3 min at room temperature.

b. Add 25 μl saturated tyrosine solution ($\approx$ 0.4 mg/ml in 0.3 M phosphate buffer).

c. Wait 5–10 min.

d. Add 100 μl Ca^{2+}-and Mg^{2+}-free PBS and then 50 μl 10% BSA in Ca^{2+}- and Mg^{2+}-free PBS.

e. Dialyze 24 hr against PBS using the same collodium bag.

f. Check the final amount of labeled protein solution recovered from the dialysis bag.

C. Bolton and Hunter Labeling Technique

Reagents and procedure

a. Protein: 20–40 μg/10–20 μl of PBS in a collodium bag at 4°C.

b. Dry the Bolton and Hunter reagent (as supplied; New England Nuclear), containing 1 mCi ^{125}I inserting a needle in the cap with a mild airstream. An iodine trap (supplied with the kit) should also be inserted in the cap. After 10 min, the reagent is completely dry. (The iodine trap should be considered highly radioactive waste.)

c. Add 100 μl of cold 0.1M borate buffer pH 8.5 to the dry B-H reagent and then add the solution to the protein.

d. Incubate, with shaking, for 15 min in the cold.

e. Add 0.5 ml of .02 M glycine in 0.1 M borate buffer and leave for 5 min in the cold.

f. Dialyze 24 hr against PBS using the same collodium bag.
g. Check the final amount of labeled protein solution recovered from the dialysis bag.

REFERENCES

Bell, G. I. (1974). *Nature (London)* **248**, 430.
Bell, G. I., and De Lisi, C. (1974). *Cell. Immunol.* **10**, 415.
Bolton, A. E., and Hunter, W. M. (1972). *J. Endocrinol.* **55**, 327.
Cotton, R. G. H., Secher, D. S., and Milstein, C. (1973). *Eur. J. Immunol.* **3**, 135.
Dembo, M., and Goldstein, B. (1978). *J. Immunol.* **121**, 345.
Ey, P. L., Prowse, S. J., and Jenkin, C. R. (1978). *Immunochemistry* **15**, 429.
Fazekas de St. Groth, S. (1979). *In* "Immunological Methods" (I. Lefkovits and B. Pernis, eds.), p. 1. Academic Press, New York.
Greenwood, F. C., Hunter, W. M., and Glover, J. S. (1963). *Biochem. J.* **89**, 114.
Köhler, G., and Milstein, C. (1975). *Nature (London)* **256**, 695.
Laemmli, U. K. (1970), *Nature (London)* **277**, 680.
Lowry, O. H., Rosebrough, N. J., Farr, L., and Randall, R. J. (1951) *J. Biol. Chem.* **193**, 265.
Mason, D. W., and Williams, A. F. (1980). *Biochem. J.* **187**, 1.
Perelson, A. S. (1979). *In* "Physical Chemical Aspects of Cell Surface Events in Cellular Regulation" (C. De Lisi and J. Blumenthal, eds.), p. 147. Elsevier North-Holland, Publ., Amsterdam.
Reynolds, J. A. (1979). *Biochemistry* **18**, 264.
Scatchard, G. (1949). *Ann. N.Y. Acad. Sci.* **51**, 660.
Shulman, M., and Köhler, G. (1979). *In* "Cells of Immunoglobulin Synthesis" (B. Pernis and H. Vogel, eds.), p. 275. Academic Press, New York.
Trucco, M. M., Garotta, G., Stocker, J. W., and Ceppellini, R. (1979). *Immunol. Rev.* **47**, 219.
Trucco, M. M., de Petris, S., Garotta, G., and Ceppellini, R. (1980). *Hum. Immunol.* **1**, 233.

2

Biochemical Characterization
of Cell Surface Antigens
Using Monoclonal Antibodies

Béla J. Takács and Theophil Staehelin

I. INTRODUCTION

The immune response involves the interaction of a number of different cell populations and their products. It is reasonable to assume that molecules on the surface of these cells might mediate some of these interactions. Surface membranes function not only as permeability barriers but also provide sites for a number of specific enzymes and other proteins that play a role in cell recognition and interaction (receptors) and in the multitude of specific transport processes. In order to describe and to

27

IMMUNOLOGICAL METHODS, VOL. II

understand these membrane functions in biochemical reactions it is essential to understand the structural organization of biological membranes.

The molecular architecture of membranes has been the subject of many discussions. For many years the generally accepted model has been that of Danielli and Davson (1935). According to this model, membranes consist of one or more biomolecular leaflets of phospholipid and neutral lipid sandwiched between two layers of globular proteins. With the advent of the electron microscope it was realized that there were numerous other membrane systems besides the plasma membrane. The morphological similarity of all membranes as observed with the electron microscope following fixation, staining, and thin-sectioning led Robertson to propose the "unit membrane hypothesis" (1962). In this model the notion of phospholipid layers being sandwiched between protein layers was retained, but the number of bimolecular leaflets of lipid was restricted to one. It was implicit in these two membrane models that the bonding between phospholipid and protein was primarily electrostatic. With the development of sophisticated biochemical and biophysical probes it became apparent that the predominant binding between membrane lipids and protein was hydrophobic rather than electrostatic, implying the deep penetration of protein into the lipid bilayer.

Benson (1966) has proposed a model in which protein extends through the entire membrane with lipids inserted into the protein network. On the other hand, Green and Perdue (1966) have suggested that membranes are composed of discrete lipoprotein subunits. These model systems imply relative rigidity of the membrane. The most recent and widely accepted membrane model was put forth by Singer and Nicolson (1973). According to this concept the membrane is fluid or dynamic. The proteins are "swimming" in or on the viscous lipid bilayer. An artist's version of this model, which accommodates most of the current information on membrane structure, is presented in Fig. 1. Any model depicting the hypothetical structure of biological membranes is greatly limited because we do not know the exact internal or external boundaries of the plasma membrane. Proteins directly or indirectly associated with the lipid bilayer are frequently differentiated into three groups depending on whether they are (1) artificially adsorbed, (2) peripheral (extrinsic), or (3) an integral (intrinsic) part of the membrane. The association of proteins belonging to the first two groups with the lipid bilayer is probably by electrostatic interactions and should be labile to treatment with isotonic salt solutions at neutral pH. In contrast, integral proteins either penetrate, are completely imbedded in, or span the lipid bilayer. These proteins are bound primarily by hydrophobic interactions, and they require the use of detergents for extraction.

Earlier studies directed at the biochemical analysis of membranes fo-

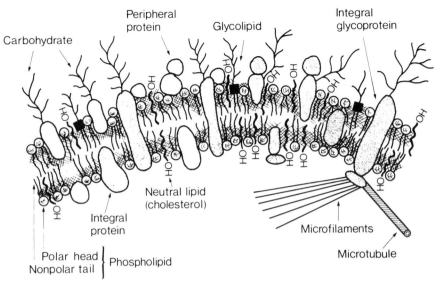

Fig. 1. An artist's representation of the plasma membrane structure.

cused largely on the lipid moieties. Techniques for the extraction and analysis of membrane lipids are therefore well worked out and are based mainly on the use of organic solvents. Lipids, which usually constitute almost half of the plasma membrane mass, serve not only as an anchoring medium for membrane proteins but may be responsible for the activity of membrane-associated enzymes. They are amphipathic and have hydrophilic and hydrophobic ends. Phospholipids comprise the majority of membrane lipids, the rest being made up of glycolipids and neutral lipids (mainly cholesterol). The glycolipid moieties seem to be restricted to the outer half of the lipid bilayer, indicating that an asymmetry exists between the two leaflets of lipid layers.

This asymmetry is also evident when we examine the distribution of membrane proteins. Most, if not all, of the intrinsic membrane proteins are glycosylated and have their carbohydrate moieties on the noncytoplasmic side of the membrane. Carbohydrate, making up approximately 10% of the membrane mass, usually consists of oligosaccharide chains covalently linked to proteins and, to a lesser extent, to lipids.

The major sugars found in membrane glycoproteins and glycolipids are glucose, galactose, fucose, mannose, galactosamine, glucosamine, and sialic acid. Sialic acid is usually terminal and provides the net negative surface charge of mammalian cells.

The array of intrinsic surface membrane proteins of human lymphocytes is very complex, and to date very few have been defined functionally. Those include the B cell receptor for antigen, a monomeric immunoglobulin M (IgM) molecule (Ada, 1970; Sulitzeanu, 1971). A smaller proportion of B cells display other classes of Ig's on their surface (Pernis et al., 1971). B lymphocytes also carry C′3 complement receptors which enable them to bind antigen–antibody–complement complexes (Bianco et al., 1970). Human T lymphocytes possess surface receptors for sheep erythrocytes (Jondal et al., 1972). A third class of lymphocytes, so-called null cells, have neither surface Ig nor receptors for sheep erythrocytes (Fröland et al., 1974). A subpopulation of all three groups, however, may bear receptors specific for the Fc portion of a certain class of Ig's (Fc receptors) (Basten et al., 1972). Serologically defined genetically polymorphic antigenic determinants present on the surface of leukocytes and other nucleated cells, referred to as major histocompatibility antigens (HLAs in humans) have been well characterized (Strominger et al., 1974). Purified HLA antigens are composed of two polypeptide chains, an alloantigenic chain with an apparent molecular size of 44,000 daltons and a 12,000-dalton polypeptide, β_2 microglobulin. The alloantigenic polypeptide is an intrinsic membrane glycoprotein and is coded for by the major histocompatibility complex (MHC) on chromosome 6. β_2 microglobulin, coded by a gene on chromosome 15, is noncovalently associated with the alloantigenic polypeptide and shows extensive homology with the constant portion of Ig light chains and heavy chains, in particular with the CH3 domain of IgG_1 (Peterson et al., 1972). The MHC region also codes for a set of antigenic specificities, called immune-associated (Ia) antigens (Snary et al., 1977).

T lymphocytes involved in either the mixed lymphocyte (MLC) reaction or in cell-mediated lysis (CML) of target cells carry cell surface receptors which enable them to recognize target cells. Attempts to characterize this T-cell receptor biochemically have given controversial results (Binz et al., 1978; Krawinkel et al., 1976).

A number of other cell surface antigens present on T lymphocytes (Anderson et al., 1979), B lymphocytes, (Humphreys et al., 1976), null lymphocytes (Ig-negative) (Humphreys et al., 1976), or the surface of neoplastic cells have also been biochemically characterized. Surface antigens of tumor cells have received perhaps the greatest attention, because the cell membrane still remains one of the most promising avenues for the attack on neoplastic disease.

The use of antibodies to characterize cell surface antigens has a number of advantages. Since antibodies cannot penetrate intact cells, the surface location of the antigen can be assessed. Furthermore, antibodies may be used to purify cell surface antigens by immunosorption or to monitor antigen purification by immunological assays. The tissue distribution of certain antigens may be assessed by antibody absorption, and appropriately labeled specific antibodies may be employed not only in the localization (Ballou *et al.*, 1979) but also in the treatment of tumors (Cosini *et al.*, 1979).

In the past the production of highly specific antisera against cell surface antigens was limited mainly because of the unavailability of sufficient amounts of highly purified antigen. For genetically polymorphic antigens this problem may be overcome in part by immunizing animals which are congenic except for the genetic locus in question (Klein, 1975). Antisera produced by xenogeneic immunization employing whole cells, cell membranes, or partially purified cell surface antigens have been of limited value, however, because of the heterogeneity of the antibody preparations. The production of specific antisera against human tumors, for example, has been hampered by the concomitant production of antibodies that also react with normal cells. This difficulty can be reduced by the use of somatic cell hybrids for immunization (Buck *et al.*, 1976), whereby the antigenic stimulus may be limited to the products of a single chromosome. The unfortunate drawback of this method is the difficulty of producing the appropriate hybrid cells. The hybridoma technique of Köhler and Milstein (1975) provides a potential answer to these problems. In this approach the multispecific response to a complex immunogen is reduced to a series of monospecific responses by cloning. Many hybridomas producing monoclonal antibodies to various cell surface antigens have been described (Trucco *et al.*, 1978); Parham and Bodmer, 1978; Kung *et al.*, 1979; Charron and McDevitt, 1979). It is hoped that by the use of monoclonal antibodies the identification, quantitation, characterization, and purification of all cell surface antigens will be possible. An antigenic blueprint of cell surface architecture would allow us not only to follow certain antigens during growth and development but could also provide a basis for the diagnosis and therapy of many neoplastic diseases.

II. PRODUCTION OF ANTIBODIES

Membrane proteins are usually good antigens because of their content of hydrophobic amino acids (Gill *et al.*, 1967) and their presence as multiple repeating units on the surface of small particles. For the preparation of either multispecific or monospecific antisera, primary immunization is usually done with either whole cells or with unfractionated membrane material. Immunization with membrane vesicles is actually preferred, because it reduces the antigenic burden on the animal and may result in the production of antibodies against minor membrane components that have been enriched in such a fraction (Bjerrum and Lundahl, 1974). Immunization with membrane material solubilized by nonionic detergents is also done. This method usually does not unmask additional antigens but can achieve higher antibody titers, possibly because of the adjuvant effect of detergents (Bjerrum and Bög-Hansen, 1976). For the immunization of rabbits (weighing 3–4 kg) with membrane material prepared from human lymphocytes, 100–500 μg of protein is administered per injection on days 0, 14, 28, and 42 in Freund's incomplete adjuvant. The injection is given subcutaneously above the scapula, and blood is withdrawn on day 15 and every 8–10 days following booster injections.

For the production of monospecific antisera the second and subsequent immunizations are done with purified antigens obtained, for example, by eluting isolated polypeptide bands after polyacrylamide gel electrophoresis in the presence of sodium dodecyl sulfate (SDS-PAGE). Alternatively, a polyvalent antibody preparation may be used to produce precipitates after crossed or lined immunoelectrophoresis, and the resulting immunoprecipitates employed for immunization. A similar schedule and antigen dose, per kilogram body weight, may be used for rabbits, pigs, and sheep. However, monoclonal antibodies have been produced using the hybridoma technique of Köhler and Milstein (1975) with mice and more recently with rats because of the existence of a number of suitable myeloma cell lines for this methodology.

A novel immunization technique developed for mice, involving a conventional preimmunization but followed by four high doses of antigen administered on each of the last 4 days before fusion, was recently presented by Stähli et al. (1980). The hybridoma technology for the production of monoclonal antibodies is described by G. Köhler in Chapter 17 of this volume. A systematic elaboration of the strategy and tactics of the method is presented in a recent article by Fazekas de St. Groth and Scheidegger (1980).

A. Analysis of Products Secreted by Hybridoma Cells

1. Radioimmunoassay

The most widely used assay system for the detection of hybridoma antibodies against cell surface antigens is the radioimmunoassay (RIA) (Goldstein et al., 1973). This method is preferred to cytotoxicity measurements because it does not depend on complement and can detect all classes of Ig's. The assay may be performed with either living or glutaraldehyde-fixed target cells (Koprowski et al., 1978). For the assay with living cells, 5×10^5 to 1×10^6 target cells (tumor cell lines, lymphoblastoid cell lines, or normal peripheral blood lymphocytes) and dilutions of antibody (culture supernatant, serum, or ascitic fluid) in a total volume of 0.5 ml of Eagle's minimal essential medium (MEM) buffered to pH 7.2 with 10 mM N-2-hydroxyethylpiperazine- N'-2-ethanesulfonic acid (HEPES) and containing 10% heat-inactivated fetal calf serum (FCS) is incubated in ∪-bottomed Linbro microtest plates for 60 min at room temperature with gentle agitation. The plates are then centrifuged at 250 g for 3 min and the supernatant aspirated. The cells are washed three times with 0.5-ml aliquots of phosphate-buffered saline (PBS) supplemented with 5% FCS and 0.02% NaN$_3$. To each well 0.05 ml of ^{125}I-labeled sheep or rabbit anti-total mouse Ig (see below) (representing approximately 50,000 cpm total counts and 8000–10,000 cpm bindable specific counts) is added, and the plates are incubated and the cells washed as above. Finally the cells are resuspended and transferred to disposable glass tubes for counting radioactivity. Target cells in medium but without test serum and target cells incubated with "normal" mouse serum (preferably from a prebleeding of immunized animals at the same dilutions as the immune serum or ascitic fluid) should be included as controls for each assay. The assay employing fixed cells is identical to the one described above for living cells. Washed target cells, at a density of 1 × 10^8 cells/ml in 0°C PBS, are fixed by the addition of an equal volume of freshly prepared 0.25% glutaraldehyde in PBS followed by agitation for 4 min at 0°C. The cells are pelleted by centrifugation in the cold and washed once with ice cold PBS and once with ice cold RIA buffer (5% FCS, 0.02% NaN$_3$ in PBS). The fixed cells are then stored in RIA buffer at 4°C. The advantage of using fixed target cells is that a large batch of cells may be prepared at one time and stored for several months without much decrease in binding efficiency.

An improved version of the RIA method was recently presented by Stocker and Heusser (1979). Target cells are attached to flexible polyvinyl chloride microtiter plates with ∪-shaped bottoms using either glutaraldehyde or anti-target cell globulin. For the glutaraldehyde method, 1 × 10^6 washed target cells in PBS are distributed to each well of the microtiter plate. The plates are then gently centrifuged at 50–100 g for 5 min. Without removing the supernatant the plate is immersed in a 1000-ml glass beaker containing ice cold 0.25% freshly prepared glutaraldehyde solution in PBS. After 5 min the plate is removed and the fixative flicked out of the wells. At all stages of the procedure removal of fluid by flicking must be done gently in order to prevent loss of the cell layer. Excess glutaraldehyde is then removed by immersing the plates consecutively in three beakers containing PBS. Finally the plate is dipped into RIA buffer and allowed to stand for 60 min at room temperature to saturate protein-binding sites on the plastic. The RIA buffer is then removed as above, and 50 μl of various dilutions of antisera or supernatants from hybridomas is added. The plate is incubated at room temperature for 60 min and washed with PBS as above. Radioactive sheep or rabbit anti-mouse Ig reagent (25 μl) in RIA buffer is then added to each well, and the plate is incubated for 60 min at room temperature. Unbound radioactivity is removed by three consecutive washes with PBS and followed by drying. The underside of the assay tray is then covered with wide adhesive tape, and the plate is pushed against an electrically heated wire suspended horizontally at the proper height. The individually cut wells are then transferred to tubes for counting radioactivity. Alternatively the dried plate may be cut with scissors.

a. Preparation of Antibodies for RIA. Sheep anti-mouse or rabbit anti-mouse Ig antibodies are first purified on an affinity column of mouse Ig's coupled to Sepharose. Hyperimmune antiserum (10–20 ml) prepared by the immunization of animals with total mouse Ig's is passed through a Sepharose column containing covalently coupled mouse Ig's (20mg/2 gm of CNBr-activated Sepharose, Pharmacia). After washing the column with PBS the specifically adsorbed antibodies are eluted with 0.2 *M* glycine–HCl buffer, pH 2.3, and neutralized by the addition of 0.3 *M* borate buffer, pH 8. The eluted antibodies are then iodinated by the chloramine-T method (Hunter and Greenwood, 1962). Free iodine is separated from the labeled antibodies by gel filtration through a Sephadex G-25 column in the presence of RIA buffer.

b. Procedure for the Iodination of Sheep Anti-Mouse IgG

i. Reagents
  Affinity-purified sheep anti-mouse IgG, ca. 2.0 mg/ml
  Potassium phosphate buffer: 0.1 *M*, pH 7.0
  Chloramine-T: 10mg/5 ml (2 mg/ml) in 0.05 *M* phosphate buffer, pH
    7.0 (freshly prepared)
  Sodium metabisulfite: 12 mg/5 ml 0.05 *M* phosphate buffer pH 7.0
    (freshly prepared)
  ^{125}I (as NaI or KI)

ii. Iodination
  1. Mix in following sequence: 0.2 ml sheep anti-mouse IgG (ca. 0.4 mg), 0.2 ml 0.1 *M* potassium phosphate buffer, ca. 2 mCi ^{125}I in 20–40 μl, and 0.1 ml chloramine-T.
  2. Incubate 20 min at 0°C
  3. Add 0.4 ml sodium metabisulfite.
  4. Add 0.1 ml 0.1 *M* KI (final volume, 1 ml).

5. Pass through Sephadex G-25 column (ca. 1 × 20 cm) equilibrated with PBS (minus Ca^{2+} and Mg^{2+}) containing 1 mg/ml bovine serum albumin (BSA) using the same buffer for elution.

6. Collect 1-ml fractions and count 1 μl of each fraction. Pool the fractions of the first peak; measure radioactivity in 1 μl; dilute with PBS containing 1–10 mg BSA/ml to obtain about 750,000–1,000,000 cpm/5 μl.

7. Store in 0.5-ml aliquots at −70°C.

8. For RIA dilute ca. 1:150 in RIA buffer. Use 50 μl per well (50,000–75,00 cpm per well).

Typical preparation: ca. 10 ml containing ca. 0.4 mg ^{125}I-labeled IgG, 1.0–1.2 mCi ^{125}I, i.e., 2–3 μCi/μg IgG. Stock aliquots may be thawed and frozen several times. We have used a preparation up to 4 months. At later times we dilute only 1:100 or less.

2. Electrophoresis

Products secreted by hybrid cells may also be conveniently assessed by SDS-PAGE analysis of culture supernatants. To define molecules that are cell-derived rather than components from the serum, metabolic labeling is necessary. This is done by simply adding 1–2 drops (10–25 μl) of [^{35}S]methionine from a No. 21 hypodermic needle to each of the cluster wells (Costar 3524) containing 0.5–1 × 10^6 hybrid cells in 2 ml of complete tissue culture medium. Because of the high specific activity of the radioactive amino acid (500–1000 Ci/mmol, 5–7 mCi/ml) it is not necessary to use methionine-free medium or to dialyze FCS. After 12–24 hr of incubation media are removed and centrifuged at 750 g for 10 min at 4°C to sediment floating cells. The supernatant is then subjected to centrifugation at 20,000 g for 15 min to sediment denatured proteins. Part of the supernatant may be directly analyzed for secreted products by SDS-PAGE followed by autoradiography (Fig. 2) However, to reduce the protein input (mainly serum albumin) it is advantageous first to enrich for secreted Ig's by either one of the following methods: (1) If the secreted Ig is of the IgG_1, IgG_{2a}, IgG_{2b}, or IgG, 1.0–1.2 mCi ^{125}I, i.e., 2–3 μCi/μg IgG. Stock aliquots may be thawed quantitatively at pH. 8.0 (Ey et al., 1978). Non-Ig serum components together with IgM, IgA, and IgE are then removed by washing three times with PBS, pH 8.0. Bound Ig's are then eluted from the absorbent with SDS sample buffer and analyzed by SDS-PAGE (Fig. 3) as described previously (Takacs, 1979). (2) All the Ig classes may be analyzed by first incubating 1-ml aliquots of the culture supernatants with 20 μl of rabbit anti-mouse total Ig antiserum at 4°C for 1–2 hr. Protein A-Sepharose (representing approximately 50 μl of settled beads) is then added, and the incubation is continued for an additional 15 min with end-to-end rotation. Washing of the

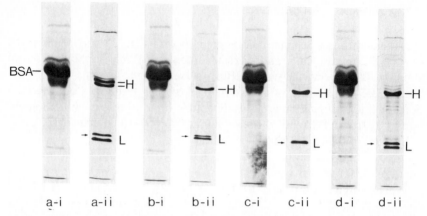

Fig. 2. Direct analysis of products secreted by hybrid cells. Hybrid cultures were derived by the fusion of spleen cells, from mice immunized with a human tumor cell line, with the mouse myeloma cell line X63-Ag8. Cultures at a density of 5×10^5 cells/ml were grown overnight in complete tissue culture medium containing 100 μCi [^{35}S]methionine/ml. Culture fluids were centrifuged at 20,000 g for 15 min. Then 100 μl of the supernatants was mixed with 50 μl of a $3 \times$ concentrate of SDS sample buffer prior to SDS-PAGE analysis. Then 50-μl aliquots were applied to each sample slot. Gels were subjected to electrophoresis at 25 mA constant current per slab gel for 3.5 hr. H and L represent heavy and light chains of Ig, and i and ii represent staining patterns and autoradiography, respectively, of the same gel track. The Ig light chains, coded by the X63-Ag8 genome, are indicated by arrows.

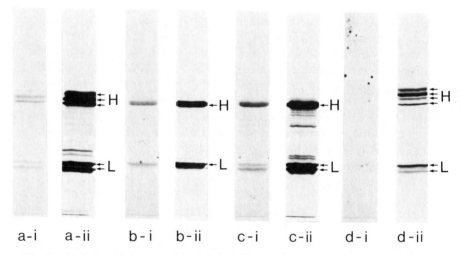

Fig. 3. Analysis of Ig's secreted by hybrid cells. Conditions for biosynthetic labeling of secreted products were identical to those described in the legend for Fig. 2. One milliliter of each culture supernatant was incubated for 30 min with protein A-Sepharose (50 μl of settled beads) at room temperature by end-to-end rotation. After washing the beads with four cycles of PBS, the specifically adsorbed Ig's were eluted with SDS sample buffer. H and L represent heavy and light chains of Ig's, and i and ii represent staining patterns and autoradiography, respectively, of the same gel track.

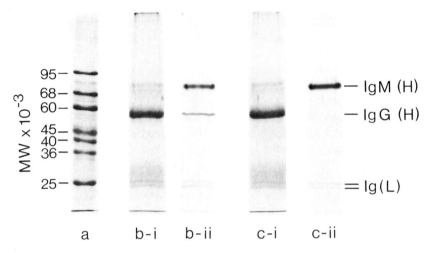

Fig. 4. Analysis of Ig's secreted by hybrid cells. Conditions for biosynthetic labeling of secreted products were identical to those described in the legend for Fig. 2. One milliliter of each culture supernatant was incubated with 20 μl of rabbit anti-mouse total Ig antiserum at 4°C for 2 hr. Protein A–Sepharose, representing approximately 50 μl of settled beads, was added, and the incubation continued for an additional 15 min with end-to-end rotation. The specifically adsorbed Ig's were analyzed by SDS–PAGE as described in the text. H and L represent heavy and light chains of Ig's, and i and ii represent staining patterns and autoradiography, respectively, of the same gel track.

adsorbent and elution of the bound immune complexes for SDS-PAGE is done as described above (Fig. 4).

B. Purification of Monoclonal Antibodies

Before attempting to purify cell surface antigens from detergent extracts of target cells by affinity chromatography with immobilized antibodies, the antibodies have to be partially purified.

Culture supernatant is centrifuged at 750 g for 10 min at 4°C followed by centrifuging at 20,000 g for 15 min in the cold. Antibodies are then precipitated by the addition of an equal volume of cold, saturated $(NH_4)_2SO_4$ while being stirred on ice. The precipitate is then allowed to stand on ice for 30 min and centrifuged at 5000 g for 10 min. The pellet is washed once with 50% saturated $(NH_4)_2SO_4$ and dissolved in $\frac{1}{20}$ of the original volume in coupling buffer (0.1 M $NaHCO_3$, 0.5 M NaCl) and dialyzed against coupling buffer for 12–16 hr in the cold.

Alternatively, antibodies are precipitated and washed with 16% (w/v) Na_2SO_4 before dissolving and dialyzing against coupling buffer.

To obtain large amounts of antibodies, hybrid cells are injected into congenic mice for the production of ascites fluid. Antibody concentration in
the ascites fluid may reach a concentration of up to 10–20 mg/ml, which is
200–500 times higher than in culture fluid.

For the purification of antibodies the ascites fluid or serum is diluted
5-to 10-fold with PBS prior to the precipitation step.

Antibody solutions in coupling buffer may be mixed directly with CNBr-
activated Sepharose (10 mg protein/ml derivatized gel) or further purified
by gel filtration or ion-exchange chromatography.

For ion-exchange chromatography the $(NH_4)_2SO_4$- or Na_2SO_4- precipitated proteins are dissolved in and dialyzed at least 6 hr against 0.01
M Tris–HCl buffer, pH 7.8, containing 0.02 M NaCl, followed by centrifugation at 20,000 g for 15 min to remove insoluble material. The supernatant fraction, derived from 10–20 ml of ascites fluid, is then applied to a
1.5 × 30 cm diethylaminoethyl cellulose (Whatman, DE-52) column
equilibrated with the same buffer. The adsorbed proteins are eluted with a
linear gradient prepared from 250 ml of 0.01 M Tris–HCl, pH 7.8, 0.02 M
NaCl, and 250 ml of 0.02 M Tris–HCl, pH 7.8, 0.5 M NaCl solutions at a
flow rate of 20–25 ml/hr at room temperature. The IgG peak elutes usually
at 0.04–0.05 M NaCl and is about 90% pure. Concentration of IgG from
pooled peak fractions is done by 50% $(NH_4)_2SO_4$ precipitation followed by
dialysis.

Alternatively, the $(NH_4)_2SO_4$- or Na_2SO_4-precipitated protein solution (2

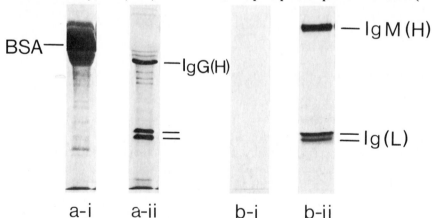

Fig. 5. Purification of IgM. Conditions of biosynthetic labeling of Ig's were identical to
those described in the legend for Fig. 2. Culture supernatant was applied to a lentil lectin–Sepharose column, and IgG and serum albumin were recovered in the effluent fraction
(a–i and a–ii). The retained glycoproteins (mainly IgM) were then eluted with 10% (w/v)
methyl-α-ᴅ-mannopyranoside (b–i and b–ii). i and ii represent staining patterns and
autoradiography, respectively, of the same gel track.

ml) in 0.1 M Tris–HCl, pH 7.5, 1.0 M NaCl buffer is applied to a 2.5 × 90 cm Sephacryl S-200 superfine column (Pharmacia) and eluted with the same buffer at a flow rate of 10–15 ml/hr.

Monoclonal antibodies of the IgM class usually contain 10–12% carbohydrate and may be purified by affinity chromatography on lentil lectin–Sepharose columns. $(NH_4)_2SO_4$- or Na_2SO_4-precipitated Ig's in PBS are applied to the column and washed with the same buffer to remove unbound material. Adsorbed proteins are then eluted with a 10% (w/v) solution of methyl-α-D-mannopyranoside in PBS. The lentil lectin–Sepharose affinity gel (Pharmacia) may bind up to 10 mg of glycoprotein per milliliter of bed volume. Purification of an IgM monoclonal antibody, with anti-human β_2 microglobulin activity, secreted by a mouse hybrid cell line using lentil lectin affinity chromatography is shown in Fig. 5.

III. LABELING PROCEDURES FOR CELL SURFACE ANTIGENS

A. Biosynthetic Labeling

For biosynthetic labeling, cells are resuspended to a density of $1.5 × 10^6$ cells/ml and incubated for 16–24 hr either in leucine- or methionine-free medium supplemented with 10% heat-inactivated FCS, antibiotics, glutamine, and 5 μCi L-[^{14}C]leucine or 50 μCi L-[^{35}S]methionine/ml, respectively. To ensure that the amino acid does not become limiting, the incubation mixture should also contain 10% (v/v) of complete medium. Incorporation of label into cells under these conditions is usually 60–80% of the added radioactivity.

B. Labeling of Cells with ^{125}I

Lactoperoxidase-catalyzed cell surface iodination according to Marchalonis et al. (1971) is described in Chapter 10 of the first volume of this series and will not be considered here.

Cells, membrane vesicles, or detergent-solubilized membrane proteins may also be conveniently iodinated using the water-insoluble chloramide, 1, 3, 4, 6-tetrachloro-3a,6a-diphenylglycoluril reagent (Fraker and Speck, 1978), available from Pierce Chemical Co. under the trade name Iodo-Gen. Films of the reagent are plated onto the walls of glass tubes by adding 1 mg of the chloramide in 100 μl of chloroform or methylene chloride to each of the 15-ml Corex centrifuge tubes and allowing the solvent to evaporate under rotation. Cells (10^7 lymphocytes), membrane vesicles, or detergent-

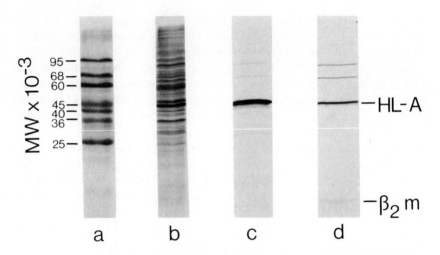

Fig 6. Purification of histocompatibility antigens (HL-A). The human lymphoblastoid cell line, WT-18, was biosynthetically labeled with [^{35}S]methionine as described in the text. A detergent extract of the labeled cells (b) was passed through an aggregated human IgG-Sepharose column to remove components that bind to Ig's (FcR, actin, and so on). The column was washed extensively with detergent-containing buffer, and the adsorbed material eluted with SDS-containing buffer (c). The effluent fractions from the aggregated Ig column were applied to an immunoadsorbent column prepared by the covalent coupling of purified monoclonal mouse anti-human β_2m antibodies to CNBr-activated Sepharose. The specifically retained components were eluted with detergent-containing buffer at pH 2.3 and analyzed by SDS-PAGE (d). Gel tracks a, b, and c represent autoradiographic patterns; track a is a Coomassie blue staining pattern of molecular-weight standards run on the same gel slab. The concentration of acrylamide was 17.5%.

solubilized membrane proteins are added in 500 µl of PBS together with 1 mCi of carrier-free ^{125}I$^-$. Iodination is continued for 20 min at 0°–2°C with gentle agitation. The iodination is terminated by withdrawal of the reaction mixture. Cells or membrane vesicles are washed free of iodine by centrifugation in PBS, followed by a 10-min incubation and wash with PBI (0.01 M phosphate buffer, pH 7.3, containing 0.15 M NaI) to displace the free ^{125}I$^-$ present. Free iodine from the detergent-solubilized membrane preparation is separated by gel filtration through a Sephadex G-25 column equilibrated with PBI and detergent.

C. Labeling of Surface Carbohydrate

Sialic acid residues of glycoproteins may be labeled by tritiated sodium borohydride (NaB^{3}H$_4$) reduction of oxidized carbohydrates (Gahmberg and Andersson, 1977). In 1 ml of PBS 1–2 × 10^7 lymphocytes are incubated for 10 min at 0°C with 1 mM sodium periodate for the formation of aldehyde groups on the sialic acid residues. The reaction is stopped by the addition of glycerol to a final concentration of 25 mM, and the cells are washed twice with PBS. The pelleted cells are resuspended in 0.5 ml of Dulbecco's balanced salt solution (DBSS), and 1 mCi of NaB^{3}H$_4$ is added to reduce the aldehyde groups to their corresponding alcohols. The mixture is incubated for 30 min at room temperature and washed twice with DBSS.

IV. PREPARATION OF CELL MEMBRANES

The choice of methods for the isolation of cell surface antigens is dictated by a number of considerations. One of these is the availability of cells or tissues as a source of antigen. Cultured cell lines provide a continuous and highly uniform source of antigen. Since the molecules recognized by antiserum or monoclonal antibodies most probably are intrinsic membrane glycoproteins, separation of the cytoplasmic membrane is chosen as an initial purification step. Since plasma membranes represent approximately 1% of the total cellular proteins, preparation of cell surface membrane alone will give approximately a 50-fold purification of surface antigens.

Theoretically membrane proteins are those necessary for the functioning of a membrane. In practice, however, proteins present in a membrane preparation are called membrane proteins. Consequently, it is essential that during membrane isolation the loss of true membrane components and, more importantly, the adsorption of extraneous contaminants to the membrane be kept to a minimum.

A. Shearing Method

Large-scale purification of membranes is best achieved by nitrogen decompression of cell suspensions, followed by differential centrifugation of the resulting homogenate (Ferber *et al.,* 1972). Vesicular membranes may then be further separated into plasma membrane and endoplasmic reticulum by isopycnic centrifugation through discontinuous Ficoll gradients (Scheme I).

Cells (5 × 10^8 to 1 × 10^9) are resuspended in 50 ml of breaking buffer [0.01 M HEPES, pH 7.5, 0.065 M NaCl, 0.25 M sucrose, 0.25 mM MgCl$_2$, 1 mM phenylmethylsulfonyl fluoride (PMSF)] and equilibrated with nitrogen gas in a Parr nitrogen cavitator (Parr Instrument Co., Moline, Illinois) for 15 min at 50 atm at 0°–4°C. Cell breakage is achieved by dropwise release of the cell suspension. After addition of ethylenediaminetetraacetic acid (EDTA, 1 mM final concentration), the homogenate is fractionated by differential centrifugation. Nuclei, unbroken cells, and debris are removed

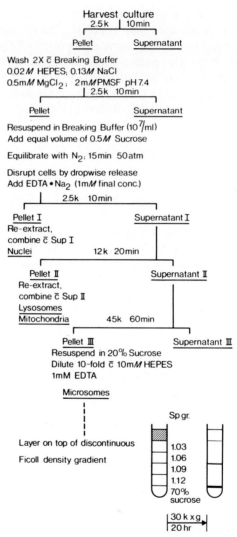

Harvest culture
2.5k | 10min

Pellet   Supernatant

Wash 2X c̄ Breaking Buffer
0.02 M HEPES; 0.13 M NaCl
0.5 mM MgCl$_2$; 2 mM PMSF pH 7.4
2.5k 10min

Pellet   Supernatant

Resuspend in Breaking Buffer (10^7/ml)
Add equal volume of 0.5 M Sucrose

Equilibrate with N$_2$; 15 min 50 atm

Disrupt cells by dropwise release
Add EDTA•Na$_2$ (1 mM final conc.)
2.5k 10min

Pellet I   Supernatant I
Re-extract,
combine c̄ Sup I
Nuclei   12k 20min

Pellet II   Supernatant II
Re-extract,
combine c̄ Sup II
Lysosomes
Mitochondria   45k 60min

Pellet III   Supernatant III
Resuspend in 20% Sucrose
Dilute 10-fold c̄ 10 mM HEPES
1mM EDTA

Microsomes

Layer on top of discontinuous   Sp gr.
Ficoll density gradient
1.03
1.06
1.09
1.12
70%
sucrose

30 k x g
20 hr

Scheme I. Scheme for the purification of subcellular components.

by centrifugation at 750 g for 15 min. The supernatant is centrifuged at 20,000 g for 20 min to pellet mitochondria and lysosomes. A crude membrane preparation is obtained by centrifugation of the supernatant at 120,000 g for 60 min. Each pelleted fraction is reextracted with breaking buffer containing 1 mM EDTA. The pelleted membranes are then washed consecutively with 10 mM and 1 mM HEPES, pH 7.5. For most experiments these membranes may be used without further purification.

However, when highly purified membranes are needed, the crude membrane preparation may be further purified by isopycnic Ficoll barrier centrifugation (Wilson and Amos, 1972). The gradient in 1 mM HEPES, pH 7.5, is prepared from 35, 25, 17.5, and 9% Ficoll representing specific gravities of 1.12, 1.09, 1.06, and 1.03 gm/cm³, respectively. After centrifugation at 30,000 g for 20 hr at 4°C, material banding at a density of 1.06 is removed and freed of Ficoll by centrifugation at 140,000 g for 60 min. The pellet is washed twice with 20 mM HEPES, pH 7.4.

B. Detergent Method

A rapid method for destabilizing cell membranes involving the weak nonionic detergent Tween 40 was recently described by Standring and Williams (1978). The method is simple to perform, and it compares favorably with other much more time-consuming procedures. A modification of this method is presented below.

Washed cells at a density of 2-4 × 10⁸/ml in isotonic buffer (0.02 M Tris–HCl, pH 7.3, 0.145 M NaCl, 1.5 mM MgCl$_2$) are mixed with an equal volume of 5% Tween 40 prepared in the same buffer. Protease inhibitor, aprotinin, 100 KIU/ml, is added, and the mixture is allowed to stand at 0°C for 15 min. Before homogenization with three or four strokes in a glass-Teflon homogenizer, concentrated sucrose solution is added to give a final concentration of 3%. The homogenate is layered onto a discontinuous sucrose gradient consisting of two equal layers of 32% (w/v) and 10% (w/v) sucrose solutions in isotonic buffer. Centrifugation is performed at 24,000 rpm for 60 min in a Beckman SW 27 rotor at 4°C. The membrane band is removed from the 32% sucrose interface and diluted 10-to 20-fold with isotonic buffer prior to sedimentation at 100,000 g for 60 min.

V. ANALYSIS OF CELL SURFACE ANTIGENS

A. Extraction of Cell Surface Antigens

Before purification of cell surface antigens, the various proteins must be extracted from the membrane matrix. The method of this extraction is extremely critical. In making a choice the investigator has to consider the nature of those components and their specific interactions in which he or she is particularly interested.

Accordingly one might employ urea, guanidine, EDTA, distilled water, organic solvents, controlled proteolysis, chaotropic agents, or manipulation of ionic strength and pH. These methods, however, do not lead to the complete solubilization of proteins strongly bound to the lipid matrix of the membrane. Therefore observations and conclusions about the molecular nature of surface proteins obtained by these extraction methods are questionable. For these proteins the use of detergents appears to provide the best extraction method. There are many detergents available for the solubilization of membrane proteins (see Helenius and Simons, 1975). For our purposes, the solubilizing agent should be able to disintegrate the membrane and keep the proteins in solution without destroying the protein's antigenic structure and interfering with antigen–antibody interactions. Neutral or nonionic detergents fulfill these requirements. The use of Nonidet P-40 (NP40) (Schwartz and Nathenson, 1971), Triton X-100 (see Helenius and Simons, 1975), Berol EMU-043 (Bjerrum and Bög-Hansen, 1976), Renex 30 (Tanaki et al., 1979), Brij (Springer et al., 1977), Lubrol PX (Converse and Papermaster, 1975), Ammonyx LO (Yu et al., 1973), and Tween (Johansson and Hjertén, 1974) are well documented. These nonionic surfactants are polyoxyethylene glycols with different hydrophile–lipophile balance (HLB) numbers. The HLB number, introduced by Griffin (1949), represents an arbitrary empirical quantity which helps to predict the usefulness or solubilizing potency of various surfactants. The effectiveness of neutral surfactants in solubilizing membrane proteins probably depends also on factors other than the HLB number. However, various studies show that almost all effective surfactants have HLB values in the range of 12.5–14.5 (Helenius and Simons, 1975).

The HLB values for some widely used neutral detergents are listed in Table I. The HLB values of mixtures of surfactants may also be approximated by simple algebraic addition. For example, a detergent blend containing 4 parts of Span 40 and 6 parts of Tween 20 has an effective HLB value of $(0.4)(6.7) + (0.6)(16.7) = 12.7$. A general guide to the use of a particular type of neutral surfactant for various membrane protein solubilizations cannot be given, because membrane proteins are solubilized to different degrees by different detergents. However, based on our own experience we prefer NP40 for the solubilization of lymphocyte plasma membranes. This detergent is a relatively mild, yet highly effective solubilizing agent for membrane proteins (Schwartz and Nathenson, 1971). At the concentration used, 0.5%, it is thought to react mainly with the hydrophobic, lipophilic portions of proteins (Lerner et al., 1971) without interfering with antibody interactions directed at the hydrophilic portions of cell surface antigens (Crumpton and Parkhouse, 1972). Furthermore, at this concentration NP40 does not solubilize nuclear membranes, an important consideration when detergent extraction of intact cells is undertaken.

Optimum conditions for solubilization with neutral surfactants include

TABLE I

Hydrophile–Lipophile Balance Values of Some Nonionic Surfactants[a]

Surfactant	Commercial value	HLB number
Sorbitan trioleate	Span 85	1.8
Sorbitan tristearate	Span 65	2.1
Sorbitan monooleate	Span 80	4.3
Sorbitan monostearate	Span 60	4.7
Polyoxyethylene (2) stearyl ether	Brij 72	4.9
Polyoxyethylene (2) oleyl ether	Brij 92	4.9
Polyoxyethylene (2) cetyl ether	Brij 52	5.3
Sorbitan monopalmitate	Span 40	6.7
Sorbitan monolaurate	Span 20	8.6
Polyoxyethylene sorbitan monostearate	Tween 61	9.6
Polyoxyethylene lauryl ether	Brij 30	9.7
Polyoxyethylene sorbitan monooleate	Tween 81	10.0
Polyoxyethylene (4.5) *p-tert*-octylphenol	Triton X–45	10.4
Polyoxyethylene sorbitan tristearate	Tween 65	10.5
Polyoxyethylene sorbitan trioleate	Tween 85	11.0
Polyoxyethylene (6) tridecyl ether	Renex 36	11.4
Polyoxyethylene (10) stearyl ether	Brij 76	12.4
Polyoxyethylene (10) oleyl ether	Brij 96	12.4
Polyoxyethylene (7–8) *p-tert*-octylphenol	Triton X–114	12.4
Polyoxyethylene (10) cetyl ether	Brij 56	12.9
Polyoxyethylene alkyl aryl ether	Renex 690	13.0
Polyoxyethylene (9) *p-tert*-octylphenol	NP40	13.1
Polyoxyethylene sorbitan monolaurate	Tween 21	13.3
Polyoxyethylene (9–10) nonyl phenol	Triton N–101	13.4
Polyoxyethylene (9–10) *p-tert*-octyl phenol	Triton X–100	13.5
Polyoxyethylene esters of mixed fatty acids	Renex 20	13.8
Polyoxyethylene (12) tridecyl ether	Renex 30	14.5
Polyoxyethylene (12–13) *p-tert*-octylphenol	Triton X–102	14.6
Polyoxyethylene sorbitan monostearate	Tween 60	14.9
Polyoxyethylene (17) cetyl-stearyl alcohol	Lubrol WX	14.9
Polyoxyethylene sorbitan monooleate	Tween 80	15.0
Polyoxyethylene (20) stearyl ether	Brij 78	15.3
Polyoxyethylene (20) oleyl ether	Brij 98	15.3
Polyoxyethylene (15) tridecyl ether	Renex 31	15.4
Polyoxyethylene sorbitan monopalmitate	Tween 40	15.6
Polyoxyethylene (20) cetyl ether	Brij 58	15.7
Polyoxyethylene (16) *p-tert*-octylphenol	Triton X–165	15.8
Polyoxyethylene sorbitan monolaurate	Tween 20	16.7
Polyoxyethylene lauryl ether	Brij 35	16.9

[a] From Becher, 1967; Helenius and Simons, 1975.

low ionic strength (less than 0.2), alkaline pH (approximately 8–8.5), and a detergent/protein ratio of at least 1.5. To prevent aggregation the protein concentration in the solubilization mixture should not exceed 3 mg/ml. Since the degree of solubilization is only slightly influenced by temperature, solubilization should be done at 0°C to reduce proteolytic degradation of the cell membrane proteins. Enzymatic degradation of the solubilized proteins can be a serious problem, and some investigators treat the solubilization mixture with a "cocktail" of protease inhibitors (Axelsson et al., 1978). Trasylol (also known as aprotinin or kallikrein inhibitor) at a concentration of 100 units/ml and PMSF at a concentration of 1 mM should be routinely included in the solubilization mixture. PMSF, which is rapidly hydrolyzed and not soluble much above 1 mM in aqueous buffers (Gold, 1967), is prepared as a 0.1–0.2 M stock solution in isopropanol. Aliquots of the stock solution are kept frozen at $-20°C$. Some investigators include ε-aminocaproic acid (1% of a saturated solution), N-α-p-tosyl-L-lysine chloromethyl ketone-HCl (10 μg/ml), and soybean trypsin inhibitor (5 μg/ml) in addition to Trasylol and PMSF.

Another problem is the formation of intermolecular disulfide bonds. Alkylation of sulfhydryl groups by including iodoacetamide (1 mM) in the lysis buffer may obviate this problem.

Certain cell surface proteins form aggregates in the presence of neutral detergents (Standring et al., 1978). This is prevented by the addition of 1–2% deoxycholate (DOC) to the neutral detergent extract after the nuclei have been removed by centrifugation. This compound is a relatively mild anionic surfactant in whose presence the proteins' quarternary structure and antigenic and enzymatic activities are preserved. However, DOC was found to interfere with antigen–antibody interaction (Rogers et al., 1979). The best remedy for problems of this sort is to exchange the surfactant for a milder one. Detergents of the Tween series, for example, although ineffective in solubilizing intrinsic membrane proteins, might have the property of preventing aggregation of membrane proteins already in solution. The detergent exchange may be accomplished by applying the membrane extract to a column of Sephadex G-25 equilibrated with the new detergent. Alternatively, membrane glycoproteins might be adsorbed to a lectin column and the detergent exchanged by washing and eluting the column with a buffer containing the new surfactant (Rogers et al., 1979).

1. Affinity Chromatography of Solubilized Membrane Proteins

a. Purification of Glycoproteins. One of the advantages of the use of neutral detergents is their lack of charge, which permits purification of solubilized membrane proteins by ion-exchange chromatography or by isoelectric focusing. However, some intrinsic membrane proteins, for example, histocompatibility antigens, display a great deal of charge heterogeneity which adversely affects their resolution by either of these techniques. These and other glycoproteins, however, may be adsorbed to immobilized lectin adsorbents in the presence of neutral detergents or salts of bile acids, particularly sodium cholate or DOC. The lectins most often used for the purification of membrane glycoproteins are concanavalin A (Con A) and *Lens culinaris* hemagglutinin (LcH). Allan *et al.* (1972) were the first to report the purification of glycoproteins from porcine lymphocyte membranes using Con A affinity columns. Later Hayman and Crumpton (1972) improved the efficiency of glycoprotein purification from the same source using immobilized lectin isolated from lentils. Both of these lectins bind to the same sugar residues of glycoproteins, but LcH binds with a 50-fold lower affinity (Stein *et al.,* 1971). This lower binding affinity facilitates a more complete elution of adsorbed glycoproteins from immobilized lectin using a competitive sugar such as methyl-α-D-mannoside or methyl-α-D-glucoside.

Lentil lectin may be prepared from commercially available lentils according to published procedures (Hayman and Crumpton, 1972) and coupled to Sepharose 4B as described (Hayman and Crumpton, 1972). Lentil lectin, coupled to Sepharose 4B, is also available commercially from Pharmacia. Before use the column (5–10 ml bed volume) should be washed consecutively with 1% (w/v) DOC in Tris–saline buffer, pH 8.0 (0.02 M Tris–HCl, 0.15 M NaCl), with 10% (w/v) methyl-α-D-mannopyranoside in 1% (w/v) DOC in Tris–saline buffer, and finally with 0.5% (w/v) DOC in Tris–saline buffer. Solubilized membrane extracts containing 10–20 mg protein are applied to the column, and the column is washed with 0.5% (w/v) DOC in Tris–saline buffer until the absorbance at 280 nm reaches a steady low level. Adsorbed material is then eluted with 10% (w/v) methyl-α-D-mannopyranoside in 0.5% (w/v) DOC in Tris-saline buffer. Elution may be more effective at an elevated temperature (45°C). Fractions of 0.2–0.5 ml are collected, and the contents of tubes with peak radioactive counts or 280-nm absorbing material are pooled. The purified glycoproteins may be concentrated by precipitation at −20°C for 48 hr with 66% (v/v) ethanol (Bridgen *et al.,* 1976) or further analyzed by affinity chromatography employing antibody bound to protein A–Sepharose or by antibody bound covalently to CNBr-activated Sepharose (Pharmacia) immunoadsorbents.

Difficulties might be encountered in trying to precipitate proteins from very dilute solutions. In this case NH_4HCO_3, to a final concentration of 50 mM, is added to the solution and the proteins coprecipitated with the bicarbonate by the addition of 9 parts of cold (−20°C) acetone.

The lentil lectin–Sepharose column is regenerated by washing extensively

with 1% DOC in Tris–saline buffer. For prolonged storage the column
should be equilibrated with 75% saturated $(NH_4)_2SO_4$. Under these conditions we have observed very little loss of binding activity.

b. Purification of Cell Surface Antigens (Scheme II). Purification of individual cell surface antigens from a complex array of molecules requires
highly specific reagents, and monoclonal antibodies meet these requirements. We will describe three approaches making use of monoclonal
antibodies in the purification of cell surface antigens.

   i. The glycoprotein fraction in the presence of NP4O is added to tubes
containing antibody bound to protein A–Sepharose (Pharmacia). The tubes
are rotated end over end for 16 hr at 4°C. Unbound material is washed
away with 0.5% NP4O in PBS, followed by washing with 0.5% NP4O in
phosphate-buffered 0.5 M NaCl solution. For the washing and elution step
the immunoadsorbent is transferred to a small column (a plastic syringe
containing a plug of glass wool to retain Sepharose) and washed with the
NP4O containing PBS until radioactivity in the wash buffer reaches
background level. Specifically bound material is then eluted with either
SDS sample buffer for SDS-PAGE analysis or with low pH (0.5% NP4O in
0.2 M glycine–HCl, pH 2.3), high pH (0.5% NP4O in 0.05 M diethyl-
amine-HCl, pH 11.5), or the chaotrop KSCN (3 M KSCN, 0.5% NP4O, in
0.02 M Tris-HCl, pH 8.0), for further analysis (see Fig. 6).
   ii. Monoclonal mouse anti-cell surface antibodies are added to NP4O-
solubilized membrane extracts (approximately 25 μl of ascites fluid per 10^7
cell equivalents) and incubated for 30 min at room temperature. An optimal amount (determined by titration) of rabbit or sheep anti-mouse Ig is
added, and the mixture incubated for 16 hr at 4°C to precipitate the immune complexes. Immune precipitates are then washed twice with 0.5%
NP4O in PBS, followed by a wash with 0.5% NP4O in phosphate-buffered
0.5 M NaCl solution. Precipitates are dissolved in SDS sample buffer by incubation in a boiling water bath for 3 min (Takacs, 1979).
   iii. Purified monoclonal antibodies are covalently coupled to CNBr-
activated Sepharose (Section II,B). NP4O-soluble membranes, glycoprotein fractions, or whole-cell extracts are added to the antibody-Sepharose
immunoadsorbent and rotated end over end in a tube at 4°C for 16 hr. The
contents of the tube are transferred to a chromatography column, and
nonspecifically adsorbed material is removed by washing as described
above. The elution of specifically adsorbed antigens with low-pH or high-
pH buffer or with a high concentration of chaotropic salt solutions is performed as described for the protein A–Sepharose column. Fractions with
radioactive peaks are pooled. Very dilute samples containing less than 500

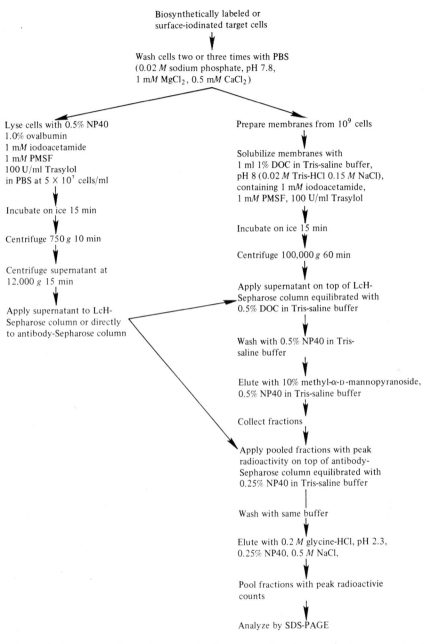

Biosynthetically labeled or
surface-iodinated target cells

Wash cells two or three times with PBS
(0.02 M sodium phosphate, pH 7.8,
1 mM MgCl$_2$, 0.5 mM CaCl$_2$)

Lyse cells with 0.5% NP40
1.0% ovalbumin
1 mM iodoacetamide
1 mM PMSF
100 U/ml Trasylol
in PBS at 5 × 10^7 cells/ml

Incubate on ice 15 min

Centrifuge 750 g 10 min

Centrifuge supernatant at
12,000 g 15 min

Apply supernatant to LcH-
Sepharose column or directly
to antibody-Sepharose column

Prepare membranes from 10^9 cells

Solubilize membranes with
1 ml 1% DOC in Tris-saline buffer,
pH 8 (0.02 M Tris-HCl 0.15 M NaCl),
containing 1 mM iodoacetamide,
1 mM PMSF, 100 U/ml Trasylol

Incubate on ice 15 min

Centrifuge 100,000 g 60 min

Apply supernatant on top of LcH-
Sepharose column equilibrated with
0.5% DOC in Tris-saline buffer

Wash with 0.5% NP40 in Tris-
saline buffer

Elute with 10% methyl-α-D-mannopyranoside,
0.5% NP40 in Tris-saline buffer

Collect fractions

Apply pooled fractions with peak
radioactivity on top of antibody-
Sepharose column equilibrated with
0.25% NP40 in Tris-saline buffer

Wash with same buffer

Elute with 0.2 M glycine-HCl, pH 2.3,
0.25% NP40, 0.5 M NaCl,

Pool fractions with peak radioactivie
counts

Analyze by SDS-PAGE

Scheme II. Scheme for the purification of cell surface antigen(s) recognized by monoclonal antibodies.

cpm/μl are concentrated for SDS-PAGE analysis by precipitation with an equal volume of cold 30% trichloroacetic acid (TCA). Precipitates are centrifuged and washed twice with cold acetone to remove excess acid. Packed TCA precipitates are often insoluble in the SDS sample buffer. This can be overcome by centrifuging the TCA precipitates in round-bottom tubes rather than conical ones and dispersing the precipitate in a small volume of buffer or 8 M urea before adding the SDS sample buffer.

Some monoclonal antibodies display a very low affinity for antigen and may not be used for antigen purification as described above. Nevertheless, the antigen(s) recognized by such antibodies may be identified by observing their retardation when passed through an immobilized antibody column. For this purpose a relatively long antibody column is used, and the detergent-solubilized membrane extract is applied in a small volume. Fractions are collected and monitored for radioactivity throughout the washing and elution cycles. Then SDS-PAGE is used to analyze appropriate fractions to assess the preferential retardation of eluted polypeptides.

B. Immunoprecipitation after SDS-PAGE Analysis

Many membrane proteins have already been characterized by SDS-PAGE which is usually the method of choice for analysis and identification of membrane proteins (Steck and Fox, 1973). Unfortunately immunoprecipitation in the presence of SDS is not possible, and many proteins are irreversibly denatured after SDS removal. However, SDS removal can result in refolding to the native conformation of enough of the polypeptides to allow the use of this high-resolution technique in combination with immunoassay (Olden and Yamada, 1977).

After conventional slab gel electrophoresis of membrane proteins (Takacs, 1979) the gel is fixed at room temperature in a solution of 25% isopropyl alcohol and 10% acetic acid for 2 hr with gentle agitation. The SDS is removed by washing the gel consecutively for 30 min each time with 10% isopropyl alcohol and 10% acetic acid, followed by 10% acetic acid and finally by PBS. The gel is cut with a razor blade, and each gel track is incubated with a 1:10 dilution of antisera or ascites fluid at 4°C for 16 hr. After washing extensively with PBS the gel tracks are incubated with iodinated antiserum directed against the first antibody for 2–3 hr at room temperature. The nonspecifically bound iodinated globulin is then removed by washing the gel with PBS, as above. The gel tracks are finally dried on filter paper (Whatman 3MM), and radioactive patterns are detected by autoradiography on medical x-ray film.

A promising new approach which also combines the high resolution of

SDS-PAGE in separating membrane polypeptides and the high specificity of monospecific antibodies in identifying antigens was recently described by Towbin *et al.* (1979). The method, first optimized for ribosomal proteins, should be adaptable for the analysis of cell surface antigens. A protein mixture is first resolved by SDS-PAGE analysis. This is followed by the electrophoretic transfer of polypeptides from the polyacrylamide slab gel onto nitrocellulose sheets. Proteins bind strongly to nitrocellulose, where they are more accessible to antibody than inside a polyacrylamide gel.

After SDS electrophoresis the gel slab is placed on a sheet of wet nitrocellulose (Millipore GSWP, 0.22 or 0.45 μm pore size), cut to the size of the gel slab, and supported by a sheet of wet Whatman 3MM filter paper. Care must be taken to avoid the trapping of air bubbles between the gel and the membrane. A second filter paper sheet is placed on the other gel surface. This sandwich is placed between two 0.5-cm-thick scouring pads (Scotch-Brite) which are in turn supported by two rigid Plexiglas plates containing holes to allow free access of electrolyte to the gel sandwich and the flow of current through the system (Fig. 7). The whole sandwich is built by starting with one of the Plexiglas supports and is finally held together firmly by rubber bands and placed between the electrodes of an electrophoretic destaining chamber containing an appropriate solvent. For ribosomal proteins (see Towbin *et al.*, 1979) electrophoresed in 8 M urea the transfer was done in 0.7% acetic acid with the nitrocellulose sheet facing the cathod. After SDS gel electrophoresis of ribosomal proteins or other soluble proteins, the electrolyte in the transfer chamber consisted of 25 mM Tris, 192 mM glycine, pH 8.3, containing 20% (v/v) methanol, with the nitrocellulose sheet facing the anode. For the transfer of cell membrane proteins after SDS-PAGE we have obtained good transfer of polypeptide bands using 6 M urea in distilled H$_2$O as transfer medium, with the nitrocellulose sheet facing the anode. In general, high-molecular-weight polypeptides are transferred less efficiently. This, however, is improved by performing the PAGE in a (5–20%) gradient gel (Takacs, 1979).

The electrodes of the transfer chamber consist of two stainless steel wire mesh sheets placed 5 cm apart. A voltage gradient of 10–20 V/cm is applied for 1–2 hr. At the end of the run, the gel is stained in 0.25% Coomassie brilliant blue in methanol–acetic acid–water, 5:1:5, at 37°C for 1 hr with gentle agitation to assess the degree of protein transfer. Part of the nitrocellulose sheet may be stained for 1 min in 0.1% amido black prepared in 45% methanol–10% acetic acid (Schaffner and Weissmann, 1973) and destained in 90% methanol–10% acetic acid to visualize the transferred polypeptide bands. The rest of the nitrocellulose sheet is washed with three changes of PBS to remove urea. This washing step is followed by incuba-

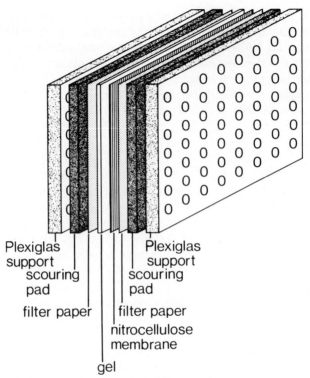

Plexiglas
support
 scouring
 pad
  filter paper

Plexiglas
support
scouring
pad
filter paper
nitrocellulose
membrane
gel

Fig. 7. Assembly for the electrophoretic transfer of SDS–PAGE-resolved polypeptides to nitrocellulose sheets.

tion of the membrane in 20% FCS in PBS for 30 min at room temperature to saturate protein-binding sites on the nitrocellulose. The membrane is washed again with PBS as above and incubated in undiluted hybridoma culture supernatant or 1:100 diluted specific antiserum or ascites fluid at 4°C for 6–16 hr. After washing with PBS as above, the membrane is flooded with iodinated sheep or rabbit antibodies directed against the first antibody for 2–3 hr at room temperature. Nonspecifically adsorbed iodinated globulin is then removed by washing the membrane with PBS as above. After drying the membrane between two sheets of filter paper, it is analyzed by autoradiography using medical x-ray film as described above, or it may be cut and the slices transferred to tubes for counting radioactivity.

Alternatively the immune complexes may be detected by using anti-Ig conjugated to horseradish peroxidase followed by treatment with O-dianisidine to localize the peroxidase (Avrameas and Guilbert, 1971).

After incubation of the nitrocellulose sheet with the specific antiserum (see above) and washing with PBS, the membrane is flooded with a solution of horseradish peroxidase-conjugated antibodies (Miles) directed against the first antibody for 2–3 hr at room temperature. The nonspecifically bound globulin is removed by washing with PBS as above. For the color reaction the membrane is incubated for 30 min with 0.0025% O-dianisidine, 0.01% H_2O_2 in 10 mM Tris–HCl, pH 7.4.

VI. CONCLUSION

The cell surface plays a crucial role in a number of well-defined cellular functions, including the immune response. In spite of the important role played by this cell organelle, our knowledge of the structural organization of biological membranes and of the mechanism of biochemical reactions operating within this structure is extremely limited. In order to increase our information at this level, we must first fractionate the membrane into identifiable subunits. Fractionation of membrane proteins and glycoproteins by conventional biochemical means has been hampered by the concomitant purification of many membrane proteins having either the same size or the same charge. Although the use of monospecific antisera to purify cell surface antigens bypasses these considerations, their highly restricted availability limits their usefulness.

The hybridoma technique of Köhler and Milstein (1975) provides a promising new approach to the production of monoclonal antibodies, potentially against every cell surface antigen. In this chapter we have described some ways of using these antibodies to purify the antigens they recognize. Our choice of methods was dictated by several considerations:

1. Whenever possible, the use of established cell lines is recommended for the purification of cell surface antigens. Cultured cell lines provide a uniform and continuous source of antigens.

2. Purification of the cytoplasmic membrane is recommended as an initial step. This not only results in enrichment of the desired cell surface antigens but also reduces contamination of the preparation by cytoplasmic proteins, in particular proteolytic enzymes.

3. Since the cell surface antigens in question represent integral plasma membrane glycoproteins, they must first be extracted from the membrane matrix in a soluble form. This solubilization step is best achieved by the use of agents that do not destroy the protein's antigenic structure. The relatively mild anionic surfactant DOC and detergents of the nonionic class meet these requirements for most antigens.

4. The glycoprotein nature of most, if not all, intrinsic membrane proteins makes possible a second enrichment step by affinity chromatography on lectin columns.

5. The final purification step is then achieved by the use of immobilized monoclonal antibody affinity columns. The use of highly specific monoclonal antibodies should allow the identification of many minor or weakly antigenic cell surface components that were missed by other methods.

The cataloging of cell surface antigens using monoclonal antibodies is progressing rapidly. The existence of an antigenic blueprint of cell surface architecture, together with a collection of monoclonal antibodies, would be invaluable not only in the diagnosis but possibly also in the treatment of many neoplastic diseases.

REFERENCES

Ada, G. L. (1970). *Transplant. Rev.* **5**, 105–129.
Allan, D., Auger, J., and Crumpton, M. J. (1972). *Nature (London), New Biol.* **236**, 23–25.
Anderson, J. K., Moore, J. O., Falletta, J. M., Terry, W. F., and Metzgar, R. S. (1979). *J. Natl. Cancer Inst.* **62**, 293–298.
Avrameas, S., and Guilbert B. (1971). *Eur. J. Immunol.* **1**, 394–396.
Axelsson, B., Kimura, A., Hammarström, S., Wigzell, H., Nilsson, K., and Mellstedt, H. (1978). *Eur. J. Immunol.* **8**, 757–764.
Ballou, B., Levine, G., Hakala, T. R., and Solter, D. (1979). *Science* **206**, 844–847.
Basten, A., Miller, J. F. A. P., Sprent, J., and Pye, J. (1972). *J. Exp. Med.* **135**, 610–626.
Becher, P. (1967). *In* "Nonionic Surfactants" (M. J. Schick, ed.), pp. 604–626. Dekker, New York.
Benson, A. A., (1966). *J. Am. Oil Chem. Soc.* **43**, 265–270.
Bianco, C., Patrick, R., and Nussenzweig, V. (1970). *J. Exp. Med.* **132**, 702–720.
Binz, H., Frischknecht, H., Mercolli, C., and Wigzell, H. (1978). *Scand. J. Immunol.* **7**, 481–485.
Bjerrum, O. J., and Bög-Hansen, T. C. (1976). *In* "Biochemical Analysis of Membranes" (A. H. Maddy, ed.), pp. 378–426. Chapman & Hall, London.
Bjerrum, O. J., and Lundahl, P. (1974). *Biochim. Biophys. Acta* **342**, 69–80.
Bridgen, J., Snary D., Crumpton, M. J., Barnstable, C., Goodfellow, P., and Bodmer, W. F. (1976). *Nature (London)* **261**, 200–205.
Buck, D. W., Gross, S. J., and Bodmer, W. F. (1976). *Cytogenet. Cell Genet.* **16**, 99–104.
Charron, D. J., and McDevitt, H. O. (1979). *Fed. Am. Soc. Exp. Biol. Proc.* **38**, 1280a.
Converse, C. A., and Papermaster, D. S. (1975). *Science* **189**, 469–472.
Cosini, A. B., Wortis, H. H., Delmonico, F. L., and Russell, P. S. (1979). *Surgery* **80**, 155.
Crumpton, M. J., and Parkhouse, R. M. E. (1972). *FEBS Lett.* **22**, 210–212.
Danielli, J. E., and Davson, H. (1935). *J. Cell. Comp. Physiol.* **5**, 495–508.
Ey, P. L., Prowse, S. J., and Jenkin, C. R. (1978). *Immunochemistry* **15**, 429–436.
Fazekas de St. Groth, S., and Scheidegger, D. (1980). *J. Immunol. Methods* (in press).
Ferber, E., Resch, K., Wallach, D. F. H., and Imm, W. (1972). *Biochim. Biophys. Acta* **266**, 494–504.

Fraker, P. J., and Speck, J. C., Jr. (1978). *Biochem. Biophys. Res. Commun.* **80**, 840–857.

Fröland, S. S., Wislöff, F., and Michaelsen, T. E. (1974). *Int. Arch. Allergy Appl. Immunol.* **47**, 124–138.

Gahmberg, C. G., and Andersson, L. C. (1977). *J. Biol. Chem.* **252**, 5888–5894.

Gill, T. J., Kunz, H. W., and Papermaster, D. S. (1967). *J. Biol. Chem.* **242**, 3308–3318.

Gold, A. M. (1967). *In* "Methods in Enzymology" (C. H. W. Hirs, ed.), Vol. XI, pp. 706–711. Academic Press, New York.

Goldstein, L. T., Klinman, N. R., and Manson, L. A. (1973). *J. Natl. Cancer Inst.* **51**, 1713–1715.

Green, D. E., and Perdue, J. F. (1966). *Proc. Natl. Acad. Sci. U.S.A.* **55**, 1295–1302.

Griffin, W. C. (1949). *J. Soc. Cosmet. Chem.* **1**, 311–326.

Hayman, M. J., and Crumpton, M. J. (1972). *Biochem. Biophys. Res. Commun.* **47**, 923–930.

Helenius, A., and Simons, K. (1975). *Biochim. Biophys. Acta* **415**, 29–79.

Humphreys, R. E., McCune, J. M., Chess, L., Herrman, H. C., Malenka, D. J., Mann, D. L., Parham, P., Schlossman, S. F., and Strominger, J. L. (1976). *J. Exp. Med.* **144**, 98–112.

Hunter, W. M., and Greenwood, F. C. (1962). *Nature (London)* **194**, 495–496.

Johansson, K. E., and Hjertén, S. (1974). *J. Mol. Biol.* **86**, 341–348.

Jondal, M., Holm, G., and Wigzell, H. (1972). *J. Exp. Med.* **136**, 207–215.

Klein, J. (1975). "Biology of the Mouse Histocompatibility-2 Complex." Springer-Verlag, Berlin and New York.

Köhler, G., and Milstein, C. (1975). *Nature (London)* **256**, 495–497.

Koprowski, H., Steplewski, Z., Herlyn, D., and Herlyn, M. (1978). *Proc. Natl. Acad. Sci. U.S.A.* **75**, 3405–3409.

Krawinkel, U., Cramer, M., Berek, C., Hämmerling, G., Black, S. J., Rajewsky, K., and Eichmann, K. (1976). *Cold Spring Harbor Symp. Quant. Biol.* **41**, 285–294.

Kung, P. C., Goldstein, G., Reinherz, E. L., and Schlossman, S. F. (1979). *Science* **206**, 347–379.

Lerner, R. A., McConahey, P. J., and Dixon, F. J. (1971). *Science* **173**, 60–62.

Marchalonis, J. J., Cone, R. E., and Santer, V. (1971). *Biochem. J.* **124**, 921–927.

Olden, K., and Yamada, K. M. (1977). *Anal. Biochem.* **78**, 483–490.

Parham, P., and Bodmer, W. F. (1978). *Nature (London)* **276**, 397–399.

Pernis, B., Forni, L., and Amante, L. (1971). *Ann. N.Y. Acad. Sci.* **190**, 420–431.

Peterson, P. A., Rask, L., and Lindblom, J. B. (1972). *Proc. Natl. Acad. Sci. U.S.A.* **71**, 35–39.

Robertson, J. D. (1962). *Sci. Am.* **206**, 64–72.

Rogers, M. J., Robinson, E. A., and Appella, E. (1979). *J. Biol. Chem.* **254**, 11126–11133.

Schaffner, W., and Weissmann, C. (1973). *Anal. Biochem.* **56**, 502–514.

Schwartz, B. D., and Nathenson, S. G. (1971). *J. Immunol.* **107**, 1363–1367.

Singer, S. J., and Nicolson, G. L. (1973). *Science* **175**, 720–731.

Snary, D., Barnstable, C. J., Bodmer, W. F., Goodfellow, P. N., and Crumpton, M. J. (1977). *Scand. J. Immunol.* **6**, 439–452.

Springer, T. A., Kaufman, J. F., Terhorst, C., and Strominger, J. L. (1977). *Nature (London)* **268**, 213–218.

Stähli, C., Staehelin, T., Miggiano, V., Schmidt, J., and Häring, P. (1980). *J. Immunol. Methods* **32**, 297–304.

Standring, R., and Williams, A. F. (1978). *Biochim. Biophys. Acta* **508**, 85–96.

Standring, R., McMaster, W. R., Sunderland, C. A., and Williams, A. F. (1978). *Eur. J. Immunol.* **8**, 832–839.

Steck, T. L., and Fox, C. F. (1973). *In* "Membrane Molecular Biology" (C. F. Fox and A. D. Keith, eds.), pp. 27–75. Sinauer Assoc., Stanford, Connecticut.

Stein, M. D., Howard, I. K., and Sage, H. J. (1971). *Arch. Biochem. Biophys.* **146,** 353–355.

Stocker, J. W., and Heusser, C. H. (1979). *J. Immunol. Methods* **26,** 87–95.

Strominger, J. L., Gresswell, P., Grey, H., Humphreys, R. E., Mann, O., McClune, J., Parham, P., Robb, R., Sanderson, A. R., Springer, T. A., Terhorst, C., and Turner, M. J. (1974). *Transplant. Rev.* **21,** 126–143.

Sulitzeanu, D. (1971). *Curr. Top. Microbiol. Immunol.* **54,** 1.

Takacs, B. (1979). *In* "Immunological Methods" (I. Lefkovits and B. Pernis, eds.), pp. 81–105. Academic Press, New York.

Tanaki, N., Tokuyama, H., Fukunishi, T., Minowada, J., and Pressman, D. (1979). *J. Immunol.* **123,** 2906–2914.

Towbin, H., Staehelin, T., and Gordon, J. (1979). *Proc. Natl. Acad. Sci. U.S.A.* **76,** 4350–4354.

Trucco, M. M., Stocker, J. W., and Ceppellini, R. (1978). *Nature (London)* **273,** 666–668.

Wilson, L. A., and Amos, D. B. (1972). *Tissue Antigens* **2,** 105–111.

Yu, J., Fischman, D. A., and Steck, T. L. (1973). *J. Supramol. Struct.* **1,** 233–248.

3

Two-Dimensional Gel
Electrophoresis

Charles Sidman

I. INTRODUCTION

When isolating, characterizing, or comparing proteins or glycoproteins, one typically attempts to utilize several biochemical and biophysical properties. Some of these properties are molecular weight, molecular dimensions, isoelectric point (charge), hydrophobicity, presence of chemical features such as disulfide bonds, and higher-order properties such as susceptibility to protease digestion or binding by specific ligands. Concerning the techniques developed to utilize these properties, certain broad generalizations can be made. First, specific ligand binding (by antibodies, lectins, or specific substrates) is a powerful separatory procedure, which allows the processing of large amounts of materials and permits purifica-

IMMUNOLOGICAL METHODS, VOL. II

tion up to 1000-fold in a single step in some cases. Often, however, depending on the starting material and the ligand used, several molecular species may be purified, resulting in the need for further analytical work. Various centrifugal or column electrophoretic and chromatographic procedures also allow the handling of bulk material but do not offer resolution sufficient for more than crude characterization and comparison of molecules. Finally, separatory procedures in polyacrylamide-based gel media offer the finest resolution and comparison capabilities for analytical purposes, often to approximately 1% of the property being measured. These procedures can also be scaled up for semipreparative purposes, but with some loss of resolution.

In this chapter, an overview is offered of several high-resolution analytical procedures for proteins and glycoproteins. These techniques are all two-dimensional; that is, they all involve two sequential separations based on different biochemical or biophysical properties. All employ electrophoresis with polyacrylamide gels in at least one dimension.

Each of these techniques was originally developed by other workers than this author. In this chapter therefore I have concentrated on the rationale for and the experimental details of how these procedures are regularly applied in our laboratory, rather than attempting a comprehensive overview of theory or principles. By thus assembling several techniques which I have found useful, and by giving the precise details of how the original procedures have been adapted and modified, I hope to enable others to utilize these methods profitably also.

II. ONE-DIMENSIONAL SODIUM DODECYL SULFATE–POLYACRYLAMIDE GELS (SDS-PAGE)

Sodium dodecyl sulfate–polyacrylamide gel electrophoresis is the major technique common to all the two-dimensional gel methods discussed in this chapter. The apparatus and basic procedures have been presented in Chapter 4 by Takacs (1979) in the first volume of this series. Here I will only note the specific procedures used in our laboratory and add a few extra details to Takacs' presentation.

A. Solutions

SDS sample buffer–reducing: 10% (v/v) glycerol, 5% (v/v) 2-mercapto-ethanol (2-ME), 2.3% (w/v) SDS, and 0.0625 M Tris–HCl, pH 6.8 (kept at 4°C)

SDS sample buffer–nonreducing: as above, but without 2-ME (kept at room temperature)

Upper SDS gel buffer (4×): 0.4% SDS in 0.5 M Tris–HCl, pH 6.8 (kept at 4°C)

Lower SDS gel buffer (4×): 0.4% SDS in 1.5 M Tris base, pH 8.8 (kept at 4°C)

30% Acrylamide: 29.2% (w/v) acrylamide, 0.8% (w/v) bisacrylamide (kept at 4°C)

30% Acrylamide with glycerol: as above, plus 10% (v/v) glycerol (kept at 4°C)

SDS running buffer: 0.025 M Tris base, 0.192 M glycine, 0.1% (w/v) SDS (kept at room temperature)

Ammonium persulfate: 10% (w/v) (stored in the dark at 4°C and made fresh every 2 weeks)

B. Apparatus

Glass plates and spacers are used as described in Takacs (1979). For greater utilization of apparatus, and to run as many samples as possible under uniform conditions, "double packs" of two notched and one un-notched glass plates are assembled, which allow two gel slabs to be run together. The plates and spacers are sealed with melted white petroleum jelly.

When using standard-sized glass plates (17 × 18 cm), 1 mm in the gradient gels described below corresponds to about 2% of the apparent molecular weight, in the range of 10K–200K. Larger glass plates (28 × 18 cm) allow resolution to less than 1% of the apparent molecular weight per millimeter of gel.

C. Gel Preparation

For routine separations of reduced proteins in the 10–200K molecular-weight range, linear 8–18% gradient gels are used. For nonreducing gels, 5–15% gels are usually employed. With the Cleveland peptide mapping technique (Section III,D), 8 and 18% (nongradient) single-percentage gels are routine. SDS-PAGE gels are prepared as follows:

1. Mix the proper amount of 30% acrylamide (with glycerol for the heavy solution of gradient gels), 4× lower SDS gel buffer (to a final concentration of 1×), distilled H_2O to the required volume, and 0.00145 vol of 10% ammonium persulfate (for gradient gels, or 0.0033 vol for single-percentage gels).

2. Degas.

3. Add 0.0005 vol of N,N,N′,N′-tetramethylethylene diamine (TEMED).

4. The gel is poured to 2 cm below the notch for two-dimensional SDS-PAGE or 3 cm below the notch for standard SDS-PAGE. (For linear gradient gels, a three-channel peristaltic pump is used, as described in Takacs (1979), to pour one or two slabs at a time. The heavy gel solution is kept cold during this process.) The acrylamide is overlaid with H_2O-saturated butanol and allowed to polymerize at least 1 hr at room temperature.

5. After the gel has polymerized, nonpolymerized acrylamide and butanol are aspirated off and the gel surface is washed with $1\times$ lower SDS gel buffer. The gel may be stored under this buffer for 1 or 2 days at room temperature.

6. The stacking gel mixture consists of 0.15 vol of 30% acrylamide, 0.25 vol of $4\times$ upper SDS gel buffer, 0.6 vol of distilled H_2O, and 0.003 vol of 10% ammonium persulfate.

7. All liquid is aspirated from the prepared separating (lower) slab gel, and any slot-forming combs are inserted to a 1.5-cm depth. (Thus at least 1.5 cm remains between the sample slots and the top of the separating gel.) The stacking gel mixture is degassed, 0.001 vol of TEMED is added, and the stacking gel solution is pipetted into the gel pack to the bottom of the notch in the glass plate. It is then overlaid with H_2O-saturated butanol and polymerized at room temperature for 30–60 min. Any combs are removed, and the stacking gel is washed with $1\times$ upper SDS gel buffer. The gel is then ready for sample application and electrophoresis (see Section III).

D. Electrophoresis

Gels can be run at constant current (in which case the voltage increases during the run) to minimize the running time, or at constant voltage (in which case the current falls during the run) to allow overnight electrophoresis. In either case the results are equivalent in quality. To minimize problems with the formation of bubbles under the gel during long runs with tall gel packs, the bottom chamber's SDS running buffer is degassed prior to electrophoresis. If a constant current is used, a maximum of 20 mA per slab is advised. At this current, the gels will become warm but will not be harmed. Electrophoresis is continued until a marker dye (bromphenol blue) or a small colored standard protein (for example, cytochrome *c,* 12,300 MW) has run to or off the bottom of the gel. The polarity in SDS-PAGE is negative at the top and positive at the bottom.

E. Processing

After electrophoresis, gels are marked by punching out and aspirating one or more holes in an available upper corner of the slab. The gels are then fixed and stained in 0.1% (w/v) Coomassie blue stain in 50% (w/v) trichloroacetic acid, for 20 min at room temperature. They are then destained using 10% acetic acid, 10% isopropanol (rocking at room temperature or at 37°C). If fluorography is necessary, EnHance solution (New England Nuclear Co.) is used to impregnate gels with the scintillant PPO (1 hr of rocking at room temperature with three times the gel volume of EnHance). The final processing step is a rinse (1 hr at room temperature) in 2% glycerol. This precipitates any PPO within the gel for fluorography and allows the gels to dry without cracking.

Processed gels are placed on 3MM filter paper and dried with vacuum alone. After drying, spots of radioactive ink are placed around the dried gel to identify the autoradiograms or fluorograms and to allow alignment of the gel and film for subsequent removal of specific bands or spots. (Pinpricks) through the film and into the gel mark the areas to be removed.) If a region's radioactivity is to be counted, gamma counts can be measured directly from an excised gel piece. For measuring beta counts, the gel slice is first permeabilized by incubation in NCS tissue solubilizer (from Nuclear Chicago Corp.) containing 10% H_2O, with 1 day of rocking at 37°C, and then adding scintillation fluid and rocking again for 1 day at 37°. The gel slice can then be counted in a scintillation counter without quenching problems.

III. TWO-DIMENSIONAL GEL TECHNIQUES

A. Isoelectrofocusing Followed by SDS-PAGE (O'Farrell Gels)

This technique, devised by O'Farrell and co-workers, is today a standard and powerful means for comparing proteins and complex protein mixtures. Proteins are first fractionated according to their isoelectric point by isoelectrofocusing (IEF) in a tubular gel of low polyacrylamide concentration. The original description of the technique (O'Farrell, 1975) called for a first separation to isoelectric equilibrium. However, this procedure was limited to proteins whose isoelectric points were neutral or acidic. Later (O'Farrell *et al.*, 1977), a modification was published which reversed the electrode polarity during the first separation and which did not run to equilibrium (nonequilibrium pH gradient electrophoresis, or NEPHGE). This modification does not resolve neutral or acidic proteins as well as the original IEF technique but has the advantage of including and separating basic proteins in addition to neutral and acidic ones. After either type of first-dimension electrofocusing separation, the tube gels are equilibrated in SDS-PAGE sample buffer and then run on SDS-PAGE. Proteins are thus separated according to isoelectric point in the first dimension, and by apparent molecular weight in the second.

1. Sample Preparation

Dry sample materials may be solubilized in the lysis buffer described by O'Farrell (1975) [9.5 M urea, 2% Nonidet P-40 (NP40), 1.6% (final) Ampholines, pH 5–7, 0.4% (final) Ampholines, pH 3–10, 5% 2-ME, kept in frozen aliquots]. However, when preparing wet samples or samples already in solution, or extracting immunoprecipitated materials from immunoabsorbent particles (my usual source of samples), the simple use of O'Farrell's lysis buffer often leads to buffer dilution and later difficulties in proper layering of solutions during sample loading for electrofocusing. I therefore solubilize wet samples in, or elute immunoprecipitated materials by, several sequential elutions at 100°C with 0.5% SDS plus 5% 2-ME (or 0.5% SDS alone for nonreducing gels). These samples may be used for SDS-PAGE or for IEF or NEPHGE. For IEF or NEPHGE, up to 50 µl (A *microliters*) of the sample in 0.5% SDS solution is combined with A milligrams of urea plus $A/4$ microliters of the following mixture (kept in the dark at 4°C for over 1 yr): 18% NP40, 35% (stock) Ampholines, pH 5–7, 9% (stock) Ampholines, pH 3.5–10, and 38% 2-ME. When mixed together, this yields samples with the same constituent concentrations as lysis buffer (the final volume is 2.3A microliters). The samples may be used immediately or frozen at −20°C.

2. Running of Isoelectrofocusing and NEPHGE First-Dimension Gels

These separations are done in a standard tube gel electrophoresis apparatus using glass tubes 12 cm long and 3.0 mm ID (6.0 mm OD). To prepare for pouring the gels, the bottoms of clean, dry tubes are sealed first with a small square of rehydrated dialysis membrane, held on by a ring of thin-walled silicon tubing, and then with a layer of Parafilm. The tubes are fixed upright and level and filled to within 1–1.5 cm of the top (depending on sample volume) with a gel mixture made as follows (for 10 ml, sufficient for 10 tubes):

a. Mix the following: 5.52 gm urea, 2.00 ml 10% (v/v) NP40 (kept at 4°C), 1.33 ml 28.38% (w/v) acrylamide plus 1.62% (w/v) bisacrylamide (kept in the dark at 4°C, 0.50 ml stock Ampholines (40%) (for IEF, 0.4 ml, pH 5–7, plus 0.1 ml, pH 3.5–10) (for NEPHGE, 0.5 ml, pH 3.5–10, or others, depending on desired range; may be mixed freely), and 1.97 ml distilled H_2O.

b. Dissolve the urea.

c. Add 10% ammonium persulfate: 10 µl for IEF or 20 µl for NEPHGE gels (basic Ampholines retard polymerization, so more ammonium persulfate and TEMED are used to compensate).

    d. Degas gently to avoid excessive bubbling and crystallization of urea on vessel walls.

    e. Add TEMED (*caution*—toxic): 7 μl for IEF, 14 μl for NEPHGE.

    f. Pipette the mixture into the prepared gel tubes.

After filling the gel tubes (with a long-tipped Pasteur pipette to avoid bubbles), overlay gently with 20 μl of overlay buffer (8.0 M urea) for IEF gels, or distilled H_2O for NEPHGE gels. Let the gels polymerize undisturbed at room temperature. The sharp interface between the gel and the overlying solution will disappear within about 30 min, and a sharp but fine interface will form at the edge of the polymerized gel within about 60 min. NEPHGE gels are ready for use after 1–2 hr of polymerization. And IEF gels, after 1–2 hr of polymerization, should have the overlay buffer removed, have 20 μl each of lysis buffer and then distilled H_2O sequentially overlaid, and be allowed to sit for another 1–2 hr. (Note: The slightest impurities in glassware, measuring utensils, and so on, can lead to premature gel polymerization in the degassing flask. Also, urea may be hard to dissolve or may recrystallize if the laboratory is too cold. A few urea crystals in a gel do not interfere, however, and disappear during electrophoresis.)

After the gels have polymerized sufficiently the Parafilm is removed and the gels rechecked for trapped air bubbles. (If any are found, the gels are discarded.) The tubes are then mounted in the gel apparatus, with the lower buffer covering the bottom 1–2 cm of the tubes. In IEF, the bottom buffer is 10 mM H_3PO_4 and the top buffer degassed 20 mM NaOH. In NEPHGE, the H_3PO_4 is on top and the NaOH on the bottom.

With IEF gels, a prerunning procedure is performed. Unpolymerized acrylamide and water are removed from the top of the gels, and 20 μl of fresh lysis buffer is added. The tubes are then carefully overlayed and filled with NaOH, and the upper buffer chamber is filled with NaOH to about 1 cm above the tubes. The gels are then prerun at constant voltage for 15 min at 200 V, 30 min at 300 V, and 30 min at 400 V (top, −; bottom, +). The upper reservoir is then emptied.

For both types of electrofocusing all solution is aspirated from above the polymerized gels and the samples are applied. (One tube can be left empty of sample to measure the final pH gradient.) Twenty microliters of overlay buffer is layered over each sample, and the rest of the tube plus the top buffer chamber are filled with upper buffer to 1 cm over the tops of the tubes.

The IEF gels are run for 10–20 hr at 400 V constant voltage (top, −; bottom, +) and then for 1 hr at 800 V constant voltage. (This variation in run length is merely for experimental convenience, as the same equilibrium is reached regardless.) The NEPHGE gels are run 4–7 hr at 400 V constant voltage (top, +; bottom, −). Here the optimal time of running must be reached empirically, depending on the pH range of maximum interest. This is because NEPHGE gels do not reach equilibrium. Basic proteins may never reach their isoelectric equilibria and so may continue to migrate into the gel as long as current is applied, while acidic proteins stop traveling when they reach their isoelectric zones but then move back toward the top of the gel (or even out) as the isoelectric zone itself migrates toward the top of the gel. In both gel procedures the current will drop throughout the run. (Note that, in IEF, negative ions move downward, so that acidic proteins lead and move furthest; while in NEPHGE, positive ions move downward, so that basic proteins lead.)

3. Handling of Isoelectrofocusing Tube Gels between Runs

After the electrofocusing run, the upper and lower chamber buffers must be disposed of with care, as they may contain much radioactivity. Sample-containing gels are marked at one end with a small injection of 0.1% bromphenol blue dye. They are then loosened by squirting warm water through a syringe needle around the inside of the tube and pushed out gently by air pressure from a syringe connected to the gel tube with plastic tubing. The tube gels are extruded directly into plastic tubes containing 5 ml of SDS sample buffer (Section II,A). They are then equilibrated for 45 min with occasional agitation, the buffer is removed and replaced with fresh SDS sample buffer, and the gels are equilibrated a second time. They may be frozen at any point during this equilibration procedure.

To measure the pH gradient formed during electrofocusing, an extra gel run without sample can be extruded onto a piece of Parafilm and sliced into 0.5-cm segments. These are then placed in 0.5-ml tubes of degassed distilled H_2O and shaken for $\frac{1}{2}$ –2 hr, and the resulting pHs measured.

4. Second-Dimension SDS-PAGE

The same apparatus used for normal SDS-PAGE is used for the second dimension of two-dimensional O'Farrell gels, with one exception. The bottom edge of the notch in the notched glass plate is beveled at an angle of approximately 45°. The gel pack is assembled with the beveled, lower edge of the notch toward the flat glass back plate, so that later the isoelectrofocusing tube gel will rest in the groove formed above the SDS-PAGE slab gel.

The lower (separating) gels for second-dimension SDS-PAGE are poured to within 1.5 cm of the bottom of the notch in the notched plate. Later, stacking gel (no comb) is poured to the bottom of the notch (Section II). After washing the upper surface of the stacking gel, an equilibrated IEF or NEPHGE gel is removed from its equilibrating buffer, transferred to a piece of foil or Parafilm, and placed above the stacking gel in the groove formed by the back plate and the beveled notch of the front plate. (The dye-injected end of the tube gel is placed in a uniform orientation.) There should be a space of 1 or 2 mm between the tube gel and the top of the stacking gel.

The tube gel is fixed above the stacking gel by running in approximately 1.25 ml per slab of melted 1% agar in SDS sample buffer. Care must be taken to avoid bubbles between the two gels. Molecular-weight standard proteins are included in the agar, which will form reference lines across the entire slab gel after Coomassie blue staining. For gels not to be impregnated with PPO for fluorography, the following mixture is prepared, aliquoted, stored at 4°C, and remelted before use: 7 mg β-galactosidase (135K MW), 7 mg phosphorylase b (93K MW), 3 mg bovine serum albumin (69K MW), 7 mg ovalbumin (45K MW), 20 mg rabbit immunoglobulin G (IgG) (50K and 25K MW), 7 mg soybean trypsin inhibitor (20K MW), 15 mg cytochrome c (12K MW), and 1 gm agar, in 100 ml SDS sample buffer. Gels which will be PPO-impregnated require about twice these amounts of protein for the reference lines to be visible. After the agar has cooled and solidified, the second-dimension SDS-PAGE gel is set up and run like a normal one. One hundred microliters of 0.1% bromphenol blue per slab can be added to the upper running buffer reservoir for tracking dye, if desired, or the progress of the colored cytochrome c band can be observed. After the run, processing is done as for normal SDS-PAGE (Section II).

Figure 1 presents examples of both types of O'Farrell two-dimensional gels (IEF and NEPHGE).

B. SDS-PAGE Followed by Isoelectrofocusing

Two-dimensional gels of the O'Farrell variety (NEPHGE or IEF followed by SDS-PAGE) can be used compare several examples of the same protein (Ig chains, for instance) if the same standards have been included in each gel. However, for a single protein component, a more economical and precise comparison is possible by first performing SDS-PAGE, which gives the optimal comparison of apparent molecular weights within the same slab gel, and then cutting out the polypeptide bands of interest. These are then rerun on IEF (or NEPHGE) slabs to obtain a side-by-side comparison of the isoelectric mobilities.

To perform this reversal of the normal O'Farrell sequence, regular SDS-PAGE is carried out and the gels dried and autoradiographed. Impregnation with PPO for fluorography should not be done in this first-dimension SDS-PAGE gel. The homologous protein bands from various tracks to be further compared are then located via the autoradiograms and excised from

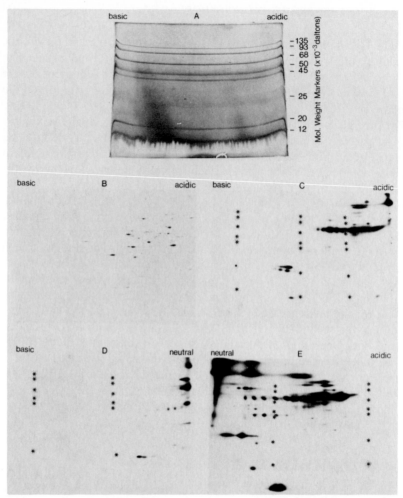

Fig. 1. O'Farrell two-dimensional gels. The total cytoplasmic and membrane proteins of thymoma line BW5147 were analyzed. (A) Photograph of a Coomassie-stained NEPHGE-type O'Farrell gel. The horizontal lines are the protein standards originally contained in the agarose used to hold the first-dimension tube gel over the second-dimension slab gel. Also visible as small spots are some of the more abundant cellular proteins. Actin is the small spot about one-third of the way from the acidic end of the gel, under the 45K-dalton OVA reference line. In (C–E) the positions of the size marker protein lines are indicated by stars. (B) NEPHGE-type O'Farrell gel of biosynthetically [35S]methionine-labeled cell lysate. (Ampholines, pH range 3.5–10; run length, 1800 V-hr.) (C) NEPHGE-type O'Farrell gel of membrane proteins iodinated by [125I]-labeled lactoperoxidase. (Ampholines, pH 3.5–10; run length, 1800 V-hr.) Note that fewer labeled protein species are seen here than in the biosynthetically labeled lysate, since lactoperoxidase iodination only labels proteins on the outer membrane surface which have available tyrosine residues. Also, the greater penetrating power of the 125I gamma emissions, compared to the 35S beta emissions, makes spots due to 125I-labeled proteins less sharp than those from 35S-labeled proteins. (D) NEPHGE-type O'Farrell gel [expanded—compare with left side of C] of the basic range of 125I-labeled membrane proteins. (Ampholines, pH 7–9; run length, 1800 V-hr.) (E) IEF-type O'Farrell gel [expanded—compare with right side of C] of the acidic range of 125I-labeled membrane proteins.

the dried gel. These are rehydrated in 0.1–1 ml of IEF–NEPHGE lysis buffer for 60 min at 20°C and then applied to the IEF slabs prepared as follows.

The IEF or NEPHGE gel mixture (Section III,A,2) is modified by using 1.67 ml acrylamide and 1.63 ml distilled H_2O per 10 ml. This yields a final acrylamide concentration of 5% instead of 4% with the standard tube gel recipe and makes the slab gel easier to handle. After degassing and the addition of TEMED, this mixture is poured into a pack of two unnotched regular slab gel plates. The gels are overlaid and polymerized like tube electrofocusing gels.

After the electrofocusing slab gel has polymerized, the gel surface is washed and the pack is disassembled, leaving the slab gel resting on one of the glass plates. This slab is mounted, gel upward, in a closable Plexiglas chamber containing water-soaked towels to maintain humidity. Carbon electrodes are laid across the two ends of the gel and are wetted with the appropriate electrode buffers (Section III,A,2). Slab IEF gels are prerun like tube IEF gels (Section III, A, 2). Next, a line of small troughs is cut into the slab gel near the appropriate starting electrode (− for IEF; + for NEPHGE). The samples (rehydrated portions of SDS-PAGE gels) are placed in these troughs in the electrofocusing slab gel, any free space is filled with lysis buffer, and a piece of plastic wrap is gently placed over the whole gel surface. The chamber is closed, and the run started. Slab IEF and NEPHGE gels are run like the tube versions, except that the combined milliamps times volts per slab should not exceed 3000. Thus the gels are run at constant voltage, with the voltage being increased gradually over the first few hours until 400 V is reached. After 400 V constant voltage is reached, NEPHGE gels are run up to 5 hr and IEF gels overnight.

After the electrofocusing run, the second-dimension electrofocusing slab gels are processed like regular SDS-PAGE slabs. The corner nearest sample No. 1 is cut off to be used later to orient the gel. Because they are soft and floppy, slab electrofocusing gels are always transferred lying on a support and placed in the new solution before the support is removed (or replaced). After processing, slab electrofocusing gels are autoradiographed or fluorographed like other slab gels.

Figure 2 shows an example of the use of this procedure to compare the light chains from a series of antigen-specific hybridoma proteins. Braun *et al.* (1979) also present a more detailed discussion of slab IEF techniques.

C. Charge-Shift Electrophoresis Followed by SDS-PAGE

Another molecular property of interest to cell biologists is hydrophobicity. Intrinsic membrane proteins are inserted into the lipid bilayer of biological membranes via an exposed stretch of hydrophobic amino acids.

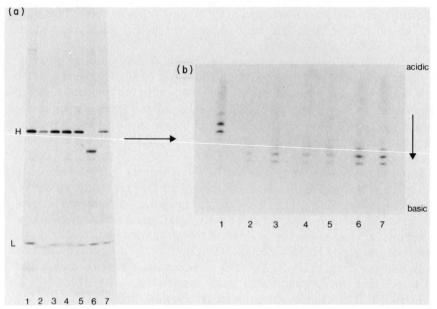

Fig. 2. SDS-PAGE followed by NEPHGE analysis of biosynthetically labeled Ig light (L) chains. Seven antigen-specific hybridoma lines (produced by C. Berek of the Basel Institute) were biosynthetically labeled with [^{14}C]leucine. The Ig secreted into the culture medium was immunoprecipitated and run on reducing SDS-PAGE (a). The isolated light-chain bands were located, excised, and rerun on a NEPHGE slab gel (Ampholines, pH 3.5–10; run length, 1800 V-hr (b). Together these procedures allow a very powerful comparison of the set of L chains. L chain 1 is both apparently larger on SDS-PAGE and more acidic in electrofocusing than the others, while L chain 2 is apparently smaller on SDS-PAGE but similar in electrofocusing to most of the others. Light chains 3–7 are indistinguishable by either criterion.

In their native state, peripheral membrane proteins or water-soluble proteins do not show such an external hydrophobic region. Several laboratories have exploited this difference in hydrophobicity, by procedures which depend on the binding of detergents, to distinguish between soluble and intrinsic membrane proteins.

One of these procedures is called charge-shift electrophoresis (CSE) and was introduced by Helenius and Simons (1977). Molecules are subjected to electrophoresis in neutral detergents or nondenaturing mixtures of neutral and charged detergents. Molecules which bind detergents via hydrophobic interactions migrate differently in all three detergent mixtures (positive, neutral, and negative), while molecules which do not bind detergents or which bind only one of the charged detergents via electrostatic rather than hydrophobic interactions migrate similarly in all three or in two of the three detergent mixtures.

The CSE technique was originally developed using purified and homogeneous proteins, or electrophoresing protein mixtures, and then applying immunodiffusion to localize specific molecules approximately. Since sample purification procedures which might denature proteins and expose internal hydrophobic regions must be avoided, SDS-PAGE before CSE is not advisable. To obtain better resolution and analysis capabilities for the electrophoresed proteins, we have adapted the CSE technique to include slicing, eluting, immunoprecipitating, and performing SDS-PAGE on fractions of the original CSE gel. This sequence combines the hydrophobicity resolution of CSE (on nondenatured samples) with immunoprecipitation and the size fractionation of SDS-PAGE and can thus be considered a two-dimensional gel technique.

1. Charge-Shift Electrophoresis

Cells (or other samples) are solubilized in CSE NP40 buffer (0.5% NP40, 0.1 M NaCl in 0.05 M glycine–NaOH, pH 9.0) for 10 min at 0°C, and the nuclei are spun out. Each sample is divided into thirds, to which are added $\frac{1}{4}$ vol (final concentration 2×) of 10× DOC (CSE NP40 buffer containing 2.5% sodium deoxycholate), CSE NP40 buffer, or 10 × CTAB (CSE NP40 buffer with 0.5% cetyltrimethylammonium bromide) (final concentration again 2×). These samples are then equilibrated at 4°C for 1–4 hr.

Gel layers on glass plates are prepared with 1% agar in CSE NP40 buffer containing no additions or 1 × DOC or CTAB. We use 7.5-cm-wide glass plates, of various lengths depending on the number of samples to be run, and pour the agar layers using 1.0 ml/7.5 cm² of area. (The bottom side of the plates is marked beforehand with the positions of the future sample troughs and the lines along which to fractionate the gel for sample elution and immunoprecipitation.) These plates are loaded into a covered electrophoresis chamber containing three separate pairs of buffer trays. One pair is filled with each appropriate detergent mixture (1×), and filter paper strips are wet and applied as electrodes. The plates are then prerun for 15 min at 4.5 V/cm (34 V in our laboratory).

After the prerun, the current is turned off. Sample slots (1 × 11 mm) are cut out down the midline of the plates, and the samples (up to 20 μl) are applied to the proper plates. A small circle 1–2 mm in diameter is also cut in each plate to hold a tracking dye sample (Gelman Co.'s RBY dye mixture, prepared in the three detergent mixtures like the other samples). The main electrophoresis is then started and continued for 2 hr at 4.5 V/cm, or other time, as appropriate. At approximately 45-min intervals during the run, the homologous electrophoresis buffer is added to each sample slot to maintain a regular electric field within the plate and avoid drying of the agar layer.

After the main electrophoresis run, the plates can be stained, destained, and autoradiographed as described in Helenius and Simons (1977). Our regular procedure is to elute and immunoprecipitate the separated proteins, however, which is described in the next section.

2. Elution, Immunoprecipitation, and SDS-PAGE
after Charge-Shift Electrophoresis

During the CSE run, immunoabsorbent beads are prepared by incubating antisera with protein A-coupled Sepharose CL-4B beads (usually 2–5 μl of antiserum per 5–10 μl of packed beads, rotating slowly for 60 min at 4°C), followed by three washes (20 min each, rotating at 4°C) in NNTA buffer (0.5% NP40, 0.5 M NaCl, 0.02 M Tris, pH 8.5, 0.1% NaN$_3$). Then 5–10 μl of packed beads prepared thus are placed into 1.5 ml portions of NNTA buffer in a series of 5-ml plastic tubes.

After the CSE run, each sample track is sliced with a razor blade into 2-mm sections (along the predrawn lines), and these sections are placed in the tubes containing immunoabsorbent beads plus NNTA. The tubes are then rotated overnight at 4°C, during which time elution and binding of the specific proteins proceeds. Since the antibody is bound to the Sepharose beads, precipitation does not occur within the slices of the CSE gel but only on the beads.

On the following day, the slices of CSE gel are removed from the tubes using a bent syringe needle as a hook. The beads are spun down, washed two or three times in NNTA, eluted, and electrophoresed as in normal SDS-PAGE. A demonstration of this technique for B-cell surface Ig is shown in Figure 3.

D. SDS-PAGE Followed by Proteolytic Peptide Mapping
(Cleveland Technique)

After isolating protein molecules as bands on SDS-PAGE, one may wish to determine whether bands of similar apparent molecular weight are really the same protein or whether bands with different apparent molecular weights are related. Cleveland *et al.* (1977) devised an economical and fast proteolytic peptide-mapping procedure based on regular SDS-PAGE methodology, which can give an initial answer to these questions. Traditional two-dimensional chromatographic separations of proteolytic peptides give better resolution than the Cleveland technique in some cases, are far more time-consuming, and are discussed by Moss (1979).

With the Cleveland technique, SDS-PAGE is run and the bands of interest are located via protein staining or by alignment with autoradiographic exposures. They are then cut out with a razor blade. A second SDS-PAGE slab gel is prepared having a higher percentage of acrylamide

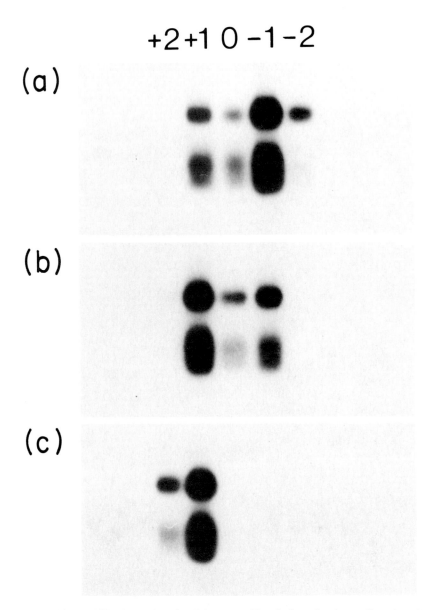

Fig. 3. Charge-shift electrophoresis of lactoperoxidase-iodinated spleen cell surface Ig. Lysates of iodinated spleen cells were equilibrated and run (see text) in CTAB plus NP40 (a), NP40 alone (b), and DOC plus NP40 (c). Slices of the CSE gels were eluted, immunoprecipitated, and displayed on SDS-PAGE as described, and the relevant portions shown here. Both Ig μ (upper) and δ (lower) heavy chains are seen to shift their CSE behavior oppositely in the two charged detergent mixtures, behavior which is characteristic and diagnostic for membrane molecules.

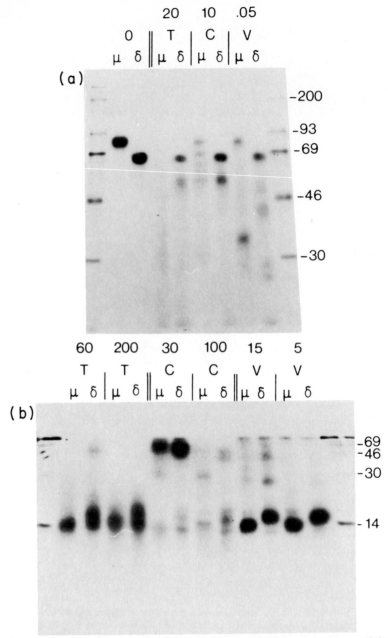

Fig. 4. Cleveland peptide mapping. Iodinated spleen cell surface Ig was immunoprecipitated and isolated on SDS-PAGE. Portions of gel containing μ and δ heavy chains were excised and rerun as described in the text, with no enzyme or various amounts of proteases added. Panel (a) was rerun on an 8% SDS-PAGE gel, and (b) on an 18% gel. The molecular weights of various standard proteins are indicated along the side of the gel. Across the top of the gel tracks are noted the number of micrograms of protease added per sample slot (C, chymotrypsin; T, trypsin; V, *St. aureus* V8 protease). Ig μ and δ chains show generally different digestion patterns but in the limit digests with trypsin show a major shared digestion product. This may be from the V region common to both classes of heavy chain.

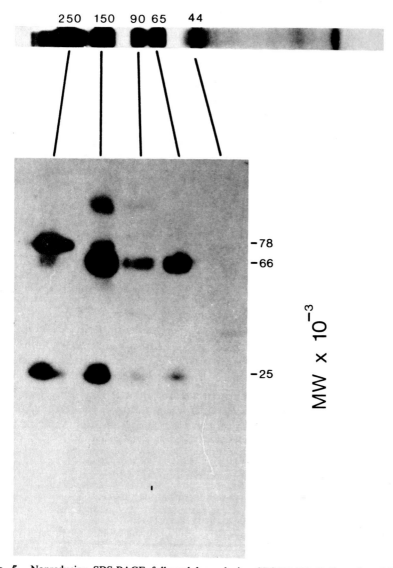

Fig. 5. Nonreducing SDS-PAGE followed by reducing SDS-PAGE. Iodinated and immunoprecipitated spleen cell surface Ig was displayed on a nonreducing 5–15% SDS-PAGE gel track. The four major and one minor bands were excised and rerun on an 8–18% gel under reducing conditions. The heaviest major nonreduced band contained mainly IgM molecules, while the other three major bands contained IgD. The minor nonreduced band did not contain any recognizable Ig class.

(usually 8–20%) in the lower (separating) gel and an upper (stacking) gel section 1 cm longer than normal. The cutout bands from the first gel are placed in the sample wells of the second slab's stacking gel. The wells are filled with SDS sample buffer, and the samples are allowed to equilibrate for 60 min (and swell if previously dried). Any bubbles are gently squeezed out, and protease solutions in nonreducing SDS sample buffer containing 20% glycerol and 0.005% bromphenol blue are overlaid above the samples. Fifty microliters containing 0.01–1 μg *Staphylococcus aureus* V8 protease, 0.01–0.2 mg trypsin, or 0.01–0.2 mg chymotrypsin per slot have given good results in our laboratory. The gels are further equilibrated for 30–60 min, and electrophoresis is begun. When the tracking dye is 1 cm above the separating gel, the current is turned off for 30 min, allowing proteolysis to proceed. Electrophoresis is then restarted, and further stages are similar to regular SDS-PAGE.

Figure 4 shows an example of the Cleveland peptide mapping technique applied to lymphocyte surface Ig heavy-chain polypeptides.

E. Nonreducing SDS-PAGE Followed by Reducing SDS-PAGE

The final two-dimensional technique mentioned here is sequential SDS-PAGE separations, first under nonreducing and then under reducing conditions. This distinguishes polypeptide chains of similar apparent molecular weight under reducing SDS-PAGE, which differ in disulfide bonding to themselves or other polypeptides, before reduction. Very simply, the first SDS-PAGE is performed using nonreducing buffers (i.e., no 2-ME), and the bands of interest are located, excised, equilibrated, and rerun as in the Cleveland peptide mapping procedure (Section III,D) using reducing SDS sample buffer (but no proteases). An example of this technique, again with lymphocyte surface Ig, is shown in Fig. 5.

REFERENCES

Braun, D. G., Hild, K., and Ziegler, A. (1979). *In* "Immunological Methods" (I. Lefkovits and B. Pernis, eds.), Vol. 1, p. 107. Academic Press, New York.
Cleveland, D. W., Fischer, S. G., Kirschner, M. W., and Laemmli, U. K. (1977). *J. Biol. Chem.* **252**, 1102.
Helenius, A., and Simons, K. (1977). *Proc. Natl. Acad. Sci. U.S.A.* **74**, 529.
Moss, B. A. (1979). *In* "Immunological Methods" (I. Lefkovits and B. Pernis, eds.), Vol. 1, p. 69. Academic Press, New York.
O'Farrell, P. H. (1975). *J. Biol. Chem.* **250**, 4007.
O'Farrell, P. Z., Goodman, H. M., and O'Farrell, P. H. (1977). *Cell* **12**, 1133.
Takacs, B. (1979). *In* "Immunological Methods" (I. Lefkovits and B. Pernis, eds.), Vol. 1, p. 81. Academic Press, New York.

4

Measurements of Antibodies
Specific for DNA

Lucien A. Aarden and Ruud Smeenk

I. INTRODUCTION

Antibodies to DNA occur spontaneously in the serum of patients with systemic lupus erythematosus (SLE) and in murine models of this disease (Stollar, 1973). These antibodies are suggested to be involved in the pathogenesis of this immune complex-mediated disease, and their presence in human serum is of considerable diagnostic value.

Interestingly enough, it has not been possible to induce these antibodies experimentally in normal animals via immunization with free or complexed DNA. The only successful approach has been polyclonal B-cell activation, by injecting lipopolysaccharide (LPS) into mice (Izui *et al.*, 1977) or by induction of a graft-versus-host reaction in a restricted number of murine parent–F$_1$ combinations. In the latter model a disease is induced that closely resembles spontaneous murine and human SLE Gleichmann *et al.*, 1978).

In the detection of antibodies to DNA the complete repertoire of immunoassays has been applied (Maini and Holborow, 1977). In our hands,

75

IMMUNOLOGICAL METHODS, VOL. II
Copyright © 1981 by Academic Press, Inc.
All rights of reproduction in any form reserved.
ISBN 0-12-442702-2

two methods are superior in terms of sensitivity and diagnostic specificity. These are the immunofluorescence technique (IFT) using *Crithidia luciliae* as substrate (Aarden *et al.*, 1975) and the Farr assay using ^{3}H-labeled circular PM2 DNA as antigen (Swaak *et al.*, 1979). The *C. luciliae* cells contain, in addition to a nucleus, a so-called kinetoplast (a giant mitochondrion) in which double-stranded DNA (dsDNA), not associated with proteins, is present. Binding of antibody to this kinetoplast reflects anti-DNA activity. In the Farr assay, we use PM2 DNA as antigen because this DNA, isolated from bacteriophage PM2, is circular. The isolation of intact circles guarantees a homogeneous molecular weight and no contamination with single-stranded DNA (ssDNA) regions.

II. ANTIGEN PREPARATIONS

A. Preparation of *Crithidia luciliae* Slides

This method is a slight modification of the original procedure (Aarden *et al.*, 1975).

1. Materials

a. Phosphate-Buffered Saline (PBS)
Na_2HPO_4–NaH_2PO_4, 0.01 M, pH 7.4
NaCl, 0.14 M

b. Culture Media
Medium I (Dissolve in about 800 ml distilled water; boil 3–4 min; filter after cooling).
$\quad$ Na_2HPO_4, 2.34 gm
$\quad$ NaCl, 4.0 gm
$\quad$ KCl, 0.4 gm
$\quad$ Glucose, 2.0 gm
$\quad$ Liver infusion (Oxoid), 1.0 gm
$\quad$ Bacto-tryptose (Difco), 15.0 gm
Medium II
$\quad$ Hemin (equine, Sigma), 20.0 mg
$\quad$ Ethanol (96%), 5.0 ml
$\quad$ Distilled water, 5.0 ml
$\quad$ NaOH, (1 M), 0.2 ml

1. Mix media I and II and make up to 1 liter. Adjust the pH to 7.4. Remove debris by centrifugation (10 min 5000 rpm) in a GSA rotor in a Sorvall RC-2 B centrifuge. Sterilize 45 min at 1 atm.
2. Use the culture medium within 2 weeks after preparation. Just before

inoculation, penicillin and streptomycin may be added to a final concentration of 100 U/ml and 100 μg/ml, respectively. This is done to avoid bacterial contamination.

Crithidia luciliae organisms can be obtained from the American Type Culture Collection, 12301 Parklawn Drive, Rockville, Maryland. All chemicals, unless otherwise specified, are Merck pro analysi (p.a.) products.

2. Procedure

About 10 × 10⁶ organisms are inoculated in 100 ml culture medium in a 500-ml Erlenmeyer flask and grown while shaking at 24°C. The doubling time of the culture is about $5\frac{1}{2}$ hr. The concentration of *C. luciliae* cultures is determined by measuring the OD at 610 nm. An OD $_{610}$ of 0.60 corresponds to a density of 20 × 10⁶ cells/ml.

After 2 days a second culture is prepared, in 100 ml culture medium in a 500-ml Erlenmeyer flask, by inoculation from the first culture.

Under conditons of vigorous aeration, cell density can reach about 100 × 10⁶ cells/ml. However, to prepare slides, cultures in the log phase are used. Therefore they are harvested by low-speed centrifugation (10 min at 600 × g) when the cell density has reached 20–40 × 10⁶/ml. After two washings with PBS, containing 1 mg/ml ovalbumin, the cells are suspended in a solution of ovalbumin (1 mg/ml) in distilled water at a density of about 10 × 10⁶ cells/ml. The distilled water causes swelling of the cells, which improves the separation between kinetoplast and nucleus. The ovalbumin greatly improves the morphology of the organisms. After 10 min, the suspension is filtered over cotton wool (in a Pasteur pipette), and about 20 μl drops are applied to glass slides. For slides we use eight-spot coated object glasses from Cooke (No. CL 800–21424). After drying under a fan the slides are fixed for 10 min in 96% ethanol; they are then dried and stored at −20°C. Slides prepared in this way may be kept for several months.

B. Preparation of PM2 DNA

Radiolabeled DNA is isolated from the bacteriophage PM2, which is grown in the presence of [³H]thymidine on its host, the bacterium *Pseudomonas* strain BAL 31. The procedure is a slight modification of the one described by Espejo and Canelo (1968).

1. Materials

a. BAL 31 Broth
Nutrient broth (Difco), 0.8% (w/v)
KCl (Merck p.a.), 0.01 M
NaCl (Merck p.a.), 0.44 M

After sterilization for 1 hr at 120°C, 10 ml of a sterile 1 M CaCl$_2$ solution and 50 ml of a sterile 0.72 M MgSO$_4$ solution are added per liter BAL 31 broth.

b. *TS Buffer*
   Tris–HCl (Merck p.a.), 20 mM, pH 8.0
   NaCl, 1 M

c. *TSE Buffer*
   Tris-HCl, 20 mM, pH 7.5
   NaCl, 0.1 M
   EDTA (BDH Chemicals), 1 mM
   [methyl-³H]thymidine (Radiochemical Centre, Ltd., Amersham, United
     Kingdom), 5 mCi of the highest specific activity available (which
     should be approximately 50 Ci/mmol)

d. *TSE-Saturated Phenol.* To 500 gm freshly distilled phenol, 70 ml *m*-cresol and 0.5 gm hydroxyquinoline are added. The phenol is saturated with TSE buffer and may be kept at − 20°C for prolonged periods of time.

e. *Miscellaneous Reagents.* Dextran sulfate (Pharmacia Fine Chemicals), polyethylene glycol (Koch Light Laboratories), sodium dodecyl sulfate (SDS; Koch Light Laboratories), CsCl, and KCl (Merck p.a.).

2. Procedure

a. *Day 0.* BAL 31 broth (20 ml) in a 100-ml Erlenmeyer flask is inoculated with *Pseudomonas* BAL 31 and grown overnight at 28°C under gentle aeration.

b. *Day 1.* The overnight culture is used to inoculate 100 ml BAL 31 broth up to an OD$_{610}$ of 0.15. Growing is continued at 28°C under vigorous aeration. Under these conditions the doubling time of the *Pseudomonas* should be about 1 hr, as followed by OD measurements at 610 nm. At OD$_{610}$ = 0.6 (corresponding to 6 × 10^7 cells/ml) the culture is infected with 2 ml of a PM2 lysate [titer 1–2 × 10^{10} plaque-forming units (PFU)/ml resulting in a multiplicity of infection (moi) of about 5]. About 3 hr after infection the culture will lyse, which corresponds to a sharp drop in the OD$_{610}$ to approximately 0.1. It is centrifuged for 15 min at 10,000 rpm (SS 34 rotor, Sorvall RC2B centrifuge). The supernatant (PM2 lysate) is kept at 4°C until further use.
   The lysate used in this procedure must be freshly prepared, because the titer of PM2 lysates decreases rather quickly. It is prepared by infecting 20 ml BAL 31 culture at OD$_{610}$ = 0.6 with 2–4 ml of an old (but never older

than 3 months) PM2 lysate.

Another 200 ml BAL 31 broth is inoculated with 1 ml overnight culture and grown overnight at 28°C under gentle aeration.

c. Day 2. Two 2-liter batches of BAL 31 broth (each in a 6-liter conical flask) are inoculated with the BAL 31 overnight culture, up to OD_{610} = 0.15. The cultures are grown at 28°C under vigorous aeration until OD_{610} = 0.6. To each culture 2.5 mCi [methyl-³H]thymidine is added. Growth is allowed to continue for 15 min. Then 40 ml PM2 lysate is added to each flask. Growing is continued until complete lysis of the cultures (about 3 hr) occurs. To each culture is added 140 ml 20% (w/v) dextran sulfate and 400 ml 44% (w/v) polyethylene glycol (PEG 6000). This is thoroughly mixed and kept at 4°C overnight.

d. Day 3. All procedures that follow are carried out at 4°C. The supernatants are carefully discarded, and the polyethylene glycol layer is centrifuged for 20 min at 8500 rpm (SS 34 rotor, Sorvall RC 2B centrifuge). Both the upper and lower phases are carefully removed, leaving the interphase. This interphase, containing the PM2 bacteriophages, is solubilized in TS buffer (total volume approximately 50 ml). A 0.5-vol of a saturated KCl solution is added and, after mixing, the solution is divided into two centrifuge tubes and centrifuged for 15 min at 12,000 rpm in a SS 34 rotor in a Sorvall RC 2B centrifuge. The supernatants contain the PM2 bacteriophages; however, since this solubilization procedure is not very effective, a large number of phages still remain in the precipitates. Therefore the precipitates are thoroughly washed, each with 10 ml TS buffer plus 1 ml saturated KCl solution, and recentrifuged for 15 min at 12,000 rpm. (Note: The supernatants are recentrifuged once to eliminate any residual debris.) The procedure of washing the precipitates is repeated four times. Supernatants are always centrifuged for a second time before being pooled. Pooled supernatants (approximately 180 ml) are then centrifuged for 1 hr at 41,000 rpm in a T 865 rotor in a Sorvall OTD-2 ultracentrifuge (or, alternatively, for 1.5 hr at 30,000 rpm in a Spinco 30 Ti rotor). The bacteriophages are precipitated by this procedure. The pellets are resolubilized in a total of 7 ml TS buffer. After complete solubilization (sometimes this takes overnight), 0.4 gm CsCl is added for each milliliter of bacteriophage solution. The solution is divided into two or three SW 65 centrifuge tubes; these are filled with TS buffer containing 0.4 gm CsCl/ml. CsCl gradients are run for 20 hr at 38,000 rpm at 8°C (SW 65 Ti rotor).

e. Day 4. The opaque bacteriophage band (about 1 cm from the top) can easily be seen in the gradients. It is isolated by puncturing the tube at the site of the bacteriophage band with a 1-ml disposable syringe and needle and gently sucking the phage band out of the gradient tube. The bacteriophage solution is dialyzed overnight against TSE buffer (two changes of 2 liters each).

f. Day 5. Bacteriophages are lysed by the addition of SDS to a final concentration of 0.5%. An equal volume of TSE-saturated phenol is added and very carefully mixed with the water layer. After 10 min of mixing, the phases are separated by centrifugation (10 min at 3000 g). The water phase is again extracted with an equal volume of phenol. Pooled phenol phases are then washed two times with 0.5 vol of TSE buffer. The combined buffer phases are then extensively dialyzed against PBS until no more phenol can be detected. (This generally takes 3 days, with frequent buffer changes.) The DNA concentration is measured at 260 nm. Ratios of A_{280}/A_{260} and A_{230}/A_{260} should be 0.54 and 0.45, respectively. The yield is about 3 mg of pure PM2 DNA, with a specific activity of 0.025 mCi/mg. The molecular weight of the DNA is 5.9×10^6. The DNA solution is kept, diluted to 100 μg/ml, at 4°C. A few drops of chloroform are added to prevent bacterial growth.

If so desired, percentages of supercoiled (component I) versus relaxed circle (component II) DNA may be determined by running an analytical 5–25% sucrose gradient (16 hr, 35,000 rpm, SW 41 Ti rotor, Sorvall OTD-2 ultracentrifuge). Usually 90% of the DNA is isolated as component I and 10% as component II; however, in time more component II emerges, probably as a result of radiation damage to the supercoiled DNA.

III. ANTI-DNA ASSAYS

A. Indirect Immunofluorescence Technique

Each slide contains eight spots of *C. luciliae.* These can be used for eight different sera or for titration of a single serum. Thirty microliters of serum diluted 1:10 in PBS is applied to each spot and incubated for 30 min at room temperature. The slide is then quickly rinsed under the tap and washed 3 times for 10 min with PBS. Each spot is then incubated for 30 min with 30 μl of the appropriate fluorescein isothiocyanate (FITC)-labeled anti-immunoglobulin (Ig) preparation, washed three times for 10 min with PBS, and mounted. As a mounting solution we use a solution of 65% (w/v) sucrose in PBS, pH 8.0, in which 0.5 μg/ml propidium iodide (Calbiochem) is dissolved. The viscosity of the sucrose keeps the cover glass in position, while the propidium iodide acts as a counterstain that intercalates into the DNA of the nucleus and kinetoplast, staining them red. It takes about 30 min for this red stain to develop fully. This counterstain facilitates location of the kinetoplast and can easily be filtered out with a KP 560 barrier filter (Leitz). Reading is done at 500 × with a standard fluorescence microscope equipped with incident illumination using a xenon arc lamp for excitation and a 50/1.00 water immersion objective.

B. Farr Assay

One hundred nanograms of ^{3}H-labeled PM2 DNA is incubated with 50 μl serum (or dilutions of serum in PBS) in the presence of 800 μg normal human Ig (Cohn fraction II) as a carrier protein. Then incubation volume is 200 μl, and the medium is PBS, pH 7.4. Incubation is carried out in large glass tubes (16 × 100 mm) for 1 hr at 37°C. The 5 ml cold 50%-saturated (1.96 M) $(NH_4)_2SO_4$ is added. The precipitate is allowed to form at 4°C for 30 min. After centrifugation for 15 min at 3000 g in a refrigerated centrifuge (4°C) the precipitate is washed twice with 5 ml cold 50%-saturated $(NH_4)_2SO_4$. After dissolving the precipitate in 1 ml Soluene 100 (Packard), 10 ml liquid scintillation fluid (Instafluor II, Packard) is added. The solution is then counted for radioactivity in a liquid scintillation counter (Packard, Model Tri-carb 2450).

From sera that bind more than 30% of the input DNA, serial dilutions in PBS are tested. Anti-DNA is expressed in units per milliliter. One unit of anti-DNA is defined as the amount of anti-DNA that binds 30% of the input DNA under the above-described conditions (Aarden et al., 1976).

Mean binding of 135 normal human sera (50 μl tested) was 5 ± 3%. This implies that sera having more than 10 units of anti-DNA per milliliter can be considered positive.

IV. CRITICAL APPRAISAL

The polymeric structure and the strong charge of DNA render it susceptible to nonspecific interactions. Under physiological conditions various constituents of normal serum, among which C1q and low-density lipoprotein are the most important, are reported to interact with DNA (Agnello et al., 1970; Smeenk and Aarden, 1980). Assays that do not comprise an inherent check on the Ig character of the DNA-binding material may therefore yield false positive results. Probably this is the major reason why anti-DNA as measured by IFT on C. luciliae is more specific for human SLE than most other assays for anti-DNA. Evidently, in this assay, only Ig binding to DNA is detected. In the Farr assay this endogenous control is not present. That is why this assay is much more susceptible to false positive reactions. Still, the Farr assay is the method of choice when radioimmunoassays are considered. This may be explained by the following. Most of the nonspecific DNA binding is based on electrostatic interactions. The 2 M $(NH_4)_2SO_4$ employed in the Farr assay as a means of separating free and bound DNA leads to disruption of these interactions. However, this is only true when the labeled DNA preparation used as antigen is purely double-stranded. Denaturation of DNA to single-stranded material enhances nonspecific binding to an intolerable degree. Even single-stranded contaminations of dsDNA preparations insignificant on a weight basis may cause considerable loss of specificity of the assay for SLE.

We have observed that, when human sera are tested, the use of PM2 dsDNA is a solution to this problem, because it can be isolated in a pure, circular, double-stranded form. In the murine situation, however, even PM2 dsDNA is bound by normal mouse serum in the Farr assay. This is probably due to C1q, as the binding activity of normal mouse serum has a sedimentation value of 11 S and this binding can be abolished by heating the sera for 1 hr at 56°C. Finally, a major advantage of the Farr assay over the IFT must be mentioned; with the Farr assay, anti-DNA can be quantitated. Especially in longitudinal studies the quantitation of anti-DNA can have important prognostic consequences (Swaak *et al.*, 1979).

REFERENCES

Aarden, L. A., de Groot, E. R., and Feltkamp, T. E. W. (1975). *Ann N.Y. Acad. Sci.* **254**, 505–515.
Aarden, L. A., Lakmaker, F., and de Groot, E. R. (1976). *J. Immunol. Methods* **11**, 153–163.
Agnello, V., Winchester, R. J., and Kunkel, H. G. (1970). *Immunology* **19**, 909–919.
Espejo, R. T., and Canelo, E. S. (1968). *Virology* **34**, 738–747.
Gleichmann, E., Issa, P., van Elven, E. H., and Lamers, M. C. (1978). *Clin. Rheum. Dis.* **4**, 587–602.
Izui, S., Kobayakawa, T., Zryd, M. J., Louis, J., and Lambert, P. H. (1977). *J. Immunol.* **119**, 2157–2162.
Maini, R. N., and Holborow, E. J., eds. (1977). *Ann. Rheum. Dis.* **36**, Suppl. 1.
Smeenk, R., and Aarden, L. (1980). *J. Immunol. Methods* **39**, 165–180.
Stollar, D. B. (1973). *In* "The Antigens" (M. Sela, ed.), Vol. 1, pp. 1–85. Academic Press, New York.
Swaak, A. J. G., Aarden, L. A., Statius van Eps, L. W., and Feltkamp, T. E. W. (1979). *Arthritis Rheum.* **22**, 226–235.

5

High-Pressure
Liquid Chromatography
of Proteins and Peptides

Vernon L. Alvarez, Carolyn A. Roitsch, and Ole Henriksen

IMMUNOLOGICAL METHODS, VOL. II

I. INTRODUCTION

High-pressure liquid chromatography (also called high-performance liquid chromatography, both terms being abbreviated HPLC) is a powerful separation technique that has recently been applied to proteins. [Two excellent reviews have been written by Rubinstein (1979) and Regnier and Gooding (1980).] This technique combines high capacity, excellent resolution, short elution times, and high sensitivity. It is especially useful as a tool for purifying the proteins and peptides that function as mediators and effectors of cellular interactions, since these are found in low concentrations and have been difficult to purify by conventional techniques. For example, both enkephalins (Bayon *et al.,* 1978) and human leukocyte interferon (Rubinstein *et al.,* 1979) have been purified by HPLC.

We have, with excellent results, applied HPLC in characterizing and purifying immunologically important compounds such as H-2 histocompatibility antigens and helper T-cell factors. Even under relatively harsh conditions isolated H-2 retains significant antigenicity, and helper T-cell factors still show biological activity.

This chapter will discuss only two types of HPLC, reverse phase and gel permeation, from a practical point of view. Several examples will be given which illustrate the diversity of the method and its applicability in immunological research.

II. GENERAL DESCRIPTION OF HPLC

A. Introduction to the System

Figure 1 illustrates the main components of a typical HPLC system. The sample to be analyzed is loaded into the sample loop with a syringe. Typical injection volumes are 50 μl to 1 ml. By a turn of the valve the loop is switched into the solvent line through which the sample is pumped to the column (the flow rate is about 1 ml/min). On the column the components of the sample are separated and then passed through a detector which measures some parameter of the sample such as light absorbance, fluorescence, or refractive index. A recorder is used to monitor the separation. The separated components can be collected in a fraction collector or directed to waste.

HPLC owes its resolving power to two factors: a high flow rate and a large number of "theoretical plates." The high flow rate is accomplished by pumping the solvent through the system at high pressure (1000–3000 psi). This requires that the chromatographic support be made of a rigid

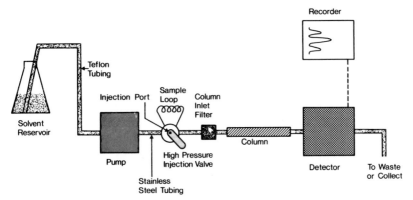

Fig. 1. Block diagram of a typical HPLC system. The individual components are discussed in the text.

material such as glass, silica, or a polymer which is then derivatized to provide the desired functional type.

The term "theoretical plates" refers to the efficiency of the system; its value depends on several factors (see Regnier and Gooding, 1980). In general, the higher the number of theoretical plates N, the better the separation. However, an extremely high N value is not necessary for all applications. The number of theoretical plates is stated on most commercially available columns; it is useful when comparing products from different manufacturers. Other important considerations are flow resistance and loading capacity, and these might require a column of lower N value.

B. Reverse-Phase HPLC

Reverse-phase chromatography is a type of chromatography in which the mobile phase is aqueous (polar) and the stationary phase is organic (non-polar). This is just the opposite, or reverse, of classic adsorption chromatography. The organic phase is made stationary by covalently linking an organic group to a solid support with a uniform particle size (usually either 5 or 10 μm). The most commonly used reverse phase consists of a saturated hydrocarbon chain containing 18 carbon atoms linked, or "bonded," to silica beads. This type is called C-18, RP-18, ODS (octadecyl silane), or some other similar name. Supports are also available with either eight carbon atoms or two carbon atoms attached to the silica; these are called RP-8 or C-8 and RP-2 or C-2, respectively. Although it is difficult to give rational guidelines on which stationary phase to use, because each separation problem must be solved empirically, it can generally be stated that longer hydrocarbon chains bind proteins tighter than shorter ones.

In reverse-phase chromatography proteins are adsorbed to the stationary organic phase and eluted with a mobile aqueous phase. Separation is achieved by differential partitioning of the proteins in the stationary and mobile phases. The separation is thus a function of (1) the nature of the protein, especially its hydrophobicity, (2) the stationary organic phase, (3) the aqueous mobile phase, and (4) the organic solvent used for elution.

Elution from the stationary phase is brought about by decreasing the polarity of the mobile phase. This is done by adding an organic solvent to the aqueous solution, which increases the hydrophobicity of the mobile phase. Typical aqueous solvents are water; 0.01–0.1 M sodium, potassium, and ammonium salts of acetate, carbonate, or phosphate; pyridine acetate; and acids such as phosphoric, acetic, and formic. The organic solvent may be, for example, acetonitrile, methanol, ethanol, or propanol. The protein elutes when the hydrophobicity of the mobile phase is sufficient to desorb it from the stationary support. It is possible to choose from many different organic solvents and thereby modulate the separation extensively. For example, acetonitrile, an organic solvent commonly used in HPLC, is substantially less hydrophobic than n-propanol, which is also used. Proteins that adsorb tightly can often be eluted with an n-propanol gradient, while proteins that bind less tightly can be separated better with acetonitrile.

The actual choice of mobile phase is somewhat arbitrary and depends on the types of proteins to be separated, their solubility and stability in the solvents used, and the detection means. There are many examples available in the literature (Regnier and Gooding, 1980; Hawk, 1979), so it is often possible to begin with an established method.

As discussed above, the elution of proteins occurs as a function of the organic solvent concentration. The eluant concentration can be either constant (isocratic) or changing (gradient). Isocratic elution is easier achieve, but it is not as flexible. A protein mixture may consist of components eluted under very different conditions. In this case an isocratic system would elute some components early and others late. This may mean that some very late-eluting components might not be detected at all. Gradient elution allows greater flexibility and generally permits faster elution of all components. Although it is technically more difficult to achieve, it generally gives better results.

C. Gel Permeation HPLC

The principles of high-pressure gel permeation chromatography (HPGPC) are the same as those of classic gel permeation chromatography (GPC). The separation is achieved by passing a mixture of proteins through a gel with a certain uniform pore size. Proteins too large to enter the pores flow around the gel and elute first from the column (the *excluded* volume), while proteins small enough to enter the pores travel a longer path and are eluted according to their size. Small molecules can enter all the pores and are eluted last (the *included* volume).

The difference between HPGPC and classic GPC lies in the gel. The gel in HPGPC must be noncompressible and able to withstand pressures up to 4000 psi. This is usually accomplished, as in reverse-phase HPLC, by using controlled-pore glass or silica. Untreated glass or silica, however, adsorbs proteins so strongly that it cannot be used. Therefore most commercial packings consist of controlled-pore glass coated (by covalent bonding) with a glycerylpropylsilane or an *N*-acetylaminopropylsilane. Nevertheless, the gel permeation columns we have worked with do not separate proteins according to their molecular weight unless the chromatography is done in 6 *M* guanidine–HCl. On the other hand, if one is looking for a purification method based not only on the principle of gel permeation, the adsorption of proteins to the column material might be an advantage.

III. COMPONENTS OF AN HPLC SYSTEM

A. Manufacturers of HPLC Systems

HPLC is now a commonly used technique for all types of separations, and many companies sell various components. The following tabulation lists several companies familiar to the authors. No attempt has been made to include all manufacturers. Most of the companies mentioned provide an excellent literature service.

Manufacturer	Principal components	Literature service
Altex	Pumps, gradient programmers, packed columns, hardware	+
Bio-Rad	Packed columns	+
Brownlee	Packed columns	+
Dupont	Packed columns, complete systems	+
Hewlett-Packard	Complete systems	
Merck	Packing material	
Rheodyne	Injection valves, hardware	+
Spectra-Physics	Complete systems	+
Waters Associates	Pumps, injection valves, detectors, gradient programmers, packed columns, packing material, hardware, complete systems	+

Below, each component of a complete HPLC system will be discussed from a practical viewpoint. The physical position of each component can be seen in Fig. 1.

B. Pumps

The pump is perhaps the most important component of an HPLC system. It should provide a stable flow rate, preferably variable over a large range. The flow should be pulsation-free, as far as possible, and the pump should be capable of maintaining its flow rate against a back pressure of at least 4000 psi. Normal operating pressures are 1000–3000 psi, but higher pressures develop occasionally.

These requirements have been met in several ways. Pump designs are of two types, piston and diaphragm. Piston pumps may contain a single piston, double pistons, or $1\frac{1}{2}$ pistons. Many levels of sophistication are available, from a simple constant-pressure pump to elaborate feedback mechanisms for controlling the flow rate exactly. It is possible to achieve good results with simple pumps, but in general the more exact the flow is regulated the more reproducible, hence "better," the chromatogram will be.

C. Valves and Filters

Strictly speaking, a valve is not necessary in an HPLC system. It is possible to inject the sample through a septum directly into the front of the column. The main limitation to this method is sample size, which must be kept small. An injection valve is much more flexible, because larger volumes can be injected.

A high-pressure injection valve diverts the flow to the column from a bypass to a sample loop. In the filling position, the mobile phase flows through a bypass to the column and the loop is connected to a filling port. The loop is then filled (completely or partially) using a syringe, and the sample is loaded onto the column by changing the position of the valve. In the loading position, the mobile phase flows through the loop to the column. The loop size can be changed to accommodate various sample volumes, and the loop need not be completely filled to be effective. It is possible, for example, to inject a sample volume of 10 μl into a 2-ml loop with no loss of resolution.

Valve designs also vary widely. Most HPLC valves on the market can withstand pressures up to 5000 psi without leaking. The biggest problem with HPLC valves is their tendency to release small particles (produced by valve deterioration) which then clog up the lines, raise the back pressure, and possibly ruin the column. In order to prevent this, it is advantageous to have a *column inlet filter* which protects the column from particles. This is a small, inexpensive item, but it should be considered essential to the HPLC system.

D. Tubing and Connectors

The tubing leading from the solvent reservoir to the pump is usually Teflon, but after the pump the system is under high pressure (1000–3000 psi). This requires stainless steel tubings, fittings, and connectors. Typical tubing dimensions are $\frac{1}{16}$-in. OD and 0.02 in. ID. In order to prevent sample spreading, the length of tubing between the valve and the column and between the column and the detector should be kept as short as possible. It is also advisable to use "low dead volume" connectors wherever possible.

E. Columns

1. General

The heart of the HPLC system is the column. An HPLC column consists of a stainless steel tube filled with the support material. One or both ends have filters to keep the packing in and to keep particles out. The ends also have connectors to which the stainless steel tubing can be joined. Figure 2 illustrates the types of columns used in our laboratory.

The *column packing,* as mentioned above, is extremely varied both in

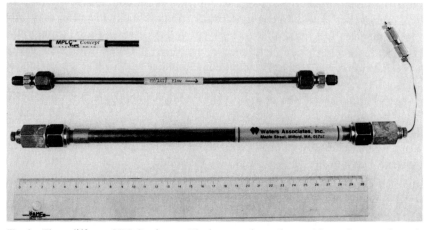

Fig. 2 Three different HPLC columns. The largest column (bottom) is a gel permeation column manufactured by Waters Associates. The other two are reverse-phase columns; the size of the middle column (HPLC Technology, Ltd.) is the one most commonly used. The smallest column (Brownlee) exhibits excellent properties for protein separation.

derivative type and manufacturer. Supposedly identical packings may show large variability from one manufacturer to another. Many companies now routinely test all columns and send test chromatograms along with the columns to show their actual separation capability. For initial experiments, choice of a particular column is somewhat arbitrary, although there are several points to consider. A good column should have (1) a high number of theoretical plates, (2) low back pressure, and (3) a test chromatogram. These requirements are not completely inflexible, because a particular application may not require such high quality.

2. Use and Maintenance

Most HPLC columns exhibit both good flow properties and a high number of theoretical plates, and they can be expected to last about a year with proper care. First, care should be taken that no air is pumped through the column. This can be prevented by purging all lines and sample loops with solvent before attaching the column. Second, the column should be protected against particles which might block the flow or cause excessive back pressure. Only HPLC-grade or filtered solvents and solutions should be used, and the column should be further protected by a column inlet filter. Third, reverse-phase columns should be cleaned after each use, since the adsorbed proteins might not all be released during an experiment. The washing is done by pumping solvent containing a high concentration of the organic component through the column. For gel permeation columns, the problems of operation and maintenance are mainly connected with corrosion. As mentioned, the solvent we use for these columns contains 6 M guanidine–HCl. The chloride ions attack stainless steel, with the result that small particles are released from solvent lines, valves, and column walls. The *entire* system should be flushed extensively with water after each use of 6 M guanidine–HCl, or serious damage could occur to all components of the system.

A technique should be developed to monitor column performance. This usually involves blank runs and standard mixtures. A blank run, in which a solution is injected without a sample, should be carried out at the start of the day and after any column disturbance (such as an extra-heavy load or a solvent change). If this is done on the same scale of detection as the analysis, it is possible to identify injection peaks, solvent peaks, "ghost" peaks, and a baseline rise due to the solvent. The actual analysis of a sample can then be compared to this blank, and the peaks identified with confidence.

It is also very important to have a standard which can be used to evaluate column performance. This is a relatively simple matter for many analytical applications of HPLC but is much more complicated for proteins. Ideally, the standard should be analyzed under the same conditions as the unknown sample and a particular peak or peaks monitored and evaluated with respect to retention time and recovery (peak height or area). For reverse-phase columns, it is difficult to obtain a standard, because commonly available proteins or peptides (such as myoglobin or insulin A chain) may not elute under the same conditions as the protein of interest. For example, insulin A chain may elute with the injection flow-through in a certain gradient, while the protein of interest is eluted after 20 min. This problem can be solved by finding an appropriate protein (by trial and error) or by injecting small aliquots of the impure mixture being separated. The latter technique is used in our laboratory; 10 μl of a known mixture is injected to monitor the column. The peaks are then compared to those of the previous day and, if they "match," the column is considered good.

Standards for HPGPC are easier to prepare, since they need only fit the molecular-weight range of the column. Any protein with a well-defined molecular weight can therefore be used.

Analysis of standard mixtures of proteins is not only important for monitoring the day-to-day performance of a particular column but can also be used to evaluate new columns. This is important because there are usually small variations among "identical" columns even when they are from the same manufacturer.

F. Detectors

The detectors used for HPLC are of several types, depending on the particular application. Ultraviolet detectors are probably the most common, although fluorescence, refractive index, and conductivity detectors are also used extensively. Virtually any detection system used with normal chromatography can be used with HPLC, usually with little or no adaptation necessary. The biggest single difference lies in the flow cell. The flow cell for HPLC must be able to withstand high pressure, and it should also have a very small volume (10–20 μl). The high resolution of the separated components from the column can be lost completely through a flow cell that is too large. Many companies now manufacture uv, fluorescence, or refractive index detectors specifically for HPLC.

For uv detection, there is a choice of a fixed- or a variable-wavelength detector. In general, a fixed-wavelength detector is more sensitive than a variable-wavelength detector because of the optical design. A variable-wavelength detector may be more sensitive, however, because the wavelength can be changed to the peak of maximum absorption.

G. Fraction Collectors

A typical HPLC system has a high flow rate (about 1 ml/min), and commonly available fraction collectors are not fast enough to catch every drop. The separated proteins are often eluted in very small volumes, and a single drop may contain most of the desired material. We use an LKB RediRac fraction collector, but there are several others which are also suitable.

H. Solvents

The HPLC system is very sensitive to impurities in the solvents. Impurities can be in the form of particles that will clog the columns, or they may be uv light-absorbing materials that will result in high background absorption and thus decrease or eliminate the high sensitivity that is one of the main features of the system. Organic solvents should therefore be purchased as special HPLC grade, if available. If this is not possible, it may be necessary to redistill a lower grade of solvent in order to obtain material of the required purity. It is most practical to make concentrated stock solutions of the aqueous buffers. They should be made from the best available grade of chemicals and water and then filtered through membrane filters before use (for example, Millipore, 1–2 μm).

HPLC pumps are very sensitive to bubbles, which will stop the flow of solvent completely. The biggest source of bubbles is the solvent itself, since it contains dissolved air that can be pulled out by the suction of the pump. This potential problem is easily eliminated by bubbling a fine stream of helium through the solutions in the reservoirs. The helium displaces all other dissolved gases, and it has such a low solubility in the liquids that there is not enough present to cause bubble problems. The organic vapors from the reservoirs should be vented into an exhaust system to prevent headaches or other health problems.

Another simple method of degassing is to evacuate the solution for 5–10 min while stirring (and perhaps heating slightly). An efficient water aspirator is often good enough for this, although a vacuum pump is better.

I. Gradient Formers

The use of solvent gradients in eluting proteins from reverse-phase columns is very important. While it is possible to use isocratic elution, the peaks are sharper and the resolution improved substantially by gradient elution. Gradients in HPLC are generally made in two ways, as illustrated in Fig. 3.

In a *low-pressure gradient* system the gradient is made before the high-

(1) Low-Pressure Gradient   (2) High-Pressure Gradient

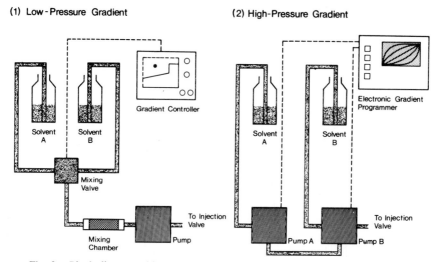

Fig. 3.   Block diagram of low-pressure (1) and high-pressure (2) gradient formers.

pressure pump. In our laboratory this is done with an LKB Ultrograd gradient maker. The gradient is formed by opening and closing two valves alternately to give the appropriate mixture. The valves must open and close quickly to minimize the time the pump is pulling against a closed system. Even though the valves may be very fast, there is always some time when the system is "closed" and bubbles may be sucked out of the solvent. If this happens, it is a serious problem because bubbles will enter the pump and the flow will stop. The risk of this can be eliminated by degassing the solvents, as described above, using helium. (*Note:* For a low-pressure gradient system, degassing solvents by evacuation is not sufficient.)

It is also important to consider the size of the mixing chamber. It is necessary for it to have a volume of 1–2 ml in order to ensure that a uniform solution passes through the column. However, this creates a dead volume in the system so that the gradient the column "sees" is 1–2 ml behind the gradient being formed at the valve. Other sources of dead volume are the pump itself, the tubing, and the sample loop. Each of these has to be accounted for in order to determine the actual concentration at which a particular component is eluted.

A *high-pressure gradient* system, as illustrated in Fig. 3, requires two pumps. In this case the gradient is made by an electronic programmer which controls the flow rate of the pumps. As an example, for a fixed flow rate of 1.0 ml/min, a mixture of 25% A and 75% B is made by pump A flowing at 0.25 ml/min and pump B flowing at 0.75 ml/min. This system is more exact and reproducible, but it is also more expensive. Both systems are used in our laboratory; each has its own particular advantages, but both work well.

J. Sample

The HPLC systems used in our laboratory, both reverse-phase and gel permeation, have a maximum capacity of approximately 2–5 mg of protein. This means that they are not suitable for the early purification steps of preparative isolation of a given protein where much larger amounts of material must be processed.

For reverse-phase HPLC, the sample can be present in almost any buffer during injection. It should always be centrifuged or filtered before injection, and compatibility with the mobile phase should be checked. If possible, the solubility of the protein mixture at the highest organic concentration to be used should be tested. High concentrations of organic solvents will denature and even precipitate some proteins. These limitations to the general applicability of reverse-phase HPLC must be evaluated in connection with specific applications. The examples of the use of HPLC in our laboratory clearly indicate that the materials we are working with retain significant antigenicity and biological activity.

Before injection, samples to be analyzed in the gel permeation system are always dissolved in the starting buffer (0.05 M Tris–HCl, pH 7.3; 6 M guanidine–HCl).

IV. EXAMPLES OF HPLC APPLICATIONS

In this section we have listed several applications of high-pressure reverse-phase chromatography and GPC in peptide and protein separations. Each application is slightly different and illustrates the versatility of this technique. In each case, all the actual running conditions are listed so that the reader can directly compare the applications.

A. Separation of Dipeptides

A good example of the resolving power of reverse-phase columns is shown by the separation of a mixture of dipeptides (Fig. 4). Notice that the peptides were monitored at 215 nm, which permits detection of all the peptides.

> Column: Zorbax ODS (Dupont), 5 μm particle size, 0.5 × 25 cm
> Solvent A: 0.07 M H$_3$PO$_4$ plus 5% ethanol

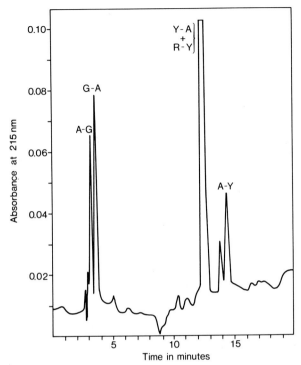

Fig. 4. Separation of dipeptides by reverse-phase HPLC. One nanomole of each dipeptide was separated using a 30-min linear ethanol gradient ranging from 0 to 50% ethanol. The aqueous solution was 0.07 M H_3PO_4. A-G, alanylglycine; G-A, glycylalanine; Y-A, tyrosylalanine; R-Y, arginyltyrosine; A-Y, alanyltyrosine.

Solvent B: Ethanol
Gradient: 0–50% B, linear, 30 min
Flow rate: 1.0 ml/min
Detection: 215 nm (multiple-wavelength detector)
Amount: Approximately 1 nmol of each dipeptide

B. Separation of Insulin A and B Chains

This chromatogram (Fig. 5) represents a different solvent than that in example A, and it also shows the separation of larger peptides. Insulin A and B chains are very difficult to separate by classic techniques, so the resolving power of the system is also demonstrated.

Column: Brownlee RP-18, packed with LiChrosorb (a tradename of E. Merck, Darmstadt, West Germany), 5 μm particle size, 0.5 × 25 cm

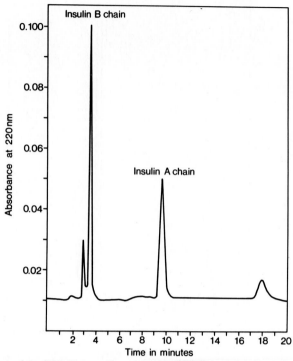

Fig. 5. Reverse-phase HPLC separation of insulin A and B chains. One nanomole of each chain was separated using a 0.01 M ammonium acetate, pH 4.5, buffer and a 30-min linear gradient of 5-30% ethanol.

Solvent A: 0.01 M ammonium acetate, pH 4.5
Solvent B: Ethanol
Gradient: 5-30% B, linear, 30 min
Flow rate: 1.0 ml/min
Detection: 230 nm (multiple-wavelength detector)
Amount: Approximately 1 nmol of each chain

C. Purification of H-2 Heavy Chains and β_2 Microglobulin

This example (Fig. 6) illustrates the use of yet another solvent system, as well as the application to much larger proteins. The heavy chains of ᴘH-2 histocompatibility antigens and β_2 microglobulin have molecular weights of approximately 38,000 and 12,000, respectively (Henriksen et al., 1978, 1979). The separation was monitored at 280 nm, and it should be pointed out that for proteins this wavelength is almost as sensitive as 220 nm.

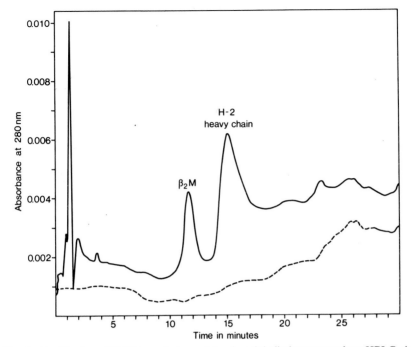

Fig. 6. Purification of H-2 heavy chains and β_2 microglobulin by reverse-phase HPLC. Approximately 200 pmol of H-2 antigen, purified by isoelectric focusing (Henriksen *et al.* 1979), was separated into H-2 heavy chain and β_2 microglobulin (β_2M) using a 30-min linear gradient of 35–80% ethanol in 0.012 M HCl.

Column: Brownlee MPLC column, packed with LiChrosorb, 10 μm particle size, 0.46 × 10 cm
Solvent A: 0.012 M HCl
Solvent B: Ethanol
Gradient: 35–80% B, linear, 30 min
Flow rate: 0.8 ml/min
Detection: 280 nm (fixed-wavelength detector)
Amount: Approximately 200 pmol of H-2 antigen purified by isoelectric focusing (Henriksen *et al.*, 1979)

The column used in this separation is noteworthy. This column (manufactured by Brownlee and called an MPLC) is the small one illustrated in Fig. 2. Its flow, capacity, and resolution characteristics are excellent. Samples of up to 6 mg have been put on this type of column. Several different reverse-phase supports are available.

The particular acid–ethanol solvent used was chosen because it allows maximum uv transmission at 220 nm and because it is volatile. The low pH (about 2) helps to dissolve proteins, and ethanol is a good eluant. These conditions are not as harsh as they might seem. The H-2 heavy chains and β_2 microglobulin retain significant antigenic reactivity, as measured with specific rabbit antisera, and the heavy chains also react with alloantisera. Fractions of about 300 μl are collected and immediately dried in a vacuum desiccator. It typically takes about an hour to dry 100–200 tubes.

D. Partial Purification of β_2 Microglobulin from a Complex Mixture of Proteins

It is often possible to obtain one component of a complex mixture of proteins in a purer form by reanalyzing a certain segment of the initial chromatogram. Figure 7 illustrates this technique, and it also demonstrates that large volumes of a sample can be loaded onto the reverse-phase column through the pump. In this case, 2 ml of a partially purified prepara-

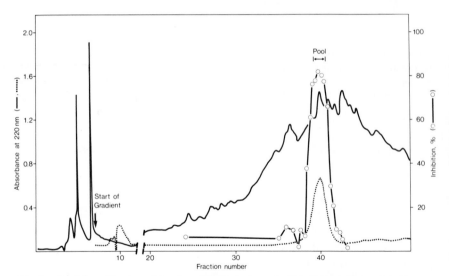

Fig. 7. Partial purification of β_2 microglobulin from a complex mixture of proteins. Approximately 2 ml of a partially purified preparation of β_2 microglobulin from mouse liver (1.3 mg protein/ml) was loaded onto a reverse-phase column through the pump. The absorbance at 220 nm was monitored (solid line), and the location of β_2 microglobulin was assessed by radioimmunoassay (not shown) (Henriksen *et al.*, 1979). The indicated fractions were pooled and reinjected into the column; the absorbance at 220 nm was again monitored (dotted line), and the presence of β_2 microglobulin established by radioimmunoassay (open circles). The proteins were eluted with a linear gradient of 10–80% ethanol in 0.012 M HCl.

tion of murine β_2 microglobulin, containing 2.6 mg of protein, was loaded through the pump. After all of the sample was loaded, the gradient was started, and the material eluted. The location of β_2 microglobulin was established by radioimmunoassay, and the appropriate fractions were pooled and reinjected into the column. It is apparent that considerable purification has been achieved. It should also be noted that the antigenic activity of β_2 microglobulin was retained (although not completely) even after repeated exposure to the low pH value of the solvent.

Column: Brownlee MPLC column, packed with LiChrosorb, 10 μm particle size, 0.46 × 10 cm
Solvent A: 0.012 M HCl
Solvent B: Ethanol
Gradient: 10–80% B in 30 min; hold at 80% B for 15 min
Flow rate: 0.8 ml/min
Detection: 220 nm (multiple-wavelength detector)
Amount: 2.6 mg of partially purified protein

E. Separation of the CNBr Peptides of H-2^a Heavy Chains

This example illustrates how GPC separates the peptides generated by CNBr cleavage of H-2^a heavy chains according to their molecular weight (Fig. 8A; Alvarez and Henriksen, 1980). Figure 8B shows that a linear elution pattern is obtained with molecular-weight standards. It is evident that this particular column is best suited for the separation of lower-molecular-weight components (less than 25,000–30,000); other columns are available which are better for the separation of proteins of higher molecular weight. As in the previous example, further purification of the individual peptides can be obtained by reinjecting them into the same column.

Column: Waters I-125 protein column, 10.8 × 30 cm, two columns in series
Solvent: 0.05 M Tris–HCl, pH 7.3, 6 M guanidine–HCl
Flow rate: 1.0 ml/min
Detection: 280 nm
Amount: CNBr digest of 2 nmol of H-2^a heavy chains

F. Partial Purification of an Antigen-Specific T-Cell-Replacing Factor and Determination of Its Molecular Weight

High-pressure reverse-phase chromatography and GPC complement each other. The first system is used to purify a biologically active com-

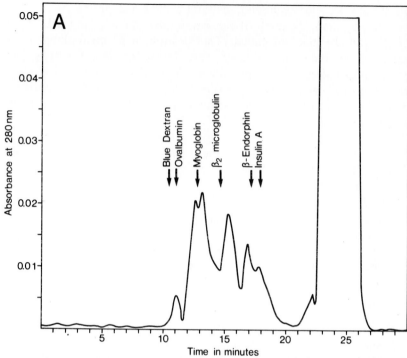

Fig. 8. Separation of the CNBr peptides of H-2^a heavy chains. Two nanomoles of H-2^a heavy chains were cleaved with CNBr and then reduced and alkylated. The incubation mixture was loaded onto a gel permeation column (A). The peptides were eluted with 0.05 M Tris–HCl, pH 7.3, 6 M guanidine–HCl, and the absorbance at 280 nm was monitored. The column was calibrated with the indicated molecular-weight markers (ovalbumin, 46,000 MW; myoglobin, 17,000 MW; β_2 microglobulin, 12,000 MW; β-endorphin, 3700 MW; insulin A chain, 2500 MW). The linear relationship between the molecular weight and the elution volume of the standards is shown in (B). K_{av} is defined as $(V_e - V_0)/(V_t - V_0)$, where V_e is the volume of solvent required to elute the molecule of interest, V_t the total column volume, and V_0 the void volume.

pound; with the second system its molecular weight can be determined under denaturing conditions (Fig. 9).

A partially purified preparation of a keyhole limpet hemocyanin (KLH)-specific T-cell-replacing factor (Henriksen *et al.*, 1980) was loaded onto a reverse-phase column, and the helper factor activity was located in the effluent by a specific plaque assay (Howie, this volume, Chapter 10). The approximate molecular weight of the active material was determined by analyzing it on a gel permeation column. Fractions corresponding to different molecular-weight ranges were pooled and reinjected onto the reverse-phase column to remove the guanidine-HCl from the active

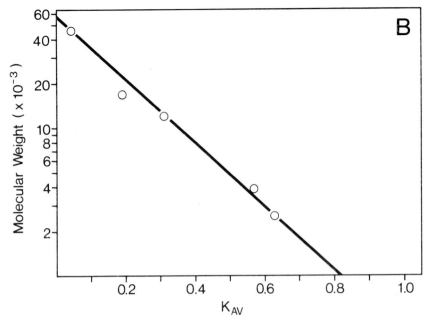

Fig. 8. *(continued)*

material. The appropriate region of the reverse-phase chromatogram was then assayed for helper activity after each injection in order to locate the particular fraction from the gel permeation column that contained the active material. This required 16 separate complete analyses.

Reverse Phase

Column: Brownlee RP-18, packed with LiChrosorb, 5 μm particle size, 0.5 × 25 cm
Solvent A: 0.012 *M* HCl
Solvent B: Ethanol
Gradient: 25–65% B, linear; at 29 min step to 80% B which is held for 20 min
Flow rate: 0.9 ml/min
Detection: 220 nm

Gel Permeation

Column: Waters I-125 protein column, 0.8 × 30 cm
Solvent: 0.05 *M* Tris–HCl, pH 7.3, 6 *M* guanidine–HCl
Flow rate: 0.4 ml/min
Detection: 280 nm

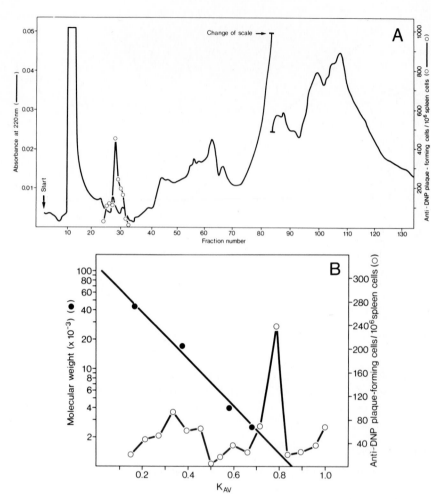

Fig. 9. Partial purification of an antigen-specific T-cell-replacing factor and determination of its molecular weight. A partially purified preparation of a KLH-specific T-cell-replacing factor was loaded onto a reverse-phase column (A). The absorbance was monitored at 220 nm, and the helper factor activity was assayed by a specific plaque assay (open circles). In order to determine the molecular weight of the active material, aliquots of the active fractions were pooled, incubated in 0.05 M Tris–HCl, pH 7.3, 6 M guanidine–HCl and injected into a gel permeation column. The column was eluted with the same buffer used for incubation. Fractions corresponding to different molecular-weight regions were pooled and reanalyzed on the reverse-phase column. The molecular-weight distribution of the active material is shown in (B). The reverse-phase column was eluted with a 29-min linear gradient of 25–65% ethanol in 0.012 M HCl. The ethanol concentration was then increased to 80% and held for 20 min. At the position indicated in the figure the full scale of the absorbance was changed from 0.05 to 0.10.

REFERENCES

Alvarez, V. L., and Henriksen, O. (1980). Isolation and partial amino acid sequencing of the cyanogen bromide peptides of H-2ª. In preparation.

Bayon, A., Rossier, J., Mauss, A., Bloom, F. E., Iversen, L. L., Ling, N., and Guillemin, R. (1978). *In vitro* release of [5-methionine] enkephalin and [5-leucine]-enkephalin from the rat globus pallidus. *Proc. Natl. Acad. Sci. U.S.A.* **75,** 3503–3506.

Hawk, G., ed. (1979). "Biological and Biomedical Applications of Liquid Chromatography." Dekker, New York.

Henriksen, O., Robinson, E. A., and Appella, E. (1978). Structural characterization of H-2 antigens purified from mouse liver. *Proc. Natl. Acad. Sci. U.S.A.* **75,** 3322–3326.

Henriksen, O., Robinson, E. A., and Appella, E. (1979). Purification and chemical characterization of papain-solubilized histocompatibility-2 antigens from mouse liver. *J. Biol. Chem.* **254,** 7651–7658.

Henriksen, O., Alvarez, V. L., Barnes, M., Bächtold, H., Frey, J. R., Hansson, E., Howie, S., Lefkovits, I., Roitsch, C. A., Söderberg, A., and Young, P. (1980). Heterogeneity of Mouse Interleukins. *FEBS Lett.* **121,** 157–160.

Howie, S. (1981). *In vitro* production and testing of antigen-induced mediators of helper T-cell function. *In* "Immunological Methods" (I. Lefkovits and B. Pernis, eds.), Vol. II, pp. 199–211. Academic Press, New York.

Regnier, F. E., and Gooding, K. M. (1980). High-performance liquid chromatography of proteins. *Anal. Biochem.* **103,** 1–25.

Rubinstein, M. (1979). Preparative high-performance liquid partition chromatography of proteins. *Anal. Biochem.* **98,** 1–7.

Rubinstein, M., Rubinstein, S., Familletti, P. C., Gross, M. S., Miller, R. S., Waldman, A. A., and Pestka, S. (1979). Human leucocyte interferon: Production, purification to homogeneity, and initial characterization. *Proc. Natl. Acad. Sci. U.S.A.* **76,** 640–644.

6

Methods in Surface Physics for Immunology

Donald F. Gerson

I. INTRODUCTION

Relevance of Surface Physics to Immunology

The immune system produces and contains a remarkable array of chemicals which act both in solution and on cell surfaces to produce physical results. Agglutination, phagocytosis, lysis, precipitation, adhesion, and recognition are all physical processes; they are described by the action of forces on objects rather than by the reconstruction of chemical bonds. On a molecular level, these processes all involve van der Waals interactions rather than covalent bonds. The methods of surface physics offer a direct route to the measurement of van der Waals forces and thus are applicable to the study of the physical consequences of immunological pro-

IMMUNOLOGICAL METHODS, VOL. II

cesses. The direct application of surface physics to immunology is in its infancy, but the utility of the approach in clarifying these seemingly complex phenomena is evident.

The methods of surface physics are not widely known and, unfortunately, are not even widely published. Surface physics has great practical importance in the manufacture and testing of surfactants, detergents, wetting agents, emulsifiers, adhesives, adhesive release agents, plastics, implantable prostheses, and contact lenses; in oil recovery, cleanup, processing, and refining; in lubrication, metal cutting, paper processing, and waste disposal; and in a host of other important industrial operations. The bulk of research and measurement in surface physics has been performed in government and industrial laboratories engaged in applied research, and while only a fraction of this work has been published, some of the greatest advances in surface physics have come from such practical research. Despite this relatively unusual situation, the basic tools of surface physics can be obtained or constructed with relative ease in a biological laboratory, and it is both the theoretical basis and the practical use of these tools and methods which will be discussed in this chapter.

It is convenient to begin with some examples of the application of surface physics to immunological phenomena. Mudd and Mudd (1926) were two of the earliest workers to discover that opsinization of bacteria by antibody directed against them altered the hydrophobicity of the bacterial cell surface. Their measure of hydrophobicity was partitioning between oil and water, which is related to the difference between the surface energies of the cells in each liquid (see below). In the case of the highly hydrophobic mycobacteria, antibody made the cell surface more hydrophilic. Van Oss *et al.* (1975) studied the effect of opsinization on the hydrophobicity of highly hydrophilic streptococci and found that specific antibody made the cells more hydrophobic. When replotted, their results demonstrate a linear function between the log of the number of bacteria phagocytized and the free energy of engulfment, calculated from surface energies, for all but the most hydrophobic bacteria, possibly reflecting the difference in response to antibody of hydrophilic and hydrophobic bacteria (see below). Using partition in biphasic mixtures formed with polyethylene glycol and dextran, Stendahl *et al.* (1977) also demonstrated that opsinization increased the hydrophobicity of *Salmonella*.

The formation of antibody–antigen complexes depends on van der Waals interactions between the molecules and usually results in precipitation of the complex. In essence, this is an example of complex coacervation, a term describing the association of soluble polymers to form an insoluble or separate phase containing virtually all of both polymers. Complex coacervation results from a change in the surface properties of the interacting polymers. Using phase partition in biphasic mixtures of polyethylene glycol and dextran, or of methylcellulose and dextran, Albertsson (1971) studied the changes in surface properties accompanying antigen–antibody complex formation for both albumin and phycoerythrin. In both cases the complex was more hydrophobic than either partner. Antigen–antibody complex formation using 3-azopyridine coupled to albumin was studied by van Oss and Newmann (1977) and van Oss *et al.* (1979a), and it was found that, by reducing the interfacial tension between the protein and the solution with ethylene oxide or dimethyl sulfoxide, it was possible both to inhibit the formation of antigen–antibody complexes and to dissociate preformed complexes. The hydrophobicity of the antigen–antibody complex may be related to the collection of this precipitate in joints and kidney tubules. The thin layer immunoassay technique and the partition affinity ligand assay depend on this phenomenon (see below).

In both of these examples, surface properties which reflect the nonspecific van der Waals interactions at cell surfaces and antigen–antibody complexes are sufficient to describe the general features of the physical processes involved. One purpose of further study of surface energies in immunological systems is to help distinguish between those aspects dominated by nonspecific interactions and those which depend on the specific recognition of an antigen by an antibody.

Some phenomena subject to analysis and study by the methods of surface physics are diagrammed in Fig. 1. Figure 1A depicts the engulfment of a bacterial cell by a phagocyte cell. The surface free energy change ΔG_s, per unit area of contact, for adhesion between the cells is given by the relation:

$$\Delta G_s = \gamma_{PB} - \gamma_{PM} - \gamma_{BM}$$

where γ is the interfacial free energy at the phagocyte–bacterium (PB), phagocyte–medium (PM), or bacterium–medium (BM) interface. Measurement of these interfacial free energies allows calculation of ΔG_s, the change in surface energy; if it is positive, the process should not occur unless other processes are driving it; if it is negative, attachment of the bacterium to the phagocyte is a spontaneous process and should occur unless other processes are preventing it. Engulfment, Fig. 1A (step 2), requires that the membrane of the phagocytic cell be sufficiently fluid to flow over the bacterium. The fate of the engulfed cell may or may not depend on surface physics. Figure 1B diagrams intercellular adhesion (step 1) and cell fusion (step 2). The same analysis applies here. Fusion, rather than long-term attachment or engulfment, requires membrane fluidity in both partners. Fusion of the nuclei within the mixed cytoplasm (mixing may not occur) is yet another problem and is not an automatic consequence of cell fusion. Figure 1C diagrams the adhesion of a cell to a solid surface, e.g., cells to nylon. Figure 1D depicts the fusion of a liposome with a cell. Both these processes involve changes in the interfacial free energies of the respective systems. Adhesion to an inert

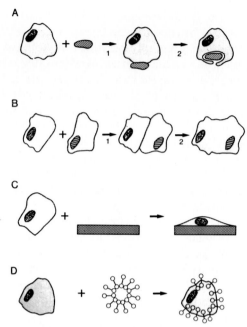

Fig. 1. Physical interactions at the cell surface involving changes in surface energy. (A) Phagocytic engulfment of other cells or of fluid droplets or particles. (B) Cell–cell contact or adhesion (step 1) and subsequent fusion (step 2). (C) Cell-surface adhesion and the spreading, or rounding of cells on a substrate. (D) Alteration of cell surface energy by the incorporation of different amphipathic constituents into the membrane from within the cell, from the solution, or from contact or fusion with liposomes, micelles, or other cells.

substrate involves a ΔG_s of a form similar to that for adhesion to the bacterium. In the case of liposome fusion, the interfacial free energy of the cell changes after fusion as a result of the incorporation of lipids from the liposome into its membrane.

Tables I–III give data on the surface energies of various substrates. Table I lists surface tensions for liquids and solutions of various types. Table II gives surface energies of various inert solids. Table III lists surface energies of cells measured against either air or aqueous solutions (see below for a further explanation).

II. REVIEW OF SURFACE PHYSICS

The study of cell surfaces constitutes a major component of cell biology and immunology. Biochemical and structural knowledge of the cell surface is well founded, however, less is known of the physical properties of the cell surface. Some new physical methods are now available which should allow expansion of knowledge in this area. One is the use of fluorescence to study

TABLE I

Surface Tensions of Liquids

Liquid	Surface tension (dyn/cm)
NaNO$_3$, 30% (w/v), aqueous	80.5
CaCl$_2$, 10% (w/v), aqueous	74.9
Water	73.0
Glycerol	
20%, aqueous	70.9
82%, aqueous	65.3
Pure	63.4
Ethylene glycol, 55%, aqueous	55.6
n-Hexadecane	27.3
Polyethylene glycol 6000	24.0
Ethanol	22.3
n-Hexane	18.4
FC-48, fluorocarbon	12.0
FC-72, fluorocarbon	10.4

the dynamics of the motion of cell surface proteins and to obtain estimates of the viscosity of the membrane in its plane (Shinitsky, 1979; Schlessinger, 1979). These measurements have helped to elucidate the early response of the cell surface to activators and hormones. Another is determination of the surface energies of cell surfaces by contact angle measurements, allowing estimations of the equilibrium constant for physical processes such as phagocytosis and cell fusion (Gerson *et al.*, 1980; Schürch *et al.*, 1980; van Oss *et al.*, 1975). The recent demonstration that phase partition in biphasic polymer mixtures can be directly correlated with cell surface energies, measured by contact angle methods, allows the use of phase partition for the determination of cell surface energies in previously calibrated systems (Gerson, 1980; Gerson and Akit, 1980; Gerson and Scheer, 1980).

Surface energy is the extra free energy term required to describe an interface between two phases, such as a cell and its growth medium. It is the net sum of all the van der Waals interactions occurring between the various components of the surfaces facing one another. Most of the processes in cell biology called interactions occur because the net free energy resulting from attachment or aggregation is negative even though covalent bonds are not restructured. The processes result from favorable changes in either ionic or surface free energies. Surface charges on cells and macromolecules have been measured extensively by electrophoretic methods, but surface energies have been largely ignored in a quantitative sense.

Qualitatively, surface energies are described as hydrophobic interactions resulting from a variety of ill-defined processes such as water exclusion and

TABLE II

Surface Energies of Solids

Substance	Surface energy (ergs/cm^2)
Platinum	$\simeq 1800$
Glass	$\simeq$ 700
Mica	$\simeq$ 350
Ice	106.0
Polyhydroxyethyl methacrylate	71.0
Phosphatidylglycerol	70.6
Gelbond, hydrophilic surface	70.1
Phosphatidylinositol	69.5
Phosphatidylcholine	67.1
Polymethoxymethyl methacrylate	60.0
Polycarbonate, Lexan	54.7
Plexiglas	53.0
Pancreatic protease	49.3
Polystyrene, irradiated	47.1
α-Amylase	45.6
Polyhexamethylene adipamide (nylon-66)	46.0
Glass, 0.6% relative humidity	45.0
Polyethylene terephthalate (Mylar)	43.0
Polymethylmethacrylate	42.0
Polyvinylidene chloride	40.0
Polyvinyl chloride	39.0
Siliconized glass	37.7
Lipase	35.4
Polystyrene	33.0
Bovine serum albumin, V	32.4
Polystyrene	33
Polyethylene	31.0
Glass, 95% relative humidity	$\simeq 31.0$
Hydroxyapatite	30.0
Polyvinyl fluoride	28.0
Keratin	27.0
Polyvinylidine fluoride	25.0
n-Hexatriacontane	21.0
Polytetrafluoroethylene	18.5
Polyperfluorostyrene	17.8
Polyperfluoropropylethylene	15.5
FC-127, fluorocarbon	12.9
Poly 1H, 1H-pentadecafluorooctyl methacrylate	10.6

TABLE III

Surface Energies of Cells and Tissues Measured by the Contact Angle Method

Organism or cell type	Surface energy (ergs/cm²)		
	γ_c	γcell–H_2O^a	Reference[b]
Thiobacillus thiooxidans	72		6
Rat neutrophil	68.3	5.5×10^{-2}	1
Guinea pig neutrophil	68.1	6.5×10^{-2}	1
Staphylococcus epidermidis	67.9	0.38	6
HeLa cells	67.8	8.7×10^{-2}	1
Mouse neutrophil	67.7	9.7×10^{-2}	1
Human erythrocyte	67.7	9.7×10^{-2}	1
BALB/c lymphocyte, Con A blast	—	0.23	6
Myeloma fusion product, FO	—	0.31	6
Cytotoxic T-cell line, DF100-6	—	0.53	6
Human erythrocyte	—	0.70	3
Mastocytoma cell line, P815	—	0.75	6
Human neutrophil	—	0.84	3
Pig pulmonary macrophages	—	0.93	3
BALB/c, transformed lymphocyte line, K	—	1.10	5
BALB/c, resting lymphocytes	—	2.53	6
BALB/c, transformed lymphocyte line, BM18-4	—	3.33	5
BALB/c, transformed lymphocyte line, ABLS-1	—	3.60	5
C57BL/nu, resting lymphocytes	—	10.11	6
Staphylococcus aureus Smith	67.3	0.14	1
Streptococcus pneumoniae 1	67.1	0.16	1
Chicken neutrophil	67.1	0.16	1
Human platelet	67.1	0.16	1
Escherichia coli 0111	67.0	0.16	1
Rabbit neutrophil	66.9	0.17	1
Haemophilus influenzae-β	66.9	0.18	1
Human fibroblasts	66.8	0.19	1
Monkey neutrophil	66.8	0.19	1
Human neutrophil	66.8	0.19	1
Human polymorphonuclear leukocytes	66.8	0.19	1
CY mosaic virus	66.5	3.7×10^{-2}	6
Staphylococcus aureus	66.5	0.22	1
Salmonella arizonae	66.4	0.24	1
Serratia marcescens	66.3	0.72	6
Salmonella typhimurium	66.0	0.30	1
Escherichia coli 07	64.9	0.48	1
Listeria monocytogenes R	63.4	0.80	1
Neisseria gonorrhoeae	63.4	0.82	1
Brucella abortus	63.2	0.85	1
Brome mosaic virus	63.1	0.43	6
Candida tropicalis	—	0.62	6
Flexibacter sp.	—	1.10	6
Pseudostugae menziesii (xylem)	59.0	—	2
Western hemlock (xylem)	56.5	—	2
Pseudomonas asphaltenicus	51.7	8.17	6
Acinetobacter calcoaceticus	50.0	—	6

(cont.)

TABLE III (*cont.*)

Organism or cell type	Surface energy (ergs/cm²)		
	γ_c	$\gamma_{cell-H_2O}{}^a$	Reference[b]
Corynebacterium lepus	48.7	10.8	6
English oak (xylem)	40.8	—	2
Human skin	38.2	—	4
Human tooth surface	30.0	—	4
Nocardia erythropolis	15.9	41.1	6
Mycobacterium butyricum	15.6	—	1

[a] γ_{cell-H_2O} is the interfacial free energy of the interface of the cell and an appropriate aqueous medium. These values are subject to the composition of the medium, and are given in milliergs/cm².

[b]References: (1) van Oss *et al.* (1975); (2) Nguyen and Johns (1978); (3) Schürch *et al.* (1980); (4) Alten (1977); (5) Gerson (1980); (6) previously unpublished results.

hydrophobic bonding. Arguments concerning the hydrophobic effect abound and are largely based on data from various types of partitioning experiments which, as will be seen below, are qualitative measures of surface energies. The abundance of noncovalent interactions giving rise to these descriptions makes it clearly worthwhile to attempt quantitative measurement of surface energies.

Quantitative measurement of surface energies has been the prime goal of surface physics for many years. This has been a technically and theoretically difficult area of study and still is, especially in the area of solid–liquid interfaces. Nevertheless, sufficient progress in the physics of interfaces has been made to allow the study of biological interfaces using the techniques developed for more orderly systems. The two most central methods of surface physics concern the measurement of either surface or interfacial tensions at liquid–air or liquid–liquid interfaces or the contact angles formed by liquid drops on plane solid surfaces. The water strider (Milne and Milne, 1978) can walk on water because of the high surface tension of the liquid and the insect's hydrophobic feet; water drops are round and stand high on the surface of a newly waxed car but spread on the oxidized and weathered paint of an old unwaxed car. It is from these phenomena that the quantitative methods of surface physics spring.

A. Surface Tension and Surface Energy of Liquids

Surface tension is the force required to part a unit length of surface. Surface energy is the energy required to create a unit area of surface. The two are dimensionally equivalent. Gibbs defined surface energy as

$$\gamma = dG/dA \tag{1}$$

where γ is the surface energy (ergs/cm^2), G the free energy (ergs), and A the area (cm^2). In liquids, measurement of the surface tension involves measuring the weight of liquid a unit length of liquid–air interface can support. In practice, the term "surface tension" is usually used for liquid–air interfaces, while "surface energy" is used for solid–air or solid–liquid interfaces. Use of the verbal terminology is not strict, but it is important to use the correct units in calculations.

The surface tensions of pure liquids range from about 10 dyn/cm for fluorocarbons to 20 dyn/cm for hydrocarbons to 63 dyn/cm for pure anhydrous glycerol and to 73 dyn/cm for water. Solutes can change the surface tension in a variety of ways. Nonionic, hydrophilic solutes generally produce a slight decrease in the surface tension of water. Glycerol at 20% (v/v) in water results in a surface tension of 70 dyn/cm, and most water-miscible alcohols, glycols, and substances like dimethyl sulfoxide produce similar effects. Salt can slightly increase the surface tension of an aqueous solution relative to that of pure water. Other substances tend to aggregate both at the air–water interface and in solution and by doing so reduce the surface tension to about 20–30 dyn/cm. Low concentrations of long-chain alcohols, fatty acids, phospholipids, and most synthetic surfactants and detergents are in this category. Typically, for such amphipathic solutes a plot of the surface tension against the logarithm of the concentration has three regions. At low concentrations, surface tension is independent of concentration and high; at a higher concentration it begins to fall with a linear slope to another concentration, the critical micelle concentration (CMC). Here, addition of further surfactant results in the production of micelles rather than in adsorption at the air–liquid interface, and thus the surface tension remains independent of moderate increases in concentration, but low. At much higher concentrations, phase changes occur which can produce minor variations in the surface tension. The formation of micelles and bimolecular lipid leaflets can be described in terms of hydrophobic interactions between the hydrophobic moieties of the molecules, or in terms of the free energies of aggregation, which can be determined from surface energies (Parsegian, 1975).

In the concentration range over which there is a linear change in γ with the logarithm of concentration, the Gibbs surface excess or absorption coefficient Γ can be determined. It is given by

$$\Gamma = (-1/RT)\,(d\gamma/d\ln C) \qquad (2)$$

where Γ is the Gibbs surface excess (mol/cm^2), R the gas constant, T the temperature (K), C the concentration, and γ the surface tension. Both Γ and the CMC are useful measures of the properties of a surfactant (Gerson and Zajic, 1979b).

B. Surface Energies of Solids

1. Young's Equation

The surface energies of solids at both air and liquid interfaces have posed what is probably the most difficult measurement problem in surface physics. Different solids clearly have different surface energies; water spreads on clean glass but forms a drop on polyethylene, while hexane spreads on both. It is this property of the spreading of some liquids on a given solid which forms the basis for measurement of the surface energies of solids.

Young (1805) described the balance of forces which determine the shape of a drop of a liquid on a solid surface. His relation is given by

$$\gamma_{13} = \gamma_{23} + \gamma_{12} \cos \theta \tag{3}$$

In the case of a liquid drop on a solid surface in air, phase 1 is the air, phase 2 is the liquid, and phase 3 is the solid. The contact angle θ is the angle at which the liquid contacts the solid (Fig. 2Bb), as measured through the liquid phase. Equation (3) refers to the equilibrium contact angle, however, in practice contact angles show a variation between an advancing

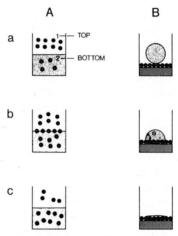

Fig. 2 The relation between the equilibrium partition of cells or particles between two liquid phases and the contact angles formed by the two liquids on a layer of these cells or particles. (A) Partition equilibrium for cells in three biphasic systems (a–c). (B) Contact angles of drops of the bottom phase on cell layers immersed in the top phase of the three biphasic systems. Partition into the upper phase is associated with high contact angles, while partition into the lower phase is associated with low contact angles.

maximum and a receding minimum (Blake and Haynes, 1973). This behavior seems to result from surface roughness or adsorption, but a clear physical explanation of this phenomenon is lacking at this time. In experimental work, the contact angle formed by a drop which has freely fallen a short distance before landing on a surface is close to the equilibrium value.

2. Critical Surface Tension for Spreading

Equation (3) contains two unknown variables, γ_{13} and γ_{23}, the interfacial free energies at the solid surface. The liquid–air or liquid–liquid interfacial free energy γ_{12}, and θ, can be measured easily. The most successful approach to the problem of determining γ_{13} or γ_{23} was first introduced by Zisman (1963, 1976) and involves finding the critical surface tension for wetting. In this method (Fig. 3), the surface energy of the solid with respect to the bulk medium is determined by finding a liquid having the maximum surface tension required for wetting the solid surface (zero contact angle). This is the critical surface tension γ_c and is a measure of the surface energy of the solid with respect to the bulk phase (phase 1). The result depends on the liquids used: Pure hydrocarbons measure only dispersive, nonpolar van der Waals interactions, while polar liquids such as water measure both

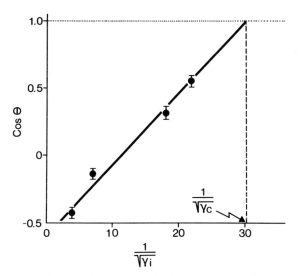

Fig. 3. The relation between contact angles and interfacial tensions for K cells (transformed lymphocytes) in biphasic mixtures of polyethylene glycol and dextran. Extrapolation to the point of complete drop spreading (cos θ = 1) gives the value of γ_c, the critical interfacial energy required for spreading.

polar and nonpolar interactions. The former are more orderly, but the latter have greater practical utility.

The critical surface tension for spreading is determined by using a series of similar liquids which will form drops on the solid under study and which have different surface tensions. Liquid–liquid pairs having various interfacial tensions can also be used. For each drop type, the contact angle and the surface tension of the liquid are measured and the relation between the cosine of the contact angle and the surface or interfacial tension is extrapolated to $\cos \theta = 1$, or to complete wetting. The corresponding surface tension is γ_c. Two linear relations have been found to describe these data with varying degrees of accuracy, and these are given by Eqs. (4) and (5). Equation (4) is Zisman's relation, while Eq. (5) was proposed by Good and Girifalco (1958; also see Good, 1975, 1977).

$$\cos \theta = a(\gamma_c - \gamma) + 1 \tag{4}$$

$$\cos \theta = a\,(1/\sqrt{\gamma_c} - 1/\sqrt{\gamma}) + 1 \tag{5}$$

where a is the slope of the respective line, γ the surface or interfacial tension at drop surface, γ_c the critical interfacial tension for wetting, and θ the contact angle.

3. Empirical Relations

Neither Eq. (4) nor (5) describes the bulk of the data very well, but the spreading of droplets on solids is a well-defined "end point," and thus γ_c can be determined with some accuracy. A more thorough understanding of solid–liquid interfacial tensions must ultimately come from a combination of the straightforward physical analysis of Young's equation and experimental correlations between contact angles and liquid surface or interfacial tensions. For hydrophobic solids such as Teflon, polystyrene, polyethlene, and other plastics, a strong correlation was found between the interaction parameter Φ (Good, 1975, 1977) given by Eq. (6) and the solid-liquid interfacial tension estimated from Eqs. (3) and (4).

$$\Phi = (\gamma_{13} + \gamma_{12} - \gamma_{23})/2\sqrt{\gamma_{13}\gamma_{12}} \tag{6}$$

Neumann (1974) and Neumann et al. (1974a,b) used this correlation to formulate an empirical equation which has been useful in the study of the interfacial free energies involved in phagocytosis (Van Oss et al., 1975), cell fusion (Gerson et al., 1980), phase partition phenomena (Van Oss et al., 1979b; Gerson, 1980; Gerson and Akit, 1980), and the adhesion of cells to hydrophobic surfaces (Neumann et al., 1979; Gerson and Scheer, 1980). However, Neumann's empirical equation fails for hydrophilic solids and liquids.

A new and more generally applicable semi-empirical relation developed in this laboratory is as follows. We found that Φ was a function of both γ_{12} and γ_{23} and that Eq. (7) is an empirical equation which closely fits all available data.

$$\Phi = \exp(\gamma_{23}(0.00007\gamma_{13} - 0.01)) \tag{7}$$

Combination of Eq. (6) with Eq. (7) gives two semi-empirical equations allowing calculation of γ_{13} and γ_{23}. Eq. (8) permits calculation of γ_{23} from γ_{12} and γ_{13}, while Eq. (9) permits calculation of γ_{13} from Θ and γ_{12}. Both Eq. (8) and Eq. (9) are easily solved numerically by computer programs which find the roots of the general function $f(x) = 0$.

$$0 = \frac{\gamma_{12} + \gamma_{13} - \gamma_{23}}{2\sqrt{\gamma_{12}\gamma_{13}}} - \exp[\gamma_{23}(0.00007\gamma_{13} - 0.01)] \tag{8}$$

$$0 = \frac{\gamma_{12}(\cos\Theta + 1)}{2\sqrt{\gamma_{12}\gamma_{13}}} - \exp[(\gamma_{13} - \gamma_{12}\cos\Theta)(0.00007\gamma_{13} - 0.01)] \tag{9}$$

C. Interfacial Free Energies and Equilibrium Constants of Physical Processes

Hydrophobic particles in aqueous suspension tend to interact to a degree proportional to their solubility, or partition coefficient, in nonpolar solvents. This constitutes the hydrophobic effect and suggests that the equilibrium constant for the aggregation of hydrophobic particles is related to the surface energies of the particles in suspension. Brønsted (1931) set out the basic relation between these measures, but there have been few direct tests of the relations he proposed (Albertsson, 1971; Walter, 1978; Gerson, 1980). The types of physical processes which can be related to surface energy differences include cell–cell adhesion, cell–substrate adhesion, cell fusion, and cell partition between immiscible liquid pairs.

Partition Coefficients

The relation of hydrophobicity to partition between immiscible liquids provides a practical approach not only to the separation of different kinds of cells or particulates (Albertsson, 1971; Walter, 1978) but also to the quantitative characterization of hydrophobicity (Zaslavsky et al., 1979; Magnusson et al., 1979; Gerson, 1980). Surfactants have been characterized in this way for many years (see Davies and Rideal, 1963) using the hydrophile–lipophile balance (HLB) scale which is a linear function of the logarithm of the partition coefficient of a surfactant between water and a hydrocarbon such as octane. The HLB of a surfactant determines which proteins the surfactant is capable of extracting from the cell surface (Storm *et al.,* 1976). Partition in biphasic aqueous mixtures of polymers is especially sensitive to small differences in hydrophobicity, and its use as an analytical tool in the study of cell surface hydrophobicity is becoming increasingly important (Walter *et al.,* 1978; Gerson, 1980).

A derivation of the relation between the partition coefficient and surface energies is given by Gerson (1980). The relation derived there is given by Eq. (10) for systems in which surface energies arising not only from van der Waals interactions but also from electrostatic interactions are important. Equation (10) predicts that, if partition is carried out between two liquid phases or between a liquid and a solid phase under various conditions having constant ionic composition but varying in hydrophobicity, the equilibrium constants will be a linear function of the hydrophobicity differences. Conversely, if hydrophobicity is constant, partition depends on the potential difference, $\Delta\Psi$, as described by the Nernst equation.

$$- \log K_{eq} = \alpha\Delta\gamma + \delta\Delta\Psi + \beta \tag{10}$$

where K_{eq} is the equilibrium constant for the partition of a particle P between two phases, 1 and 2, $[P]_2/[P]_1, \Delta\gamma = \gamma_{2P} - \gamma_{1P}, \Delta\Psi = \Psi_{2P} - \Psi_{1P}$, and α, β, and δ are empirical constants which include all nonidealities in the parameter with which they are associated.

Thus partition measures hydrophobicity for a series of biphasic mixtures of polymers in an aqueous solution created with constant salt and buffer composition but variable nonionic polymer concentrations. Partition can also measure surface charge if the salt composition or concentration varies but the polymer concentration is constant. In some situations, however, both properties change (e.g., systems with phosphate and polyethylene glycol), and in these cases complete knowledge of both the surface energies and charges is required. These two approaches have been used with considerable success to study separately van der Waals and electrostatic effects (Walter, 1978; Gerson, 1980). Adhesion of cells to hydrophobic solid surfaces also obeys Eq. (10) (Gerson and Scheer, 1980).

As experimentally direct approach to the relation between K_{eq} and $\Delta\gamma$ has been given by Gerson (1980). Partition coefficients of cultured cells in immiscible liquid–liquid systems were related to the difference between the surface energies of the cells in each phase. This difference is directly measured experimentally by the contact angle formed by a droplet of the dense liquid phase resting on cells immersed in the light phase. Young's equation then gives $\Delta\gamma$, if the interfacial tension between the two phases γ_{12} is known:

$$\Delta\gamma = - \gamma_{12} \cos \theta \tag{11}$$

The empirical relation between the equilibrium constant for the partition of cells between two phases, K_{eq} and the contact angle formed on the cells by a drop of one liquid immersed in the other is given by Eq. (12) (Gerson, 1980). The relation between the equilibrium constant and contact angle for conditions of constant γ_{12} but with different solid particles is diagrammed in Fig. 2 (Gerson, 1980).

$$\log K_{eq} = \alpha\gamma_{12} \cos \theta + \beta \tag{12}$$

III. METHODS OF MEASUREMENT

A. Surface Tensions at Air-Liquid Interfaces

Surface tension is the force required to part 1 cm of liquid surface, and the usual methods measure this directly. Determination of the surface tension of a liquid takes advantage of the complete wetting of certain solids by the liquid to be measured to form a linear segment of air-liquid interface. The force required either to break or to renew continually this interfacial line is then measured with a sensitive but conventional balance.

Two methods are commonly employed for the determination of surface tensions. The duNouy method (Moore, 1972) involves measurement of the force required to pull a horizontally positioned platinum wire ring of known circumference through a liquid interface. The Wilhelmy method (Moore, 1972) involves measurement of the static or steady-state downward force on a thin, wettable plate of known width immersed in the liquid. Both methods directly measure the weight of liquid which can be supported by the surface tension of the liquid and thus potentially can be as accurate as the balance employed.

The duNouy method tends to be the least troublesome and is the most frequently used. A platinum ring, typically 6 cm in circumference, is held horizontally by a frame (visible below the balance in Fig. 4) and is attached to the balance by a small hook. Such rings are available from Cahn-Ventron (7500 Jefferson Street, Paramount, California). The ring is first submerged in the liquid, and then the liquid container is slowly lowered while the force on the ring is continuously recorded. The maximum force on the ring in dynes per centimeter is the surface tension.

The Wilhelmy method is probably more accurate than the duNouy method because of the more uniform geometry of the interfacial line. To measure surface tension, the plate is suspended from the balance so that its lower edge is horizontal and parallel to the liquid surface. The liquid container is slowly raised toward the plate until contact is made, and the liquid exerts a strong downward pull on the plate. As movement upward continues, the force decreases slightly as a result of the displacement of water

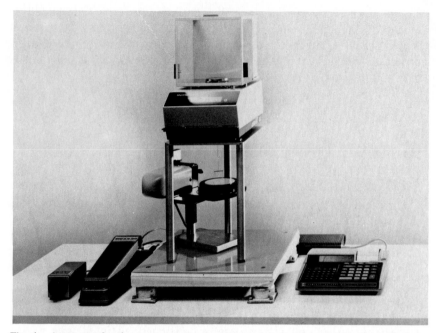

Fig. 4. Apparatus for the measurement of surface or interfacial tension by the duNouy or Wilhelmy method. A sensitive electrobalance (Mettler A30) measures the force exerted from below by the duNouy loop (in place) or a Wilhelmy plate suspended at the liquid interface. Digital data from the electrobalance is transmitted through a BCD interface to a Hewlett-Packard 97S calculator which computes the surface or interfacial tension in dynes per centimeter from the weight measurement in grams. The sample is elevated to immerse the ring or plate, and then lowered to make a measurement, by a Wild motorized microscope stage with an added fine-speed control.

by the plate. Extrapolation of this linear trend to the point of initial contact gives the surface tension. Alternatively, the plate is partially submerged and then steadily withdrawn, and the linear trend is extrapolated to the point of detachment. If the plate is perfectly wettable, the two values should give the same result. Hysteresis in the contact angle made by the liquid on the plate causes the two results to differ.

Some practical details which aid in the execution and improve the accuracy of each method are as follows. In all cases, it is advisable to have as wide a liquid container as possible to avoid errors due to adhesion of the surface to the wall of the container (Furlong and Hartland, 1979). For aqueous solutions, a container which is not wettable is an advantage, and plastic petri dishes or 200-ml Teflon beakers work very well. Large diameters are needed if the vessel is glass. If platinum rings or plates are used, they must be cleaned in acid periodically and heated to a yellow-white color between measurements. Glass coverslips etched with hydrofluoric acid also can be used in the Wilhelmy technique. However, the material of choice is high-grade filter paper (Gaines, 1977). A suitable and convenient filter paper is Whatman No. 1, available in 1- or 3-cm-wide rolls.

Equipment for measuring surface tension is available from many supply houses. Most of it is of archaic design and should not be used. Two suitable commercial setups are (1) the Fisher Autotensiomat, produced by Fisher Scientific, and (2) the Cahn–Ventron electrobalance with a surface tension accessory. The Fisher Autotensiomat is a complete unit designed primarily for the duNouy technique, although it is suitable for the Wilhelmy method as well. It is sensitive and has the best sample table arrangement available. The Cahn–Ventron equipment is slightly more sensitive, and the zero is adjusted with much greater ease, but the sample table is poorly designed and has a limited range.

An arrangement which combines the sensitivity of an electrobalance with a sample table having a wide speed and distance range is shown in Fig. 4. A Mettler A30 balance is supported above a Wild Type 374548 motorized microscope stage. The Mettler balance is digital, reads to 0.1 mg, and may be attached to a Hewlett-Packard 97S calculator to provide continuous digital recordings with direct conversion of the output from milligrams to dynes per centimeter. The motorized microscope stage is adapted for use by providing an external 10-turn 10K potentiometer in place of the foot-pedal-operated speed control. Slower speeds can be achieved by altering the gears in the drive unit. The entire assembly is protected from mechanical shock and vibration by a multilayered table of lead and sheet silicone rubber mounted on shock absorbers. A similar arrangement can be obtained with any of the various strain gauge balances now on the market, provided there is access to the balance pan from below. It is also convenient to have direct analog output of the force–displacement curve.

B. Interfacial Tensions at Liquid–Liquid Interfaces

1. duNouy and Wilhelmy Methods

Liquid–liquid interfacial tensions (e.g., oil–water) are of greater utility for many problems in cellular biophysics than liquid–air surface tensions, since most cells and tissues exist in an aqueous medium. There are three methods which are useful for measuring liquid–liquid interfacial tensions on a routine basis: (1) the duNouy or Wilhelmy method, (2) the hanging drop method, and (3) the spinning drop method.

Application of the Wilhelmy or duNouy method simply involves immersing the sensing plate or ring in the denser of the two liquids and then layering on the less dense liquid in the same way that a discontinuous density gradient is formed. The upper liquid layer must be deep enough to prevent its air–liquid interface from interfering with the measurement. Results obtained with this method are usually quite accurate down to the range of 0.1–1.0 dyn/cm. Several practical problems are often encountered which deserve comment. If the interfacial tension is high, as when one of the liquids is aqueous and the other is a hydrocarbon or fluorocarbon, the meniscus where the liquid–liquid interface meets the container is large enough to interfere significantly with measurements. The best solution to this problem is a wider container, preferably made of a material which will minimize meniscus formation. Siliconized glass (Siliclad, Clay-Adams, or Repelcoat, Hopkins and Williams, Great Britain) can often be useful, but great care must be taken to remove all unbound silane prior to use. Teflon and polypropylene beakers are also useful but are opaque.

Unfortunately, the low liquid–liquid interfacial tensions most relevant and useful to investigations of biological surfaces are below the range measured by the direct techniques described above. Both the duNouy and Wilhelmy techniques also depend on the wetting of a solid material, which by surface adsorption may alter the results obtained if the interfacial tension is small. The two techniques of choice for the measurement of low interfacial tensions are the pendant drop and spinning drop techniques. Both rely on the dependence of drop shape on interfacial tension when the drop is suspended in a force field. The various pendant drop methods use the gravitational field; the spinning drop method uses a centrifugal field.

2. Pendant Drop Technique for Measuring Liquid–Liquid Interfacial Tensions

The pendant drop technique is an extremely accurate and experimentally easy method for determining the interfacial tension between two immiscible liquids. It is the method of choice for many of the liquid–liquid pairs most useful in determinations of interfacial tensions at cell and protein surfaces. Measurements are performed by forming a drop of the denser liquid on the tip of a small capillary immersed in the less dense liquid and measuring certain dimensions of the drop. Since a complete mathematical solution to drop shape is available, interfacial tension can be determined from the effective density of the drop and its shape parameter.

The equipment required for photographing small droplets can probably be assembled from microscopes available in any biological laboratory. All that is required is a microscope of relatively low power and a camera attachment for it. An arrangement suitable for relatively large drops has been described by Bagnall (1978), which simply uses a macro lens and bellows on a standard, 35-mm, single-lens reflex camera, with the drop illuminated by a columnated light beam. It is much easier to put a standard laboratory microscope on its back, as shown in Fig. 5. Either older-style microscopes which swivel at the base, or the most modern ones which have flat backs parallel to the optical axis, are best. Older ones have the advantage that the optical parts, rather than the stage, move for focusing. Of course, it is advantageous to use the more modern planar objectives even on an old microscope body, since a uniform linear representation of the field of view must be obtained. For this, it is also important to adjust the condenser to provide optimal illumination. A typical result is given in Fig. 6. For samples in which both liquids are transparent and colorless and the refractive index difference is small, differential interference-contrast (e.g., Nomarski optics, as in Fig. 5) or phase-contrast optics are extremely useful in providing greater definition at the maximum diameter of the drop.

Difficulties encountered in photographing these small drops lead to a desire for more sophisticated equipment. The smaller the interfacial ten-

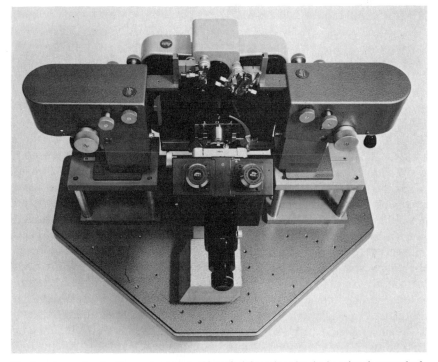

Fig. 5. Apparatus for the measurement of interfacial tensions by the hanging drop method. A fine capillary is held by the micromanipulators (left and right), and a drop of the more dense liquid is formed under the surface of the less dense liquid held in the small chamber on the microscope stage. The drop is observed by interference-contrast microscopy, photographed, and measured.

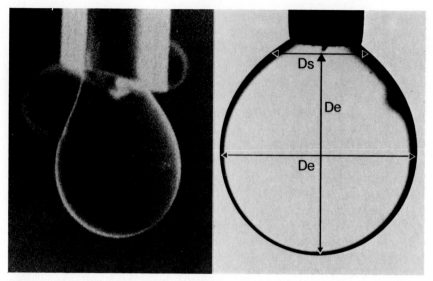

Fig. 6. A drop photographed with the apparatus shown in Fig. 5. The drop is formed from the more dense phase of a biphasic liquid system and is surrounded by the less dense phase. Symbols refer to Eq. (13) in the text.

sion, the smaller the drop must be (see below), so magnification must be increased, resulting in a loss of working distance. For large drops and low magnifications, spectrophotometer cuvettes of various sizes are useful containers. Circular, water-jacketed ones are often useful, but plastic cuvettes 1 × 1 × 3 cm have the advantages of low cost, disposability, and ease of modification (e.g., Starstedt, No. 67741). For small drops and higher magnifications, very good cuvettes can be made from microscope slides and coverslips. Two coverslips are glued to the slide, one on each side, so that a small chamber is formed that is the width of the thickness of the slide (~ 2 mm). The best glue is silicone RTV (Dow Corning), which is available in a transparent form and cures in an hour or so when warmed. The open ends of the chamber can also be sealed with silicone, and it is sometimes advantageous to seal in a hypodermic needle at each end. Many chambers can be made at one time and then disposed of following use. While curing, the silicone releases acid, and thus chambers should be washed before use.

The next most frequent difficulty is vibration either from the building or the photographic equipment. Vibration-damping tables tend to be large and relatively expensive, but excellent ones are available (e.g., Micro-g tables, TMC, Woburn, Massachusetts). Common cement balance tables work quite well. The general principle of construction is that a relatively heavy tabletop must be supported by vibration dampers. A large but excellent solution to the problem is a stone or cement slab mounted on inner tubes from small tires (e.g.,minibike or Vespa inner tubes). An alternative which is less cumbersome is to make the tabletop of several alternating layers of metal and dense rubber (e.g., three to five aluminum and sheet silicone rubber layers each 3 mm thick); reflection of the pressure waves at each interface provides a considerable increase in the effective vibration absorption per kilogram of tabletop. (This is the principle of the design of the cranium.) Vibrations from the photographic equipment can be minimized by locking the mirror in place prior to opening the shutter and by using flexible or contact-free couplings to the microscope tube. The latter are available from most camera and microscope manufacturers.

To obtain consistent liquid drops easily, a micrometer syringe is necessary (Gilmont, Great Neck, New York). A step-drive attachment on a small-volume microliter syringe (e.g., those available from Hamilton) is also useful in many instances. The syringe can be either directly attached to the capillary or indirectly connected by a relatively rigid (e.g., Teflon) plastic tube. The latter reduces vibrations but should not distend under moderate pressure. For relatively high interfacial tensions, syringe needles without sharpened ends are useful. [These are available commercially for use in intravenous or perfusion arrangements. Intramedic tubing (Clay-Adams) is designed to fit snugly into and onto these needles and is very useful.]

For low interfacial tensions, such as those between immiscible aqueous polymer mixtures, small capillary diameters are required. In the determination of interfacial tensions between 10^{-2} and 10^{-4} dyn/cm, we have used glass capillaries between 300 and 10 μm. These are prepared with microelectrode pullers used by neurophysiologists and thus are usually available in the academic environment. The only requirement is that the broken tip be level and relatively smooth. Tips can be ground using the methods of Ogden et al. (1979) and Corson et al. (1979), but breaking by a sharp axial pull usually yields a good edge. Choice of tip size can be somewhat of a problem when both the effective density and interfacial tension of a drop are low, but glass capillaries of about 100 μm are often the right size to start with. Figure 7 gives estimates of tip diameters for drops having convenient relative dimensions (see below).

The calculation of interfacial tension from the measurement of drop shape proceeds as follows. The shape parameter S is the ratio of Ds to De, the maximum diameter of the drop (Fig. 6):

$$S = Ds/De \qquad (13)$$

The value of S cannot be used for direct calculation of the interfacial tension γ_i but must be used to find a second parameter $1/H$ from tables or cor-

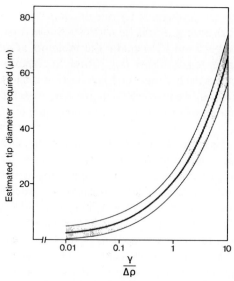

Fig. 7. The relation between the ratio of the interfacial tension γ and the difference in density $\Delta\varrho$ between the drop and the surrounding medium, and the capillary tip diameter required to form a stable drop of easily measured dimensions.

relations calculated from the equations for drop shape. Misak (1968) has derived semiempirical equations which allow calculation of $1/H$ from S for values of S between 0.4 and 1.0. These equations are of the form of Eq. (14), and the coefficients are given in Table IV. It is relatively important to use all the significant digits given.

$$1/H = aS^b + cS^3 + dS^2 + eS + f \qquad (14)$$

Once $1/H$ has been calculated, the interfacial tension between the two liquids γ_i is obtained from

$$\gamma_i = g\,\Delta\varrho De^2(1/H) \quad \text{dyn/cm} \qquad (15)$$

TABLE IV

Values of the Coefficients of Misak's Equation [Eq. (2)] for Determining the Coefficient $1/H$ from the Shape Parameter S of a Pendant Drop

Range of S		a	b	c	d	e	f
0.401	to ≤ 0.460	0.32720	-2.56651	0	-0.97553	0.84059	-0.18069
>0.460	to ≤ 0.590	0.31968	-2.59725	0	-0.46898	0.50059	-0.13261
>0.590	to ≤ 0.680	0.31522	-2.62435	0	-0.11714	0.15756	-0.05285
>0.0680	to ≤ 0.900	0.31345	-2.64267	0	-0.09155	0.14701	-0.05877
>0.900	to 1.000	0.30715	-2.84636	-0.6166	1.08315	-0.18341	-0.20970

where $g \doteq 960.4$ cm/sec^2, $\Delta\varrho$ is the difference in density between the two liquids (gm/cm^3), and De the actual maximum diameter of the drop.

3. Spinning Drop Technique for Measuring Interfacial Tensions at Liquid-Liquid Interfaces

The spinning drop technique allows the determination of interfacial tensions from the dimensions of a droplet suspended by centrifugal force at the axis of a rapidly rotating tube. Typically, a glass tube is rotated around its cylindrical axis at a high speed (1000–4000 rpm or more). One end of the tube has a rubber seal similar to that of a serum cap. To measure interfacial tensions, the tube is initially completely filled with the more dense liquid, and rotation is commenced at a slow speed. A small drop of the less dense liquid is then introduced with a microliter syringe. Usually, this drop centers itself, and at low speed it remains more or less spherical. The rate of revolution is then gradually increased until the drop assumes the shape of a cylinder with rounded ends having an axial ratio of about 3 or 4. Measurements of the length and width (corrected for refraction) of this elongated drop, plus knowledge of the speed of revolution and the density difference between the two liquids, allow calculation of the interfacial tension.

This method can be useful in measuring interfacial tensions, but the equipment required is not as generally accessible as that required for the pendant drop technique. Also, in practice the method is plagued by a multitude of little problems which cumulatively limit its use for routine measurement. Nevertheless, it has several attractive features which may make it worthy of careful consideration; the foremost of these is the ease with which low interfacial tensions can be measured in liquids of small density difference.

The method as presently used was first described by Princen et al. (1967) and later simplified by Cayias et al. (1975) and Slattery and Chen (1978). A detailed description of a sophisticated experimental apparatus is given by Cayias et al. (1975), but simpler devices also capable of giving good results are described by Silberberg (1952) and Ryden and Albertsson (1971). One problem is to obtain smooth rotation at relatively high speeds of revolution. For this purpose we have used air turbine drills of the type used by either tool and die makers or by dentists. The former operate well at speeds between 7000 and 20,000 rpm, while the latter will operate at 60,000–200,000 rpm. Both drills have adjustable chucks which can be used to hold short glass tubes. At low speeds, Teflon bearings can be used at the far end of the tube; a completely satisfactory solution to this problem for the high speeds obtainable with the dentist's drill has not yet been found (S. Schürch and D. F. Gerson, unpublished results).

To determine interfacial tension from drop shape, Eq. 16 is used. This equation assumes an axial ratio of 4 or greater; for smaller axial ratios, more complex equations must be used (Cayias *et al.*, 1975; Slattery and Chen, 1978).

$$\gamma = 1.234 \times 10^6 \, (\Delta\varrho \, d^3/p^2) \tag{16}$$

where γ is the interfacial tension (dyn/cm), $\Delta\varrho$ the density difference between the two liquids (gm/cm^3), d the actual diameter of the cylindrical drop formed spinning, provided its axial ratio exceeds 4 (the measured diameter must be divided by 1.332 to correct for refraction), and p the period of rotation of the tube (msec/rev).

C. Contact Angles and Solid–Liquid Interfacial Free Energies at Cell Surfaces Using Immiscible Liquid Phases

The measurement of contact angles formed by liquid drops on planar solid surfaces is the only satisfactory route to the determination of solid–liquid interfacial free energies. While partition coefficients (see above) can provide a comparative measure of interfacial energy at the cell surface, only the application of data obtained from contact angle measurements can produce a direct quantitative measure of this interfacial energy. The equations describing the physics of the contact angle method and the analysis of the data obtained are given above; the following concerns the techniques used to obtain consistent, accurate measurements of contact angles on layers of living cells.

The method consists of the following steps: (1) obtaining a uniform, planar layer of the cells to be measured, (2) obtaining a suitable liquid–liquid two-phase system capable of giving accurate measurements and for which the interfacial tension has been measured using the methods described above, and (3) measuring contact angles of drops of one liquid on layers of cells immersed in the other liquid.

1. Cell Preparation

Cell suspensions from tissue culture, blood, or tissue macerates are collected on cellulose acetate, Teflon, or polycarbonate microporous filters, by suction, to a cell density of $2\text{--}5 \times 10^3$ cells/mm^2. It is important to wash the cells to remove fetal calf serum or other compounds of the medium which may obscure or coat the cell surface. For mammalian cells, Dulbecco's modified phosphate-buffered saline has been found useful, but any similar solution can be used provided it is compatible with, and preferably the same as, the medium used to form the two-phase system used for measurement (see below).

The cells are then placed in the filter apparatus, and the liquid is slowly removed by suction. We have found the Millipore filter apparatus (XX10025000) to be the most satisfactory, although any such unit could be used. Filters with a pore diameter of 0.45 or 0.8 μm are generally satisfactory. No differences in the results occur when cells are collected on filters of different materials or from different manufacturers provided the entire surface of the filter is covered by a multiple layer of cells. To obtain a compact layer of cells which will stay on the filter when it is immersed in the bulk fluid of the measuring system, the filtration is continued until the surface of the filter, which is covered by cells, first becomes matte in appearance. Filtration should then be stopped immediately to prevent drying of the cells; the sintered-glass filter support retains sufficient fluid to keep the cells moist for the short period between the filtration step and immersion in the measuring fluid. Alternatively, the cells can be centrifuged onto the surface of the filter or any other suitable surface.

Bacterial or other types of cells or cellular fragments can of course be collected in the same manner, but some care must be taken to wash the cell surface free of any surface-active components of the medium (protein, undefined extracts, and so on). In addition, bacteria, fibroblasts, or other adhesive cells can be allowed to adhere to glass or plastic coverslips, filters, or other surfaces for a period of time, and these cell-coated objects used for the determination of cell surface energies. One convenient means of doing this is to use Costar Leighton tubes (No. 3393) which provide a smooth low-energy (polymethylpentane) surface to which many cell types adhere easily and which are presterilized (Trusal *et al.*, 1979).

2. Liquid–Liquid Systems for Measuring Interfacial Tensions at Cell Surfaces

Although in some early studies bacteria and neutrophils were collected on a filter and then air-dried prior to the measurement of contact angles (van Oss *et al.*, 1975), this clearly is not suitable for most situations and cell types. We have developed two approaches to this problem which keep the cells completely immersed in a physiological saline medium throughout measurement. The first is to measure the contact angles formed by drops of fluorocarbon or hydrocarbon liquids on cells immersed in a physiological salt solution or, conversely, to flood the cell layer with a long-chain liquid hydrocarbon such as tetradecane and place drops of saline on the cell layer (see Neufeld *et al.*, 1980). This has the advantages of ease and rapidity while maintaining a physiological environment [linear alkanes larger than decane have few if any toxic effects, and fluorocarbons are sufficiently nontoxic to be used as plasma and whole-blood replacements (Maugh, 1979)]. This first approach, however, has the mixed blessing that it provides a measure of only the dispersive or hydrophobic component of the van der Waals energy at the cell surface. Sometimes this can be of direct interest (Gerson and Zajic, 1977; Neufeld *et al.*, 1980; Andrade *et al.*, 1979), however, for many purposes it is desirable to measure both the polar and dispersive components of the surface free energy.

Hydrophobic fluids useful for measurements at cell surfaces must be free of surface-active components. We have detected no problems with fluorocarbons. (The FC series produced by the 3M Company are especially useful, and FC40 is available from Sigma, St. Louis, Missouri. Perfluoroalkanes can also be used.) Hydrocarbons are usually impure when purchased. They can be cleaned by extensive washing with analytical grade sulfuric acid, followed by washing with distilled water and dilute base. Several iterations are often necessary. The hydrocarbon then should be dried by passing through anhydrous Na_2SO_3. Trace contaminants can then be removed by filtration through activated alumina. The ultimate test of purity, for the purposes outlined here, is that the interfacial tension against good quality distilled water should be close to the values given in the *CRC Handbook of Chemistry and Physics*. The final material should be saturated with water before use but must be stored dry to prevent microbial degradation with the concomitant production of surfactants (Gerson and Zajic, 1979a,b).

The second approach we have developed is much more sensitive, by a factor of up to 10^{-5}, and measures the low interfacial tensions between aqueous media and hydrophilic polymers. In order to do this, we have employed the aqueous two-phase systems which form spontaneously on the mixing of water-soluble hydrophilic polymers such as polyethylene glycol and dextran, Ficoll, xanthan, pullulan, methylcellulose, and the like. The first use of these mixtures in the determination of cell surface energies was with protoplasts formed from *Zea mays* and *Aureobasidium pullulans* (Gerson *et al.*, 1980). The method has since been applied to lymphocytic cell lines, yeast, numerous bacteria (Gerson, 1980; Gerson and Akit, 1980; Gerson and Scheer, 1980), and a variety of other blood cell types (Schürch *et al.*, 1980).

Albertsson (1971) has described a multitude of aqueous polymer systems which form two or more phases and which potentially are useful in the determination of interfacial free energies at cell surfaces. However, it is also necessary to know the interfacial tension between the two phases in order to make calculations based on the contact angle data. Ryden and Albertsson (1975) measured interfacial tensions for biphasic systems composed of polyethylene glycol (6000 MW) and dextran (500,000 MW) using the spinning drop technique. Schürch *et al.* (1980) have measured interfacial tensions for the biphasic system composed of polyethylene glycol

(20,000 MW) and dextran (500,000 MW) using the pendant drop technique. Thus far, these are the only systems characterized sufficiently to allow their use in the determination of cell–medium interfacial tensions by the contact angle method. The compositions of the mixtures and the interfacial tensions between the resulting phases are given in Table V.

Preparation of these mixtures proceeds most easily if polyethylene glycol and dextran are prepared separately at twice the desired final concentration and then combined. On mixing, a cloudy emulsion of the two phases forms, and greater consistency in the final results is obtained by mixing this emulsion for 15–30 min at the temperature at which it will ultimately be used prior to separation of the phases. Phase separation will occur with most of these mixtures by simply allowing settling for about 24 hr. Alternatively, the emulsion can be centrifuged, at the final ambient temperature,

TABLE V

Interfacial Tensions between the Two Phases of Aqueous Mixtures of Dextran and Polyethylene Glycol (PEG)

	Composition[a]		Interfacial tensions ± SEM
I[b]	Dextran, 500,000 MW (%, w/w)	PEG, 20,000 MW (%, w/w)	(γN/m)
	5.0	5.0	22.8 ± 1.42
	4.5	4.5	17.0 ± 1.11
	4.3	4.3	6.41 ± 0.561
	4.0	4.0	3.47 ± 0.260
	3.5	3.5	1.11 ± 0.0721
	3.0	3.0	0.643 ± 0.0562
	Composition		Interfacial tension ± SEM
II[c]	Dextran, 500,000 MW (%, w/w)	PEG, 6000 MW (%, w/w)	(γN/m)
	8.0	6.0	65.5 ± 1.5
	7.0	4.4	20.0 ± 5.0
	6.0	4.0	7.4 ± 0.2
	5.0	4.0	3.1 ± 0.05
	5.2	3.8	2.1 ± 0.05
	5.0	3.5	0.46 ± 0.03

[a] The composition is expressed as percent of dextran and PEG per total weight of the mixture.

[b] Data from Schürch *et al.* (1980).

[c] Data from Ryden and Albertsson (1971).

until the phases are completely separated. Separation of the phases at a temperature different from that used for measurement results in disequilibrium between the phases and anomalous results.

Salts appear to have some influence on the interfacial tension between the phases. While this has not yet been measured thoroughly, it seems to be the basis for the phase separation results obtained by Walter *et al.* (1978) and by Zaslavsky *et al.* (1979). Polyethylene glycol appears to interact with phosphate, resulting in an increase in the interfacial tension of polyethylene glycol–dextran mixtures made in phosphate buffers and in the precipitation of calcium and magnesium salts from solution. There is only a small effect of 0.9% NaCl on these polymer systems.

3. Measurement of Contact Angles in the Determination of Liquid–Solid Interfacial Free Energies

In this method, small drops of a liquid are placed on a planar surface, for example, a layer of cells on a microporous filter or of protein on an ultrafiltration membrane. The contact angle is measured between the surface (through the drop) and the tangent to the drop at the point where the drop and surface meet (Fig. 8). The apparatus required for the measurement of contact angles is similar to that required for the measurement of interfacial tension by the hanging drop technique. The same apparatus can be used, but usually a lower-power objective lens of greater working distance and aperture is required.

Figure 9 shows an apparatus constructed specifically for the purpose of measuring contact angles. The components are mounted on an optical rail and consist of a focusable light source, an *X-Y-Z* micromanipulator stage with fine control in the *X-Y* plane, the zoom lens body from a Wild M405 stereomicroscope, and a prism for reflecting the projected light beam onto a ground-glass screen for measurement. The zoom lens system from a Wild

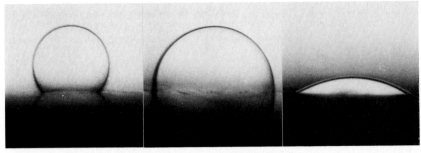

Fig. 8. Contact angles observed for drops of the dense phase of a liquid–liquid pair on solids of different surface energies immersed in the light liquid phase.

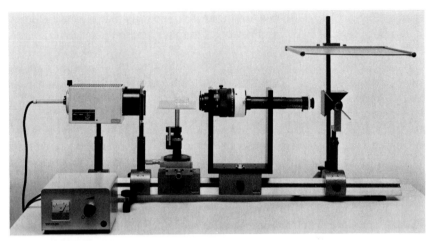

Fig. 9. Apparatus for the measurement of contact angles. From left to right, a columnated light source illuminates the sample chamber resting on an X-Y-Z micromanipulator stage. The drops are observed through the lens head of a Wild M405 stereomicroscope with a monocular viewing tube having a goniometer eyepiece. The image is projected through a prism onto a ground-glass screen for measurements.

M405 microscope provides the advantages of both variable magnification and a large aperture, giving a bright, easily seen image on the ground-glass screen. The lens assembly is similar to that of a macro lens for a camera but, for the purpose of forming a stereo image, its virtual image is observed through two smaller lens systems. For the purpose of measuring contact angles, a monocular lens holder was constructed which provided parfocal adjustment throughout the magnification range. The eyepiece was a Wild 10 or 15× goniometer eyepiece. Thus the drop under observation, the cursor, and the protractor scale were all focused together on the ground-glass screen.

As was the case for the apparatus for measuring hanging drops, simple, inexpensive, and yet highly effective optical systems can be constructed with old microscope parts commonly found in biological laboratories. Slide projectors make excellent light sources, and small laboratory jacks and microscope stage micromanipulators provide sufficiently accurate positioning of the sample.

To measure contact angles with air as the bulk fluid (top phase, Fig. 2Bb), small drops of relatively uniform size are placed on the sample and the angle of contact with the surface is measured relatively quickly. Problems resulting from the use of air as the bulk fluid generally result from evaporation, which can be limited by placing a housing over the sample table. The effect of drying on the surface of mammalian cells or other tissues on cells may be severe, and thus it is generally better to use a liquid bulk phase for cells. Air can be used as the bulk phase for plastics or other such inert surfaces.

To measure contact angles with two immiscible liquid phases, suitable sample chambers are required. These can be constructed from glass microscope slides and cover glasses of various sizes using silicone RTV transparent cement, much as aquaria are constructed. These chambers are inexpensive and utilitarian and provide an excellent optical image. It is also possible to use plastic rectangular tissue culture flasks which have had their upper surface removed by a hot wire cutter. These have the advantages of cleanliness, disposability, and minimal meniscus formation. The junction between the lower surface and the walls of these flasks usually results in optical distortion which can be avoided by placing the specimen on a microscope slide in the culture flask. With some bulk phases, the filter on which the cells have been collected will tend to float, but its edges can be held down with small (2–5 mm) stainless steel weights.

Placing drops of the sensing fluid on the layer of cells immersed in the bulk fluid requires some care. Generally, drops between 1.0 and 0.1 mm in diameter are desirable; these are most easily formed by a Pasteur pipette drawn out to a tip diameter of about 0.5–0.1 mm. With hydrocarbon sensing fluids, the filter holding the cell layer must be mounted upside down, suspended between two pieces of microscope slide, and held in place by another on top of it, and the drops applied from below by a hook-shaped pipette. With both hydrocarbon and fluorocarbon liquids, drops must be formed below the surface of the aqueous phase, since they will rarely penetrate the air–water interface if dropped from above. This is also the case for biphasic aqueous polymer systems.

The use of biphasic aqueous polymer systems provides the most realistic measure of cell–medium interfacial tensions available at this time. Preparation of these mixtures has been described above, and their use in contact angle measurements on cell layers will now be described. One characteristic of these mixtures is that the interfacial tension between the phases is an exponential function of their composition. This is useful, since it allows a wider range of interfacial tensions to be investigated, but also leads to handling problems. The slightest evaporation will sufficiently change the composition to affect the interfacial tension radically, and thus water loss must be carefully avoided in order to obtain consistent results. Stock solutions of each polymer at twice its final concentration must be kept in the cold or frozen, but mixed when at room temperature; all condensation from the sides of the bottles must be mixed back into the solution before use. Sterility is essential, since many polymer-utilizing microbes produce endodepolymerases, and the resulting change in molecular weight also radically alters the interfacial tensions. During settling or centrifugation, all separation funnels, graduated cylinders, and centrifuge tubes must be dry before use and kept covered throughout. At the time of measurement, the sample chamber containing the bulk liquid must be covered whenever possible, especially during observation, because of heat from the light source. The pipette used to deliver the droplets of the dense phase is best used quickly and only once to avoid the effects of rapid drying of its contents at the tip.

The dense phase of a biphasic aqueous polymer system is generally more viscous than its counterpart. The most reproducible method of applying a drop to a cell layer is to release it from the pipette well above the cell layer, but below the surface of the bulk fluid, and to allow it to gently settle to the surface. As it does so, the drop deforms gradually, makes contact with the cells, and slowly settles to a final equilibrium shape. For the dextran–polyethylene glycol systems described above, equilibrium requires 15–20 min, and anomalously high values will be obtained if measurements are taken before equilibrium is reached. Generally, the contact angle is stable from 15 min to 2 hr after application of the drop to the surface.

Typically, the contact angles measured are variable within a limited range, and the distribution within the range is relatively flat. The statistical strategy we have adopted is to measure both edges of at least 20–25 drops on a given sample of cells and to repeat this process three to four times for each cell type. The mean and standard deviation (or median and confidence intervals) of such a group of measurements can usually be reproduced with considerable accuracy at another time, provided of course the cells have not changed.

A set of such measurements made with four to five of the biphasic mixtures in a dilution series provides the data for the construction of a Good-Girifalco plot (Good and Girifalco, 1958; Good, 1975, 1977) which allows determination of the critical interfacial tension of the cell surface. In this plot, the cosine of the contact angle is plotted against $\gamma 12^{-\frac{1}{2}}$, and the result is usually a straight line. The interfacial tension which corresponds to $\cos \theta = 1$ is the critical interfacial free energy of the cells, γc. Figure 3 gives the results obtained with cell line FO. Use of Eq. (8) and Eq. (9) allows direct calculation of the cell–liquid interfacial free energies for both liquids of the biphasic mixture from the contact angle, Θ, and the interfacial tensions between the liquids, γ_{12}.

IV. THIN LAYER IMMUNOASSAY TECHNIQUES

Elwing and co-workers (1977, 1980) have developed a thin layer immunoassay technique which depends on the change in hydrophobicity which accompanies antigen–antibody complex formation. In this technique, protein antigen or virus particles (Holmgren *et al.*, 1980) are absorbed onto a polystyrene petri dish, and the surface is exposed to a dilution series of antibody. The change in the hydrophobicity of the surface is measured qualitatively by observing the condensation of water droplets on the surface and is measured quantitatively by using contact angles of water drops in air on the surface bearing the antigen–antibody complex. There is a linear relation between the log of the quantity of antigen absorbed to the polystyrene surface and the cosine of the contact angle formed by a water drop on the surface in air. This is in accord with the relation between the equilibrium constant and the contact angle described earlier. The relation between the cosine of the contact angle and the amount of antibody added to a surface bearing adsorbed antigen is typical of an adsorption isotherm, and thus allows calculation of the amount of antibody or antigen in a sample from previously determined calibration curves. In the case of bovine serum albumin (BSA) and BSA-antibody, the complex was more hydrophilic than the antigen. Clearly, some antigens may be more hydrophobic than the complex, but in most situations, a change in surface hydrophobicity towards that of the antibody is to be expected following complex formation. The partition affinity ligand assay (Mattiasson and Ling, 1980) is based on similar principles.

V. CONCLUSIONS

The methods described in this chapter allow measurement of the surface energy of living cells, proteins, and inert solids. The free energy of a physical interaction can then be calculated as the difference between the final and initial surface energies of the system. These free energies are fundamental to cell–cell interactions, the actions of cell adhesion proteins, protein conformation and self-assembly (Kellenberger *et al.*, 1979), and protein–lipid and lipid–lipid interactions (Parsigian, 1975).

Two ancillary methods which undoubtedly should be used to complete studies of cell surface physics are cell electrophoresis (Sherbet, 1978) and phase partition (Walter, 1978). Surface charge contributes to the total surface energy of a cell; it dominates at long distances but can be overcome by van der Waals interactions once intimate contact is made. Phase partition in biphasic polymer solutions can be made to depend on cell surface energy (Gerson, 1980) and thus provides a route to a qualitative measurement of cell surface energy which uses only standard biochemical techniques.

There is now an indication that the first attachment step of killer T cells to their targets depends on cell surface energy, and it is hoped that measurements of surface energy will aid in the elucidation of other phenomena in immunology.

REFERENCES

Albertsson, P. A. (1971). "Partition of Cell Particles and Macromolecules," 2nd ed. Wiley (Interscience), New York.

Alten, H. (1977). *Am. Chem. Soc. Div. Org. Coat. Plast. Chem., Pap.* 37(1), 587–593.

Andrade, J. D., Ma, S. M., King, R. N., and Gregonis, D. E. (1979). *J. Coll. Interface Sci.* 72; 488.

Bagnall, R. D. (1978). *Ealing Rev.* Nos. 1/2; p. 11.

Blake, T. D., and Haynes, J. M. (1973). *Prog. Surf. Membr. Sci.* 6; 125.

Brønsted, J. N. (1931). *J. Phys. Chem. A* (Festband) p. 257.

Cayias, J. L., Schechter, R. S., and Wade, W. H. (1975). *ACS Symp. Ser.* 8, 234.

Corson, D. W., Goodman, S., and Fein, A. (1979). *Science* 205, 1302.

Davies, J. T., and Rideal, E. K. (1963). "Interfacial Phenomena," 2nd ed. Academic Press, New York.

Elwing, H. (1980). *FEBS Letters* 116, 239.

Elwing, H., Nilsson, L. A., and Ouchterlony, O. (1977). *J. Immunol. Meth.* 17, 131.

Furlong, D. N., and Hartland, S. (1979). *J. Cell. Interface Sci.* 71, 301.

Gaines, G. L. (1977). *J. Cell Interface Sci.* 62, 191.

Gerson, D. F., and Zajic, J. E. (1977). *Dev. Ind. Microbiol.* 19, 577.

Gerson, D. F., and Zajic, J. E. (1979a). *Antonie van Leeuwenhoek* 45, 81.

Gerson, D. F., and Zajic, J. E. (1979b). *Process Biochem.* 14 (7), 20.

Gerson, D. F., and Zajic, J. E. (1979c). *ACS Symp. Ser.* 106, 29.

Gerson, D. F., Meadows, M. G., Finkelman, M., and Walden, D. B. (1980). *In* "Advances in Protoplast Research" (L. Ferenczy and G. L. Farkas, eds.), p. 447. Akademiai Kiado, Budapest.

Gerson, D. F. (1980). *Biochim. Biophys. Acta* 602, 269.

Gerson, D. F., and Akit, J. (1980), *Biochim. Biophys. Acta* 602, 281.

Gerson, D. F., and Scheer, D. (1980). *Biochim. Biophys. Acta* 602, 506.

Good, R. J. (1975). *In* "Adhesion Science and Technology" (L. H. Lee, ed.), p. 104. Plenum, New York.

Good, R. J. (1977). *J. Coll. Interface Sci.* 59, 398.

Good, R. J., and Girifalco, L. A. (1958). *J. Phys. Chem.* 62, 1418.

Homgren, J., Svennerholm, L., Elwing, H., Fredman, P., and Strannegard, O. (1980). *Proc. Natl. Acad. Sci. U.S.A.* 77, 1947.

Kellenberger, E., and Kistler, J. (1979). *In* "Unconventional Electron Microscopy for Molecular Structure Determination" (W. Hoppe and R. Mason, eds.), p. 49. Vieweg, Braunschweig.

Magnusson, K. E., Kihlström, E., Norlander, L., Norquist, E. A., Davies, J., and Normark, S. (1979). *Infect. Immun.* 26, 397.

Mattiasson, B., and Ling, T. G. I. (1980). *J. Immunol. Meth.* 38, 217.

Maugh, T. H. (1979). *Science* 206, 205.

Milne, L. J., and Milne, M. (1978). *Sci. Am.* 238(4), 134.

Misak, M. D. (1968). *J. Coll. Interface Sci.* 27, 141.

Moore, W. J. (1972). "Physical Chemistry," 4th ed. Longmans, Green, New York.

Mudd, S., and Mudd, E. (1926). *J. Exp. Med.* 43, 127.

Neufeld, R. J., Zajic, J. E., and Gerson, D. F. (1980). *Appl. Environ. Microbiol.* 39, 511.

Neumann, A. W. (1974) *Adv. Colloid Interface Sci.* 4, 105.

Neumann, A. W., Good, R. J., Hope, C. J., and Sejpal, M. (1974a). *J. Coll. Interface Sci.* 49, 291.

Neumann, A. W., Gillman, C. F., and van Oss, C. J. (1974b). *J. Electroanal. Chem.* 49, 393.

Neumann, A. W., Absolom, D. R., van Oss, C. J., and Zingg, W. (1979). *Cell Biophys.* 1, 79.

Nguyen, T., and Johns, W. E. (1978). *Wood Sci. Technol.* **12**, 63.

Ogden, T. E., Citron, M. C., and Pierantoni, R. (1979). *Science* **201**, 469.

Parsegian, V. A. (1975). *In* "Physical Chemistry" (H. van Olphen and F. J. Mysels, eds.), p. 27. Theorex, La Jolla, California.

Princen, H. M., Zia, I., and Mason, S. G. (1967). *J. Coll. Interface Sci.* **23**, 99.

Ryden, J., and Albertsson, P. A. (1971). *J. Coll. Interface Sci.* **37**, 219.

Schlessinger, J. (1979). *In* "Physical Chemical Aspects of Cell Surface Events in Cellular Regulation" (C. DeLisi and R. Blumenthal, eds.), p. 89. Elsevier/North-Holland Publ., Amsterdam.

Schürch, S., Gerson, D. F., and McIver, D. J. L. (1980). *Biochim. Biophys. Acta* (in press.).

Sherbet, G. V. (1978). "The Biophysical Characterization of the Cell Surface." Academic Press, New York.

Shinitzky, M. (1979). *In* "Physical Chemical Aspects of Cell Surface Events in Cellular Regulation" (C. DeLisi and R. Blumenthal, eds.), p. 173. Elsevier/North-Holland Publ., Amsterdam.

Silberberg, A. (1952). Ph.D. Thesis, University of Basel, Basel. Switzerland.

Slattery, J. C., and Chen, J. D. (1978). *J. Coll. Interface Sci.* **64**, 371.

Stendahl, O., Tagesson, C., Magnusson, K. E., and Edebo, L. (1977). *Immunology* **32**, 11.

Storm, D. R., Field, S. O., and Ryan, J. (1976). *J. Supramol. Struct.* **4**, 221.

Trusal, L. R., Baker, C. J., and Guzman, A. W. (1979). *Stain Technol.* **54**, 77.

van Oss, C. J., and Neumann, A. W. (1977). *Immunol. Commun.* **6**, 341.

van Oss, C. J., Gillman, C. F., and Neumann, A. W. (1975). "Phagocytic Engulfment and Cell Adhesiveness." Dekker, New York.

van Oss, C. J., Absolom, D. R., Grossberg, A. L. and Neumann, A. W. (1979a). *Immunol. Commun.* **8**, 11.

van Oss, C. J., Absolom, D. R., and Neumann, A. W. (1979b). *Colloids Surfaces* **1**, 45.

Walter, H. (1978). *Trends Biochem. Sci.* **3**, 97.

Walter, H., Krob, E. J., and Moncla, B. J. (1978). *Exp. Cell Res.* **115**, 379.

Young, T. (1805). *Philos. Trans. R. Soc. London* **95**, 65.

Zaslavsky, B. Y., Miheeva, L. M., and Rogozhin, S. V. (1979). *Biochim. Biophys. Acta* **588**, 89.

Zisman, W. A. (1963). *Ind. Eng. Chem.* **55**, 10, 18.

Zisman, W. A. (1976). *ACS Adv. Chem. Ser.* **43**, 1.

7

Hapten-Modified Antibodies Specific for Cell Surface Antigens as a Tool in Cellular Immunology

Salvatore Cammisuli

I. INTRODUCTION

Recognition processes at the cell surface are of paramount importance in the adaptation of a cell to its environment. Interaction of cells during embryonic development, species- and organ-specific cell recognition, contact

IMMUNOLOGICAL METHODS, VOL. II
Copyright © 1981 by Academic Press, Inc.

inhibition of growth, and the histocompatibility requirement for cellular cooperation in the immune system are some of the phenomena that can be dictated by cell membrane interactions. These phenomena are of major importance in cell biology, since they relate to the question of cell differentiation: how a cell responds to its environment and how this response alters expression of the cell genes.

To understand the common principle underlying these phenomena, it is essential to understand the nature of the cell surface receptors and to be able to monitor the effect induced by selectively perturbing them.

In small lymphocytes, structurally distinct receptors have been shown to be selectively associated, as evidenced by their coordinate movement under capping or patching conditions and by the fact that antisera directed against one may inhibit ligand binding to another (reviewed by Loor, 1977). The study of these specialized interactions, which may play a major role in the process of lymphocyte differentiation, has been hampered by the fact that a general technique of double labeling suitable for the investigation of these phenomena has not been available.

This chapter describes the hapten sandwich labeling (HSL) system, a methodology which lends itself to the simultaneous detection and study of any given pair of cell surface antigens independently of their location on the same cell or on different cells.

The methodology described here has been devised for antigen visualization with fluorescence, electron microscopy, and autoradiography, but it can be easily adapted for receptor-specific cell separation and for the induction of selected bridging events between receptors present on the same or on different cells.

II. HAPTEN SANDWICH LABELING

A. Background

1. Fluorescent Antibody Technique

A major tool for the study of cell membrane antigens is the fluorescent antibody (FA) technique developed by Coons and colleagues in 1941 (reviewed by Goldman, 1968). This technique involving fluorochrome-conjugated antibodies combines histochemical and immunological methods and pinpoints specific antigens present in tissue sections or cellular smears. Because of its versatility, specificity, and simplicity, the FA method has acquired an important place in cell biology. The sensitivity of this procedure can be increased by the use of the indirect (sandwich) method. In this case, the unmodified specific antiserum is applied to a test specimen, allowing the antibody and antigen to combine. The specimen is then washed free of excess reagent and treated with a fluorescein-labeled antibody against the immunoglobulin (Ig) of the species of the initial antisera.

Other fluorochrome markers emitting energy at different wavelengths than fluorescein have been devised, allowing fluorescence double labeling. The basic principles involved in using modified antibodies to detect surface antigens have been extended from fluorescence to electron microscopy, autoradiography, and enzymatically mediated staining techniques, all based on the conjugation of antibodies to appropriate markers.

2. Limitation of the Fluorescent Antibody Technique

In general, the conventional direct and indirect FA techniques are not adequate for the type of studies previously indicated. This limitation derives from the fact that the majority of differentiation antigens are only detectable as alloantigens, thus requiring alloantisera for their detection. Since alloantisera are generally of low titer they require amplification by an indirect procedure, but the use of second-layer anti-Ig is inadequate because it would result also in the labeling of cells bearing endogenous Ig. Simultaneous labeling of two alloantigens would not be possible for analogous reasons. Even in the rare cases where high-titer alloantisera or monoclonal alloantibodies are available, the use of sandwich procedures is necessary when it is desirable to induce a relocation (capping or patching) of selected alloantigens, since these antigens cannot often be redistributed by cross-linking with a single antibody layer.

For the reasons noted above, cross-species sandwiching is unsuitable unless special precautions are taken to avoid staining all cells with surface Ig. In some such procedure, endogenous Ig can be "capped off" (endocytosed and/or shed away) with anti-Ig prior to labeling with the alloantisera and its anti-Ig amplifier (reviewed by Loor, 1977). While this technique may overcome the ambiguity due to labeling endogenous Ig, it creates the more subtle possibility of an undiscerned cell membrane alteration. Investigation of the behavior or association of different markers after Ig removal is probably questionable because of artifacts that may be created by the stripping process. These problems have been bypassed at times by the use of less conventional sandwiching procedures. One such procedure involves the use of antiallotypic antisera rather than anti-Ig. In this case, amplification is achieved by antibodies directed against allotype determinants on the antisurface antibodies but not on the endogenous surface Ig. This system demands the developing of specific antiallotypic antisera (a difficult achievement) and moreover would be virtually impossible for simultaneous labeling of two alloantigens, since this would require a double set of developing antiallotypic antisera. Developing antisera directed against the γ chain of IgG have also been used, the rationale being that endogenous IgG is expressed in only a marginal fraction of B lymphocytes. In this case also study of more than one alloantigen at a time is not possible and, moreover, we have found that the sensitivity of this technique at least for some antigens is far from satisfactory.

B. Principle of Hapten Sandwich Labeling

The HSL method is a modification of the conventional indirect antibody technique (Lamm *et al.,* 1972; Wofsy *et al.,* 1974; reviewed by Wofsy *et al.,* 1978). Immunoglobulins with specificity for a particular antigen are chemically modified so that several hapten groups are covalently attached under conditions permitting retention of antibody activity. Antigen detection may then be amplified with a two-layer technique by using the haptenated Ig's in conjunction with anti-hapten antibodies coupled to fluorescent, electron microscopic, enzymatic, or radioactive markers (Fig. 1).

The same methodology can be easily adapted to cell surface ligands that are non-Ig in nature, for example, hormones, enzymes, and mitogens. Heitzmann and Richards (1974) have used a similar approach with the avidin–biotin complex technique, in which biotynil residues function as haptens and avidin carries the marker.

The HSL procedure, while conceptually similar to the indirect FA technique, does not have the limitations discussed before and therefore is especially useful in the following circumstances: (1) where alloantibodies are required, thus barring employment of conventional procedures for amplified antigen detection with second-layer anti-Ig from another species, and (2) where multiple cell surface antigens are under study and a conventional procedure is needed for the simultaneous labeling of any

First layer: Second layer:

Hapten-conjugated   Marker-conjugated
anti-cell surface antibody   anti-hapten antibody

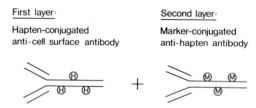

Fig. 1. Hapten sandwich labeling. A single hapten-conjugated anti-cell surface antibody preparation may be used in conjunction with its anti-hapten amplifier in its native form or appropriately marked to permit (1) labeling for fluorescent and electron microscopy, (2) autoradiography, (3) isolation of membrane antigens, (4) physical separation of selected cell subpopulations, (5) complement-mediated killing of selected cell subpopulations, or (6) generation of selected bridging events between receptors present on the same or on different cells.

given pair. Moreover, since cell surface antigens can readily be capped by appropriate hapten sandwich procedures, these reagents may be well suited to studies on the removal ("capping off") and reappearance in the membrane of selected antigens that do not cap with a single antibody layer. Similarly hapten sandwich reagents are very useful in studying antigen redistribution and whether two antigens may be associated on a cell surface.

C. Hapten-Coupling Procedures

The methodology of HSL depends on the availability of a reaction procedure which allows a high number of hapten molecules to be conjugated to a cell membrane ligand without altering its binding properties.

We have obtained satisfactory results using the amidination reaction, a reaction shown to have only a minor effect on protein biological properties. The reaction of imido esters with amino acids and peptides in water has been characterized by Hunter and Ludwig (1962) who have found that under mild conditions of temperature and pH only primary amino groups are amidinated. Wofsy and Singer (1963) have demonstrated that the three-dimensional structure of proteins is retained even after amidination of all lysines. These authors have also demonstrated that extensive acetamidation has only marginal effects on antibody-binding activity and on protein antigenicity. Similar results have been obtained with hormones and enzymes: Although their biological activity is extremely dependent on protein conformation, it appears that amidination has little effect on them except when an amine is vital to the active site (cf. Whiteley and Berg, 1974).

To adapt amidination to the coupling of haptens to proteins, we have synthesized the bifunctional reagents methyl *p*-hydroxybenzimidate (HB) and methyl 3,5-dihydroxybenzimidate (DHB) (Fig. 2) (Cammisuli and Wofsy, 1976). These compounds have a phenol ring available for an electrophilic attack by a diazonium reagent, and they also have the great ad-

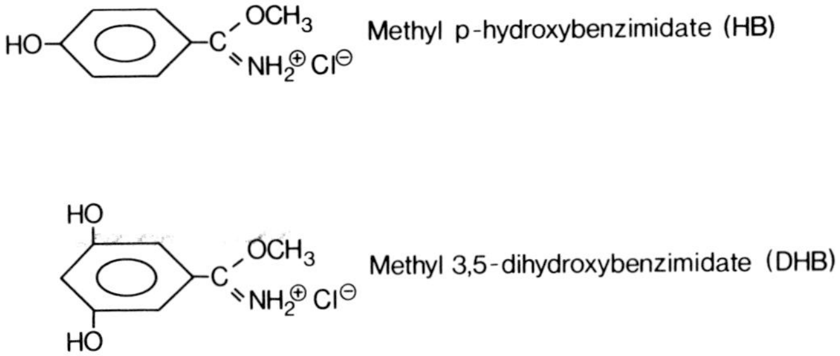

Fig. 2. Imido esters used as bifunctional reagents to couple haptens to proteins.

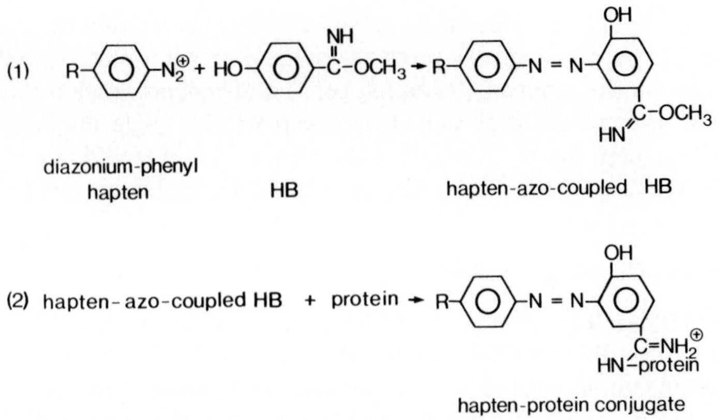

Fig. 3. Preparation of hapten–protein conjugates. (1) Diazotized hapten is reacted with HB (or DHB). (2) The azo-coupled hapten–HB (or hapten–DHB) is then reacted with the protein preparation to yield the hapten–protein conjugate. R, Hapten determinant group.

vantage of being soluble in aqueous solution while being very resistant to hydrolysis [the half-life of the related methyl benzimidate exceeds 50 hr at 39°C and pH 8.5 (Hunter and Ludwig, 1962)]. This last characteristic has been exploited by first modifying the imido ester by a diazonium reaction and, after quenching the excess diazonium, adding the reaction solution, without isolation of intermediates, to the antibody or other protein to be modified. By this method, protein amino functions are converted to hapten-linked amidine groups (Fig. 3).

We have taken advantage of this reaction to conjugate up to 30 hapten molecules per molecule of Ig with only marginal losses (< 13%) in antibody-binding activity. Extensively hapten-amidinated antibodies can be used in the HLS technique, permitting a level of sensitivity and specificity equal to or greater than that obtained with conventional indirect immunospecific labeling techniques; they have the added advantage of versatility required for double labeling and the observation of alloantigens.

III. PREPARATION OF HAPTEN SANDWICH LABELING REAGENTS

A. Synthesis of Amidinating Reagents

Methyl *p*-hydroxybenzimidate hydrochloride and methyl 3,5-dihydroxy-benzimidate hydrochloride are synthesized according to the method of Pinner (cf. Hunter and Ludwig, 1962). In both cases it is practical to carry out the reaction over a molecular sieve to ensure strictly anhydrous conditions. When stored at − 70°C over Drierite, HB and DHB are stable indefinitely. *p*-Hydroxybenzimidate can be obtained commercially from Pierce Chemicals, Rockford, Illinois.

Reagents

3,5-Dihydroxybenzonitrile: MW 135 (Gallard-Schlesinger, Carle Place, New York)

p-Hydroxybenzonitrile: MW 119 (Aldrich Chemical Co., Milwaukee, Wisconsin)

HCl (gas): MW 36.5

Methanol, absolute: MW 32.0, density 0.79 gm/ml, kept anhydrous by storage over a molecular sieve

Ether anhydrous: kept anhydrous by storage over a molecular sieve

Molecular sieve: 4 Å (Merck, Darmstadt, West Germany)

1. Synthesis of p-Hydroxybenzimidate

p-Hydroxybenzonitrile [50 mmol (5.950 gm)] is dissolved in 75 mmol (3.1 ml) of dry methanol in a two-necked 50-ml flask containing 20–30 pellets of molecular sieve. One neck of the flask is fitted with a gooseneck filled with Drierite, while the other is fitted with a stopcock. The mixture is cooled to 0°C in an ice bath. Through the stopcock ∼ 75 mmol (2.8 gm) of dry HCl is introduced into the reaction mixture. [As an alternative to the weighing of HCl it is possible to pass the gas into the reaction mixture to saturation. We have found that in this case some free HCl is carried in with the HB preparation. In this case, during the preparation of hapten–HB (Section III,B) great care must be taken to correct the pH immediately.] After 1 hr at 0°C the reaction mixture, which has crystallized to a solid mass, is resuspended in cold anhydrous ether, filtered on sintered glass, and washed with 100 ml of cold anhydrous ether. The white, needle-shaped crystals so obtained are dried over P_2O_5 under vacuum and stored over Drierite at − 70°C. They have a melting point, with decomposition, at 164°C.

2. Synthesis of Methyl 3,5-Dihydroxybenzimidate

3,5-Dihydroxybenzonitrile [50 mmol (6.750 gm)] and dry methanol [50 mmol (2.1 ml)] are dissolved in 25 ml of anhydrous ether in a two-necked flask containing 20–30 pellets of molecular sieve. One neck of the flask is fitted with a gooseneck filled with Drierite, while the other is fitted with a stopcock. The mixture is cooled to 0°C in an ice bath. Through the stopcock ∼ 75 mmol (2.8 gm) of dry HCl is introduced, and the reaction is allowed to proceed at 4°C. After 18 hr the straw-colored crystals obtained at the bottom of the flask are washed with 100 ml of anhydrous ether on a sintered-glass filter. The crystals are dried over P_2O_5 under vacuum and stored at $-70°C$. They have a melting point, with decomposition, at $275°-280°C$.

B. Preparation of Hapten–Protein Conjugates

Aminophenyl haptens are coupled by diazotization to the phenolic ring of HB or DHB. The resulting hapten–azoimido ester reaction mixture is directly used to modify proteins. The hapten of choice is arsanilic acid (ars), because it is easily available and produces conjugates with good solubility with both HB and DHB (Section III, C). When double labeling is required, other suitable non-cross-reactive haptens are *p*-aminobenzoylglycine and *p*-aminobenzoylglutamic acid (Wallace and Wofsy, 1979).

Reagents

Arsanilic acid: MW 217 (Aldrich Chemical Co., Milwaukee, Wisconsin)
p-Aminobenzoylglutamic acid: MW 266 (Sigma Chemical, St. Louis, Missouri)
p-Aminobenzoylglycine: MW 194 (ICN Nutritional Biochemicals, Cleveland, Ohio)
HCl: 1 *M*
NaOH: 5 *M*
Borate buffer: pH 8.6, 0.34 *M* (21.4 gm H_3BO_3 plus 4 gm NaOH in 1 liter H_2O)
p-Hydroxybenzimidate: MW 187
3,5-Dihydroxybenzimidate: MW 203
Imidazole: MW 68

1. Diazotization of Aminophenyl Haptens

This reaction is carried out according to Tabachnick and Sobotka (1959). First, 1.8 mmol of *p*-aminophenyl compound is dissolved in 4 ml of 1 *M* HCl. The mixture is cooled to $0°C$ in an ice bath, and 1.8 mmol (0.124 gm) of $NaNO_2$ in 1 ml of water is added to the cooled mixture with stirring. The reaction is allowed to proceed for 20 min at $0°C$. The 0.36 *M* diazo reagent can be used directly or stored at $-20°C$ for several months.

2. Modification of Proteins with Hapten–Azo-HB

a. Coupling of Diazotized Hapten to HB. Diazo reagent is reacted with HB in a 3:1 molar ratio to ensure that all HB molecules are hapten-conjugated (Section III,C). [A recent report (Wallace and Wofsy, 1979) suggests a reaction at a HB/diazonium molar ratio of 1:5. The storage life reported for the hapten–HB conjugate is in this case much lower (2 weeks).] Then 0.6 mmol of HB (0.112 gm) are resuspended with stirring in 3 ml of ice cold borate buffer adjusted to pH 9.2. To this suspension 1.8

mmol of diazo reagent in 5 ml is slowly added (5-10 min). The pH of the reaction is maintained by the addition of 5 N NaOH. The pH should not be left for any extended amount of time above 9.5 or below 7.5, since at these pH values HB is easily hydrolyzed. After all the diazonium has been added, the reaction is allowed to proceed for 2 hr at room temperature at pH 9.2 $\pm$ 0.2. The excess diazonium is then quenched with 1.8 mmol (0.124 gm) imidazole. After 30 min the reaction mixture is brought to pH 8.6 with HCl and diluted to a final volume of 10 ml with borate buffer. This 0.06 M hapten-azo-HB reagent can be used directly to modify protein or can be stored at $-70°C$ and used in the next 6 months.

b. Modification of Protein with Hapten-Azo-HB. Because of the extreme sensitivity of HSL, it is suggested that highly purified preparations be modified (Section IV, A,4). We have obtained our best results with protein A- or DEAE-purified Ig preparations.

To 2 parts of a protein solution (1-10 mg/ml) in borate buffer is added 1 part of 0.06 M hapten-azo-HB. The reaction is allowed to proceed for 16-20 hr at room temperature. Under these reaction conditions Ig is modified with about 22 hapten groups per molecule. The colored modified protein is separated from excess reagent by gel chromatography over an appropriately selected gel [i.e., Bio-Gel 100 (BioRad, Richmond, California) for Ig, Bio-Gel 60 for Con A], using as eluant 0.017 M borate buffer, pH 8. According to their solubility (section III,C) hapten-amidinated proteins can be equilibrated by dialysis in PBS or left in the borate buffer used for their elution. The modified protein is stored like the original protein.

3. Modification of Proteins with Hapten-Azo-DHB

a. Coupling of Diazotized Hapten to 3,5-Dihydroxybenzimidate. The diazonium reagent is reacted with DHB at a 1.5:1 molar ratio to ensure that all HB molecules are hapten-conjugated. The reaction is performed under nitrogen to minimize quinone formation. First, 0.6 mmol of DHB (0.122 gm) is resuspended with stirring in 3 ml of ice cold borate buffer adjusted to pH 8.5. To this suspension 0.9 mmol of diazonium reagent in 2.5 ml is slowly added (5-10 min). The pH of the reaction is maintained by the addition of 5 N NaOH. After the diazonium has been added, the reaction is left to proceed for 1 hr at pH 8.2-8.5. The excess diazonium is then quenched with 0.9 mmol (0.06 gm) imidazole. After 30 min, the reaction mixture is adjusted to pH 8.5 and diluted to 10 ml. This 0.06 M hapten-azo-DHB reagent can be used directly to modify protein or can be stored at $-70°C$ and used in the next 3 months.

b. Modification of Protein with Hapten-Azo-DHB. To 1 part of a protein solution (3-15 mg/ml) in borate buffer 2 parts of 0.06 M hapten-azo-DHB are added. The reaction is allowed to proceed for 6-8 hr at room temperature, and 2 parts of 0.06 M hapten–azo-DHB are added again. The mixture is allowed to react overnight at room temperature.

The modified protein (about 12 hapten groups per molecule of protein in the case of Ig) is separated from excess reagent by gel chromatography on Bio-Gel using PBS as eluting buffer. The modified protein is stored like the original protein. At physiological ionic strength and pH we have not detected any solubility problems.

C. Effect of Hapten Amidination on the Solubility of Proteins

Hapten-amidinated antibodies, while apparently undergoing no significant denaturation or inactivation over a wide modification range, show markedly diminished solubility. The solubility of the amidinated Ig's decreases with a decrease in pH and an increase in ionic strength and is dependent on the kind of hapten and imido ester used.

Native HB and DHB produce very insoluble proteins; for this reason it is important that all the imido ester molecules used during the reaction with proteins be coupled with the diazo reagent. This can be achieved by carrying out the reaction between the diazo reagent and imido ester in the presence of a molar excess of diazonium.

Solubility problems are encountered when proteins with intrinsically low solubility are modified with hapten–HB. No solubility problems have been observed with small, soluble proteins [i.e., concanavalin A (Con A), RNase, prolactin, Fab fragments, bovine serum albumin (BSA)]; however, certain preparations of hapten–HB–Ig tend to precipitate on prolonged storage under physiological conditions of pH and ionic strength. In this case the precipitate can be resolubilized by dialysis in borate buffer (0.017 M, pH 8.0) and then stored in the same buffer. Before use for cell labeling, the solution is brought to physiological conditions by additions of $\frac{1}{10}$ vol of 10 × phosphate-buffered saline (PBS). We have obtained excellent cell labeling with similar poorly soluble hapten–HB–Ig preparations.

Certain haptens, for example, p-aminophenyllactoside (lac) and p-aminophenylglucoside (glu), when coupled to proteins via HB, give rise to conjugates of unsatisfactory solubility which cannot be safely used under physiological conditions of pH and ionic strength. In this case the solubility problems can be bypassed by using DHB. Indeed DHB is the reagent of choice in all cases where hapten–HB modification produces protein conjugates of insufficient solubility.

D. Preparation of Anti-Hapten Antibodies

Anti-hapten antibody can be produced using different immunization protocols. In this section we will describe a simple immunization schedule which allows us to obtain anti-arsonate (anti-ars) antibody in a month. The same procedure can be applied in producing anti-hapten antibodies of different specificities.

1. Preparation of Ars-KLH

Reagents
Borate buffer: 0.5 M, pH 8.5
Keyhole limpet hemocyanin (KLH) (Calbiochem-Behring, San Diego, California)
Diazotized ars: 0.36 M (prepared as described in Section III,B,1)

Two milliliters of a 50 mg/ml KLH solution previously equilibrated by dialysis in 0.5 M borate buffer, pH 8.5, is added to a vial. The vial is placed in an ice bath, and to the ice cold solution 0.36 ml of the diazonium reagents is added drop by drop with magnetic stirring. The pH of the reaction mixture must be kept between 8.5 and 9.0 using 5 M NaOH. After 1–2 hr of stirring, the reaction is allowed to go to completion at 4°C overnight. The ars-conjugated KLH is purified by gel chromatography on Sephadex G-25 equilibrated with 0.05 M borate buffer, pH 8.0. The colored first peak is eluted, sterilized by Millipore 0.45-μm filtration, and stored either at 4°C or frozen.

2. Emulsification of Ars-KLH with Complete Freund Adjuvant

Complete Freund adjuvant (CFA) is mixed with an equal amount of ars-KLH appropriately diluted with saline (1 mg/ml for rabbit and 0.5 mg/ml for chicken immunization) in order to obtain a stable water-in-oil emulsion. A drop of the emulsion should float on water without any spreading. Optimal emulsions are obtained with a high-speed electric homogenizer by slowly adding the ars-KLH solution to the CFA.

3. Rabbit Anti-Ars

Adult rabbits are injected intramuscularly with 1 ml of a 500 μg/ml ars-KLH–CFA emulsion. The antigen dose is divided between the two thigh muscles. After 2–3 weeks the same immunization protocol is repeated. Ten days after boosting, the rabbit can be ear-bled (30–50 ml according to the animal's size). Subsequent boostings are done with 200 μg of ars-KLH emulsified with incomplete Freund adjuvant. It is possible to repeat several cycles of boosting and bleedings.

4. Chicken Anti-Ars

Adult chickens are injected intramuscularly with 0.4 ml of a 250 μg/ml ars-KLH–CFA emulsion. The antigen dose is divided between the two breast muscles. After 1 month, the treatment is repeated. Ten days after the boosting, the chicken can be bled (15–30 ml according to the chicken's size). Bleeding can be repeated after 1 week. After a 2- to 3-week rest, the boosting and bleeding can be repeated. Similar cycles can be repeated several times. Before isolation of anti-arsonate antibody by affinity chromatography, the lipoprotein present in the chicken serum or plasma must be precipitated. To each milliliter of chicken serum add 40 μl of a 10% dextran sulfate solution and 100 μl of 1 M $CaCl_2$. After 30 min at room temperature the lipoprotein precipitate is spun down and discarded.

5. Purification of Anti-Ars Antibodies

Anti-ars antibodies are isolated by affinity chromatography on ars-modified Sepharose 4B as described by Wofsy and Burr (1969).

a. Preparation of Ars-Coupled Sepharose 4B

Reagents
    CNBr-activated Sepharose 4B (CNBr–Sepharose): CNBr–Sepharose can
        be obtained commercially from Pharmacia, Uppsala, Sweden, or pre-
        pared according to a standard procedure (Axén et al., 1967)
    Arsanilic acid: MW 217, 4 × 10^{-2} M in 0.1 M $NaHCO_3$, pH 9.0
    $NaHCO_3$ buffer: 0.1 M, pH 9.0

To 10 ml preswollen CNBr–Sepharose resuspended in 10 ml $NaHCO_3$ 1 ml of 4 × 10^{-2} M ars is added. The solution is mixed gently for 24 hr at 4°C. The gel is then washed on a sintered-glass funnel with 1 liter ice cold H_2O and 1 liter $NaHCO_3$ buffer.

Ars–Sepharose 4B is stored in the refrigerator in the presence of 0.02% NaN_3 as a preservative. Since upon storage some hapten may leak out from the gel, ars–Sepharose must be equilibrated with fresh buffer before use.

b. Isolation of Anti-ars Antibodies

Reagents
    Ars–Sepharose 4B column: 1 ml of gel can retain 15–20 mg of anti-ars
        antibodies
    Benzenearsonic acid: MW 202, 0.3 M solution in borate-buffered saline
        (BBS).
    Borate-buffered saline: 0.17 M borate, 0.12 M NaCl, pH 8.0 (10.3 gm
        H_3BO_3 and 7.3 gm NaCl in 1 liter H_2O, adjusted to pH 8 with NaOH)
    Trichloroacetic acid (TCA): 10% solution
    Acetic acid: 0.1 M.

The antiserum, clarified by centrifugation at 10,000 g for 10 min, is passed through an ars–Sepharose column. The column is then washed extensively with BBS until the effluent is protein-free ($OD_{280} < 0.01$). The column is then saturated with 0.3 M benzenearsonic acid in BBS. After a 15–30 min incubation at room temperature, the antibodies are eluted with 0.3 M benzenearsonic acid. Elution is continued until the effluent is protein-free, as detected by TCA precipitation (1 drop of effluent placed in 0.5–1 ml 10% TCA should not show any turbidity). The TCA-positive eluate is pooled, concentrated to $\frac{1}{4}$ vol of the original antiserum passed through column, and dialyzed against several changes of PBS. Antibody concentration is determined by spectrophotometry. The extinction coefficient of a solution containing 1 mg/ml Ig is 1.47 at 280 nm. The column is washed with 1 vol 0.1 M acetic acid to free gel from high-affinity antibodies.

E. Preparation of Labeled Anti-Hapten Antibodies

Anti-hapten antibodies used as a second layer in HSL can be coupled to a variety of markers according to their intended usage. In this section we will describe procedures for coupling anti-ars antibodies to sheep red blood cells (SRBCs) and to protein markers. The same procedures can be used with other anti-hapten antibodies.

1. Preparation of Fluorescent Anti-Ars

For conjugation of fluorescein isothiocyanate or tetramethyl rhodamine isothiocyanate to the purified anti-hapten antibodies, the reader is referred to Chapter 9 in the first volume of this series, or to any standard procedure for the conjugation of fluorescein and rhodamine to antibody (Goldman, 1968).

2. Conjugation of Anti-Ars Antibody to Other Protein Markers

Selected protein markers can be efficiently conjugated to antibody. The conjugated antibodies retain their binding activity and can be used as second-layer reagents in HSL. In this section we describe the conjugation of KLH to anti-ars according to the method of Nicholson and Singer (1971). Kishida *et al.* (1975) have described an alternative procedure for preparing ferritin–antibody conjugates.

Reagents
KLH (Calbiochem-Behring, San Diego, California)
Glutaraldehyde: EM grade
$(NH_4)_2CO_3$: 0.1 M
Phosphate buffer: 0.1 M, pH 6.8
Phosphate buffer: 0.05 M, pH 7.5

Five milligrams of antibody and 25 mg of KLH in a 1-ml volume are equilibrated by dialysis in 0.1 M phosphate buffer, pH 6.8. To this solution 0.1 ml of 0.5% glutaraldehyde is added slowly and with stirring. The mixture is allowed to stand for 1 hr at room temperature. The reaction is then quenched by dialysis against cold 0.1 M (NH$_4$)$_2$CO$_3$ for 3–4 hr. The reaction mixture is then dialyzed overnight in 0.05 M phosphate buffer, pH 7.5. The conjugate KLH–anti-ars is then separated from unreacted anti-ars and anti-ars polymers as the first peak in gel chromatography on Ultragel ACA 22 (LKB, Bromma, Sweden) or Sepharose 6B (Pharmacia, Uppsala, Sweden).

3. Conjugation of Anti-Ars to Sheep Red Blood Cells

Reagents

Sheep red blood cells (SRBCs)
Anti-ars antibody: 2–5 mg/ml in saline
CrCl$_3$ · 6 H$_2$O: 2.5 × 10^{-4} M in saline, prepared immediately before use
Fetal calf serum (FCS): heat-inactivated (30 min at 56°C). RPMI 1640:
  with 10% heat inactivated FCS (RPMI–FCS)
Phosphate-buffered saline
Saline: 0.85% NaCl

The SRBCs are washed four times with saline. To 1 ml packed SRBCs is added 0.5–1 ml of anti-ars antibody and 10 ml of 2.5 × 10^{-4} M CrCl$_3$ solution. The suspension is rotated gently at 30°C for 1 hr. The reaction is then quenched with 20 ml of PBS. The SRBCs are then washed twice more with PBS and once with RPMI–FCS and then resuspended at 1–2 × 10^9 cells/ml in RPMI–FCS. Conjugated SRBCs should resuspend as single cells with no evident clumps.

IV. SELECTED EXAMPLES OF THE APPLICATION OF HAPTEN SANDWICH LABELING REAGENTS

A single preparation of hapten-modified ligand to a cell surface marker can be used, either directly or conjugated with anti-hapten antibody, for different approaches in the study of lymphocyte antigens. In this section we will give the methodology used for (1) fluorescent visualization of cell surface antigen, (2) antigen-specific separation of differing lymphoid cell populations, and (3) studies on lymphocyte activation. Other possible applications of HSL will be briefly outlined. The application of HSL reagents in electron microscopy has been described by Wofsy *et al.* (1974) and Carter and Wofsy (1976).

A. Fluorescent Labeling

Fluorescent labeling has been already discussed in the first volume of this series. Here we will focus on the application of the HSL methodology in the fluorescence labeling of alloantigens. Hapten sandwich reagents have been successfully used for single labeling and in labeling two lymphocyte antigens simultaneously, whether present on the same or on different cells.

As in the case of conventional fluorescence labeling, hapten sandwich reagents must be ultracentrifuged before use to eliminate aggregates and complexes which allow nonspecific staining. Usually $\frac{1}{2}$ hr centrifugation at 100,000 g minimizes this problem. Nonspecific staining due to Fc binding can be excluded by using Fab preparations; chicken anti-ars antibodies can be used instead of Fab fragments of rabbit antibodies.

1. Single Labeling

Reagents
    FCS, heat-inactivated (30 min at 56°C), 0.45-μm Millipore-filtered
    PBS, 5% FCS, 0.1% NaN$_3$, pH 7.3 (PBS-FCS-NaN$_3$)
    PBS, 5% FCS, pH 7.3 (PBS-FCS)
    Hapten-modified anti-cell surface antibodies in PBS
    Fluorescein or rhodamine-conjugated anti-hapten antibodies

Staining is carried out in a 5-ml plastic tube. About 5×10^6 lymphocytes suspended in 50–100 μl of PBS-FCS-NaN$_3$ are gently mixed with an equivalent volume of the hapten-modified anti-cell surface antibody and then incubated for 20 min at 0°C. It is necessary to predetermine the antibody concentration which gives optimal staining and minimum background. The cell suspension is then underlayered with 1–2 ml of FCS and spun at 300 g for 7 min at 4°C. The pellet is resuspended in 2.5 ml of PBS-FCS-NaN$_3$ and centrifuged for 7 min at 200 g. The PBS-FCS-NaN$_3$ wash is repeated one more time. The pellet is then resuspended in 50–100 μl of buffer and gently mixed with an equivalent volume of a predetermined concentration of fluorescent anti-hapten antibody. One FCS gradient and two PBS-FCS-NaN$_3$ washes are repeated, as for the first layer. The cells are then ready for microscopy.

Staining can also be done under "capping conditions" (reviewed in Loor, 1977) to induce redistribution of the antigen under study. This labeling procedure must be carried out in the absence of NaN$_3$. Cells are treated as described above up to the 20-min incubation on ice with the fluorescent anti-hapten antibody. After that the cell suspension is kept in a 37°C water bath for 10–20 min. The cells are then washed three times, as described before, with the cold buffer containing NaN$_3$.

2. Double Labeling

The HSL reagents can be readily used to label any given pair of alloantigens simultaneously. In this case the two anti-surface antibodies must be modified with two non-cross-reacting haptens (Fig. 4). We have had success with ars-HB and lac-DHB (lac-HB conjugates are poorly soluble) (Cammisuli and Wofsy, 1976). It has been recently reported that excellent results are obtained with ars-HB and *p*-aminobenzoylglutamic acid–HB (Wallace and Wofsy, 1979). The staining procedure is identical to the single labeling. It is possible to add in the first step the two anti-cell surface Ig preparations amidinated with the two non-cross-reacting haptens. Excess reagent is eliminated with a FCS gradient and two PBS-FCS-NaN₃ washes. The pellet is then resuspended and incubated with a mixture of the two anti-hapten antibodies bearing either fluorescein or rhodamine. After one FCS gradient and two PBS-FCS washings, the cells are ready for microscopy. At times, better results are obtained when the cells are labeled sequentially for the two antigens.

Sequential labeling is, on the other hand, mandatory in "cocapping" experiments, where the physical relation of two antigens is under study (Section I). In this case the antigen to be capped is stained first under capping conditions as described in Section IV,A,1. The cells are then washed in ice cold medium with azide. The second antigen is labeled in the presence of azide as described in Section IV,A,1.

3. Microscopy

Cells are resuspended in FCS at a concentration of ~ 10⁷/ml. They can be prepared for fluorescent microscopy as either wet or dry mounts. Obviously microscope light sources, filters, and objectives must be selected to

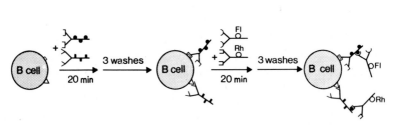

Fig. 4. Double labeling. Two alloantigens, each coupled with a different non-cross-reactive hapten (represented as closed circles and rectangles), are used in conjunction with the two respective anti-hapten antibodies conjugated either with fluorescein (Fl) or rhodamine (Rh) to label simultaneously two alloantigens (represented as open squares and open triangles) present on the same cell surface.

permit optimal visualization of fluorescein while excluding rhodamine staining, and vice versa.

4. Sensitivity of Hapten Sandwich Labeling

The sensitivity of HSL has been investigated by comparing the fluorescence intensity of spleen cells stained using rabbit anti-mouse brain Ig or goat anti-mouse Ig either with hapten sandwich reagents or with the conventional indirect antibody technique. While no difference was found in the fraction of lymphocytes detected by the two procedures, a qualitatively higher intensity of staining was achieved with our reagents.

In an attempt to quantitate the amplification obtainable with our system, we have shown that ars-HB-amidinated anti-galactoside (gal) antibodies (22 ars groups per mole), when bound to a gal–Sepharose affinity column, can in turn bind a 12:1 molar ratio of anti-ars antibodies. This value compares with the 7:1 ratio detected in precipitates formed in extreme antibody excess by antibody directed against another Ig antigen, which is frequently used to estimate the maximum effective antigenic valence of the Ig molecule. Using indirect FA, Pressman et al. (1958) estimated the maximum ratio of antibody to another Ig antigen to be in the range of 4–12. In this case, the extent of amplification was calculated by determining the maximum dilution of the anti-surface antibody preparation capable of detecting the specific antigen. The estimated antibody/Ig antigen ratios were lower than those indicated in our system probably because an antiserum from one species against Ig from another species may not contain effective titers of antibodies against every potential antigenic determinant; further, the native antigenic determinants are distributed unevenly, so that the maximum theoretical amplification according to strictly steric considerations may not generally be obtainable with conventional indirect labeling. The utilization of antibodies extensively coupled with hapten–HB (~20 haptens per Ig molecule) in the hapten sandwich method minimizes these limitations. In principle the limit for amplification with hapten-amidinated antibodies is steric, since the number of haptens that can be attached without significantly inactivating antibody is in excess of the number of second-layer antibodies that can fit around a 7 S Ig molecule. In any case, the higher amplification ratio achieved with hapten–HB-modified antibodies provides the basis for greater labeling sensitivity than is possible with conventional reagents. Hapten–DHB-modified antibodies (10–14 haptens per Ig molecule) can also be used in HSL to achieve excellent visualization of alloantigens.

The enhanced sensitivity obtained with hapten-amidinated antibodies is especially apparent when alloantigens are under study, since in this case the use of anti-Ig for amplification is not possible for the reasons indicated earlier.

5. Specificity of Hapten Sandwich Labeling

Hapten-amidinated anti-cell surface antibodies, amplified by anti-hapten antibodies as a second layer, have been used to achieve high sensitivity and specificity in labeling a variety of mouse alloantigens (Ia, H-2K^K, and Thy-1.2) usually difficult to label effectively with conventional procedures. The specificity of labeling has been assessed by testing lymphocytes of mouse strains either negative or positive for a particular marker.

Because of the high sensitivity of HSL, it is essential to hapten-modify only preparations which have been carefully absorbed to eliminate unwanted background activities which would otherwise result in decreased levels of labeling specificity. In general, this background can be removed by two sequential absorptions of the Ig preparations with an equal volume of packed cells of the appropriate negative control strain. At times, when this absorption is incomplete, it may be necessary to absorb further already modified preparations.

It is also necessary to hapten-modify protein A- or DEAE-purified Ig preparations, since reagents prepared by hapten amidination of an $(NH_4)_2SO_4$-precipitated Ig fraction may give rise to somewhat higher levels of nonspecific staining, possibly because of the modification of some non-Ig serum components which may tend to stick to the cell membrane and be amplified in HSL.

B. Hapten Sandwich Labeling Rosetting

It is possible to use hapten-modified ligands to cell membrane antigens in conjugation with erythrocytes conjugated to anti-hapten antibody to perform specific rosetting of differing lymphoid cell populations (Wofsy *et al.*, 1978; Slomich *et al.*, 1980).

The HSL rosetting procedures are based on the work of Parish and colleagues (1974) who, in analogy with the conventional indirect antibody technique, used erythrocytes coated with antibody raised against rabbit Ig to form rosettes with lymphocytes reacted with rabbit anti-surface antibody. This is the technique of choice when lymphocyte subpopulations are to be separated on the basis of alloantigen differences, for the reasons described in Section II,A,2. An added advantage of the HSL rosetting procedure is that the rosettes formed among ars-labeled lymphocytes and anti-ars-conjugated SRBCs are extremely stable. This is a direct consequence of the high number of haptenic determinants which can be bound to a lymphocyte using ars-amidinated anti-surface antibodies and which permit extensive multipoint binding by anti-ars-SRBCs.

Reagents

Fetal calf serum: heat-inactivated (30 min at 56°C)
Hapten-modified anti-surface antibodies
RPMI 1640 without bicarbonate
RPMI 1640, 5% FCS (RMPI-FCS)
Anti-ars-coupled SRBCs: see Section III,D,3 (anti-ars-SRBCs)
Ficoll–Hypaque: 1.09 gm/cm^3
Crystal violet: 1% in H$_2$O

Rosetting is carried out with lymphocyte preparations with as few dead cells as possible. High viability can be easily achieved by gradient centrifugation on Ficoll–Hypaque. Five milliliters of the cell suspension is layered over 4 ml of Ficoll-Hypaque in a polycarbonate tube (16 × 125 mm), equilibrated at 20°C, and spun for 20 min at 2000 g in a centrifuge prewarmed to 20°C. The centrifuge, equipped with a swinging-bucket rotor, should be capable of reaching the desired speed in about 30 sec. Dead cells and red blood cells will pellet on the bottom of the tube. Cells are labeled with haptenated anti-surface antibody as described in Section IV,A,1 for fluorescence labeling, but using RPMI-FCS as buffer. Also, in this case concentration of anti-surface antibodies should be predetermined to achieve the maximal number of rosettes without clumping of labeled lymphocytes. Cells are then resuspended at 2–10 × 10^7 cells/ml in RPMI-FCS and added dropwise with gentle shaking to the appropriate volume of anti-ars-SRBCs. The ratio of lymphocytes to anti-ars-SRBCs should range between 1:20 and 1:50. The mixture is incubated on ice with occasional gentle shaking. After 20 min, rosettes are ready for inspection. Microscopic visualization of rosettes is improved by adding 1 drop of 1% crystal violet per milliliter of cell suspension and reading after 5 min.

Rosettes are isolated from the cell preparation adjusted to 10^7 lymphocytes/ml by gradient centrifugation on Ficoll–Hypaque as described previously for the removal of dead cells. Rosettes and red blood cells will pellet at the bottom of the tube.

C. Studies on B-Cell Activation

1. Rationale

Hapten-conjugated antibodies can be considered "bifunctional" because (1) they can be recognized by specific soluble or membrane-bound anti-hapten antibodies, and (2) they can recognize their homologous antigen.

We have exploited this bifunctionality in adapting HSL methodology to the study of B-cell activation. The HSL reagents can be used to attach selectively to the desired receptor on the B-cell membrane a carrier molecule which in turn mediates cooperation among labeled B cells and carrier-primed T cells (Fig. 5) (Cammisuli *et al.*, 1978; Cammisuli and Henry, 1978; Cammisuli and Cosenza, 1980). With this experimental system it is possible to investigate the role of selected receptors in the co-operative events between helper T and B cells.

Another related approach is to use hapten-conjugated anti-cell surface antibodies to mediate a bridging event between the antigen-binding receptors of hapten-specific lymphocytes and, according to the specificity of the haptenated antibody, selected cell surface antigens present either on the same (Fig. 6A) or on a different cell (Fig. 6B).

The advantages of this approach are found again in the fact that most antigens involved in the processes of B- and T-cell cooperation are only detected with alloantibodies, so that in order to create selected bridgings or disturbances at these receptors a conventional technique cannot be used.

Obviously, this experimental system must be adapted to the individual problem under study. In the next section we will describe an example of the application of HSL reagents in the study of B- and T-cell cooperation.

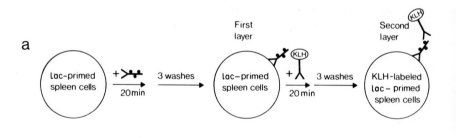

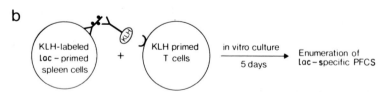

Fig. 5. Cooperation of T helper cells with B cells bridged through a selected receptor. (a) The carrier molecule KLH is bound to lac-primed spleen cells using ars-HB–anti-H2 antibodies in conjunction with the conjugate KLH–anti-ars. (b) The KLH-labeled B cells are cultured *in vitro* with KLH-primed T cells. With this experimental system we have shown that it is possible to elicit a T cell-dependent immune response in the absence of interaction at the B-cell receptor.

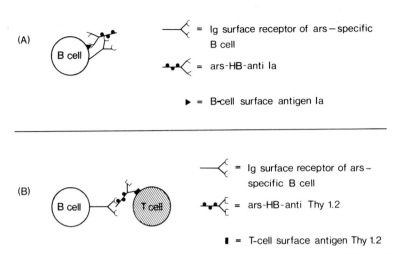

Fig. 6. Schematic representation of the use of hapten sandwich reagents to induce selected bridging events at the cell surface level. (A) Ars–HB–anti-cell surface antibodies are used to cross-link the B-cell Ig receptor with a selected antigen present on the same cell surface. In the figure the cross-linking between Ig receptor and Ia antigen is depicted. (B) Ars–HB–anti-cell surface antibodies are used to bridge B cells with T cells. In the figure the bridging of an ars-specific B cell with a Thy-1.2-positive cell is depicted.

2. The Bridging of T Helper Cells and B Cells through a Selected Receptor

We have successfully used HSL-mediated bridging to induce an idiotype-restricted anti-phosphorylcholine response bridging helper T cells selectively to idiotype positive B cells (Cammisuli and Cosenza, 1980), or to induce an anti-phosphorylcholine response (Cammisuli and Cosenza, 1980), or an anti-lactoside response (Cammisuli *et al.*, 1978) in the absence of interaction at the B-cell Ig receptor.

Spleen cell suspensions are depleted of T cells by sequential treatment with anti-Thy-1 and agarose-absorbed guinea pig complement. This cell suspension is used as a source of B cells. A carrier molecule [i.e., KLH or chicken gamma globulin (CGG)] is attached to the selected B-cell membrane antigen by using a labeling technique analogous to that used for fluorescence labeling. Obviously the whole procedure has to be sterile. B cells resuspended in RPMI and 5% FCS at a concentration of 5×10^7/ml are incubated for 20 min in the presence of the appropriate ars-modified anti-surface antibody. The concentration of the anti-surface antibody must be predetermined. When the carrier molecule is focused on the B-cell membrane via the H-2 or Ia antigens, we have found that the optimal concentration is about $\frac{1}{20}$ of the concentration giving optimal fluorescence labeling. When we have focused a carrier molecule via the Ig receptor, we have found that relatively higher concentrations of antibody are required. The cells are then washed three times with RPMI and 5% FCS, resuspended at 5 × 10⁷ cells/ml, and then incubated for 20 min with an appropriate concentration of the carrier molecule conjugated to anti-ars antibodies (Section III,D,2). We use KLH–anti-ars at approximately 100–500 μg/ml of original anti-ars. When the carrier molecule used is CGG, we use purified chicken anti-ars at a concentration of 100 μg/ml. The cells are then washed three times with RPMI and 5% FCS and resuspended in the culture medium. Labeling of the cells is carried out at 0°–4°C to avoid loss of label. Cells are stored in an ice bucket.

T cells specific for the carrier molecule are obtained according to any standard procedure, resuspended in the culture medium, and added at an optimal concentration to the cold B cells. The cell mixture is then distributed into dishes and cultured. We have used both standard Mishell–Dutton 1-ml cultures with 1.5 × 10⁷ cells/ml and 0.2-ml microtiter cultures with 1–3 × 10⁶ cells/ml. In our experiments we have enumerated plaque-forming cells (PFCs) to assess T helper cell-dependent B-cell activation.

D. Other Suggested Applications of Hapten Sandwich Labeling

Results obtained with the HSL technique suggest additional applications of hapten-conjugated proteins to problems in cell biology. One possibility is the use of hapten-modified ligands such as hormones, toxins, enzymes, and mitogens in conjugation with labeled anti-hapten antibodies to detect specific membrane receptors. When indirect labeling is necessary for their detection, HSL makes it possible to bypass the problem of raising monospecific antisera against the specific ligands. This is advantageous in cases where a considerable titer of specific antibody cannot be raised because the molecule under study is not strongly antigenic, because of its cross-reactivity with other endogenous molecules, or because only a limited amount of the ligand is available.

Because of the mildness of the hapten amidination procedure, it is possible to modify several ligands with retention of their biological activity. It has been shown that ovine prolactin (three ars groups per molecule) binds to mouse mammary epithelial cells with a high retention of biological activity. We have also ars-amidinated Con A and the glucosamine groups of lipopolysaccharide (LPS) derived from a mutant strain of *Salmonella typhimurium* with virtually complete retention of mitogenic activity. Both LPS-ars and Con A-ars have been successfully used in conjunction with fluoresceinated anti-ars antibodies to label lymphocyte membranes.

The HSL reagents can be successfully used to obtain C'mediated cytotoxicity in cases where the surface antigen-binding ligands are not C'-fixing. These ligands can be used to focus on the cell surface membrane C'-binding anti-hapten antibodies which will mediate C'-mediated killing. We have successfully used noncytotoxic ars-modified anti-Ia antibody in conjunction with rabbit anti-ars antibody to kill Ia-positive lymphocytes.

For isotopic labeling, it is possible to use HSL reagents where cell membrane ligands cannot be directly tagged at high specific activity and an indirect amplifying technique is necessary. Hapten-amidinated antibodies, enzymes, and hormones can be stored in stable form (nonradioactive) and used as required with amplification by radioactive anti-hapten antibodies (whole or Fab) which are easily monitored and purified by affinity chromatography.

V. CRITICAL APPRAISAL

The HSL methodology here described is an extension and not a mere duplication of the conventional indirect antibody technique. The advantages provided by HSL are evident in the study of alloantigens, where the conventional indirect FA technique has its major shortcomings.

It should be noted that, because of the extreme mildness of our hapten conjugation procedure, the same methodology can be used not only with hapten-conjugated antibodies but also with other hapten-conjugated ligands to cell surface antigens (Section IV,D).

It is advantageous that a single preparation of hapten-conjugated ligands can be used in conjunction with appropriate anti-hapten antibodies for several purposes ranging from antigen visualization, to separation of membrane components and of cell subpopulations, to cell-to-cell bridging. When working with several alloantibodies, an added advantage is that a stock preparation of labeled anti-hapten antibodies can be used with all hapten-modified preparations. The advantage is evident when working with autoradiography where the easily obtainable purified anti-hapten antibodies carry the isotope.

The most obvious disadvantage of HSL is that some chemistry is required for the preparation of hapten-conjugated proteins. The chemistry involved, however, is quite straightforward and can be easily carried out in any immunology laboratory.

Because of the high sensitivity of the system, great care should be taken in the preparation of reagents (Section IV,A,5) and in assessing the solubility properties of the hapten-modified proteins (Section III,C). These requirements must be satisfied to achieve excellent levels of specificity.

ACKNOWLEDGMENT

The methodology reported in this chapter originated at the University of California, Berkeley, in Dr. L. Wofsy's laboratory. Part of the methodology discussed here has also appeared in "Selected Methods in Cellular Immunology" (Freeman, San Francisco, California, 1980), edited by B. Mishell and S. Shiigi. This chapter contains exerpts from the doctoral thesis, "Bifunctional Reagents for Coupling Haptens to Antibodies: A General Procedure for Double Labeling Membrane Antigens," 1976, by S. Cammisuli, University of California at Berkeley.

REFERENCES

Axén, R., Porath, J., and Ernback, S. (1967). *Nature (London)* **214**, 1302.

Cammisuli, S., and Cosenza, H. (1980). *Eur J. Immunol.* **10**, 299.

Cammisuli, S., and Henry, C. (1978). *Eur. J. Immunol.* **8**, 662.

Cammisuli, S., and Wofsy, L. (1976). *J. Immunol.* **117**, 1685.

Cammisuli, S., Henry, C., and Wofsy, L. (1978). *Eur. J. Immunol.* **8**, 656.

Carter, D. P., and Wofsy, L. (1976). *J. Supramol. Struct.* **5**, 139.

Goldman, M. (1968). "Fluorescence Antibody Methods." Academic Press, New York.

Heitzmann, H., and Richards, F. M. (1974). *Proc. Natl. Acad. Sci. U.S.A.* **71**, 3537.

Hunter, M. J., and Ludwig, M. L. (1962). *J. Am. Chem. Soc.* **84**, 3491.

Kishida, Y., Olsen, B. R., Berg, R. A., and Prockop, D. J. (1975). *J. Cell Biol.* **64**, 331.

Lamm, M. E., Koo, G. C., Stackpole, C. W., and Hämmerling, U. (1972). *Proc. Natl. Acad. Sci. USA* **69**, 3732.

Loor, F. (1977). *Prog. Allergy* **23**, 1.

Nicholson, G. L., and Singer, S. J. (1971). *Proc. Natl. Acad. Sci. U.S.A.* **68**, 942.

Parish, C. R., Kirov, S. M., Brown, N., and Blanden, R. V. (1974). *Eur. J. Immunol.* **4**, 808.

Pressman, D., Yagi, Y., and Hiramoto, R. (1958). *Int. Arch. Allergy Appl. Immunol.* **12**, 125.

Slomich, M., Kwan, E., Wofsy, L., and Henry, C. (1980). *In* "Selected Methods in Cellular Immunology" (B. Mishell and S. Shiigi, eds.) p. 212. Freeman, San Francisco, California.

Tabachnick, M., and Sobotka, H. (1959). *J. Biol. Chem.* **234**, 1726.

Wallace, E. F., and Wofsy, L. (1979). *J. Immunol. Methods* **25**, 283.

Whiteley, N. M., and Berg, H. C. (1974). *J. Mol. Biol.* **87**, 541.

Wofsy, L., and Burr, B. (1969). *J. Immunol.* **103**, 380.

Wofsy, L., and Singer, S. J. (1963). *Biochemistry* **2**, 104.

Wofsy, L., Baker, P. C., Thompson, K., Goodman, J., Kimura, J., and Henry, C. (1974). *J. Exp. Med.* **140**, 523.

Wofsy, L., Henry, C., and Cammisuli, S. (1978). *Contemp. Top. Mol. Immunol.* **7**, 215.

8

HLA-DR Typing by Complement-Dependent B Lymphocyte Lysis

Gianni Garotta and Tauro M. Neri

I. INTRODUCTION

The DR antigen system is expressed predominantly on B lymphocytes and is controlled by the HLA region located on the short arm of chromosome 6 (Francke and Pellegrino, 1977). These antigens, which may be homologous to mouse immune-associated (Ia) antigens, are coded by an allelic series of genes belonging to a locus mapped between HLA *B* and *D* loci very close to the latter (Sociu-Foca *et al.,* 1980). DR antigens were described by van Rood's group in 1975, but the first comprehensive

IMMUNOLOGICAL METHODS, VOL. II

TABLE I

DR Gene Frequencies in Different Ethnic Groups[a]

Allele	Caucasian	Mongoloid	Negroid
DR1	8.29	5.60	6.49
DR2	13.34	19.73	17.82
DR3	11.05	1.43	17.82
DR4	11.43	22.98	5.11
DR5	10.39	2.98	14.97
DRW6	2.50	5.35	6.49
DR7	12.55	1.62	10.75
DRW8	3.68	8.86	7.89
DRW9	2.07	14.21	3.10
DRW10	1.50	NT	5.10
Blank	23.21	17.24	4.46

[a] Derived from VIII International Histocompatibility Workshop predata analysis. Values are percentages. NT, Not tested.

serological analysis of these markers was undertaken at the VIIth International Histocompatibility Workshop (Bodmer *et al.,* 1977). Seven specificities were defined, DRW1, DRW2, DRW3, DRW4, DRW5, DRW6, and DRW7, but not all the specificities within this locus were identified. In Caucasians, the estimated gene frequencies gave 34.9% blanks. The VIIIth International Histocompatibility Workshop defined 10 specificities; DRW6, DRW8, DRW9, and DRW10 were considered provisional specificities, while DR1, DR2, DR3, DR4, DR5, and DR7 were upgraded to full HLA status (Albert *et al.,* 1980) (Table I). During this workshop the existence of supertypic, cross-reacting specificities was confirmed, and for the combinations DR1 + DR2 + DRW10 + (DRW6), DR3 + DR5 + DRW6 + DRW8, and DR4 + DR7 + DRW9 were proposed the designations MT1 (DC1), MT2, and MT3, respectively (Park *et al.,* 1980). In Caucasians the newly estimated gene frequencies gave 26.78% blanks. This value is overestimated, because it is comprehensive of the DRW9 and DRW10 gene frequencies.

II. PRINCIPLE OF THE TEST

The cytotoxicity test consists of incubating living lymphocytes with antisera containing anti-HLA-DR antibodies in the presence of complement, with the National Institutes of Health (NIH) standard procedure (Ray *et al.,* 1974). When the antibodies are bound to the lymphocyte surface antigens, the complement is activated and the cell is killed. Eosin solution added to the reaction stains the dead cells and reveals positive reactions.

The main source of typing alloantisera are volunteers immunized according to a planned program or multiparous women. Because of the limited supply of antisera, the basic lymphocyte cytotoxicity test has to be a microtechnique like that successfully introduced by Terasaki and McClelland (1964) and then developed by Terasaki's group (1978).

III. DETAILS OF THE TEST

A. Lymphocyte Separation Technique

For B-cell preparation plastic ware or siliconized glassware have to be used, because these cells adhere to glass. About 20 ml of 100 U/ml heparinized venous blood is diluted 1:2 with balanced saline solution (BSS) [e.g., phosphate-buffered saline (PBS), Hanks' BSS, Earle's BSS] and layered onto a lymphocyte separation medium (LSM, a Ficoll–sodium metrizoate solution of density 1.077) at 2 vol of diluted blood on 1 vol of LSM. Yields of peripheral blood lymphocytes (PBLs) may occasionally be less when large tubes (50 ml) are used, and it may be preferable to employ smaller replicate tubes (10 or 13 ml). Any BSS can be used, but calcium-free buffered saline may have the advantage of minimizing the cell clumping that occasionally occurs after passage on LSM. The tubes are centrifuged for 15 min at 20°C with an interphase (blood–LSM) force of 1000 g. The cells of the interphase are collected carefully and pooled, and their suspension is diluted at least five times with BSS and centrifuged at 400 g for 15 min at 20°C. A further washing at the same force (400 g) for 10 min is required. After PBL harvesting from the interface, half of the top layer of the plasma–BSS mixture is saved and kept on ice.

A time-saving procedure for PBL separation can be employed using a Fisher centrifuge. Cells collected from Ficoll, in the minimum volume that is possible, are transferred to Fisher tubes (one tube per interface) and spun for 1 min at 4000 g in the Fisher centrifuge. The supernatant is discarded, and the pellet is resuspended in BSS and centrifuged in the Fisher centrifuge for 1 min at 1000 g.

In both procedures, PBL cells are then treated with thrombin to remove platelets and residual granulocytes. The PBL cells from 20 ml of venous blood are transferred to two to four Fisher tubes, and 1 drop of thrombin solution (100 U/ml) is added. The capped tubes are rotated on a vertical wheel at 8–10 rpm. Platelet and granulocyte clumps form in 3–5 min and are removed by spinning the tubes for 3 sec at 1000 g in the Fisher centrifuge and transferring the supernatant to clean Fisher tubes. The suspension is washed for 1 min at 1000 g and resuspended, and the pellets are

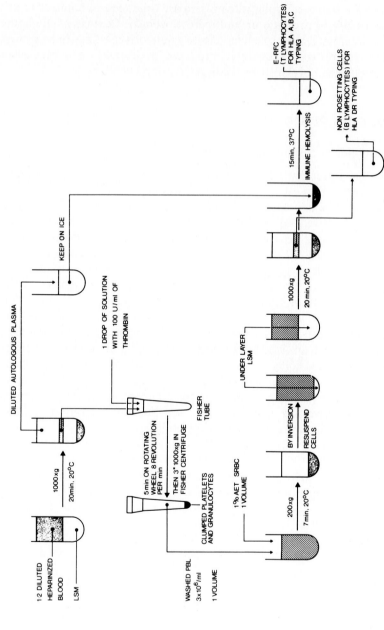

Fig. 1. Flow diagram for the T- and B-lymphocyte separation procedure.

pooled from the same sample in 2–3 ml of McCoy's medium supplemented with heat-inactivated 30% fetal bovine serum (FBS). The cells are counted and diluted to 3 × 10⁶ cells/ml in McCoy's medium with 30% FBS.

The average yield of PBLs is 48.9% (range 36–82%) or an average of 0.82 × 10⁶ lymphocytes/ml venous blood. There is no selective loss of lymphocyte subpopulations, the viability ranges over 97–98%, and no contamination of platelets or granulocytes is observed.

B. Isolation of T and B Lymphocytes

Human T and B lymphocytes are characterized by surface markers; i.e., besides DR antigens, B cells carry surface membrane immunoglobulin (SmIg), while T cells carry a receptor for sheep red blood cells (SRBCs), which allows the formation of E rosettes, and lack both SmIg and DR antigens (Aiuti *et al.*, 1974). The B-lymphocyte enrichment for DR typing can be achieved by depleting PBLs of E-rosette-forming T lymphocytes (E-RFC). After incubation at 37°C, the mixture of PBLs and SRBCs is centrifuged and held overnight on ice. The pellets are gently resuspended, and the suspensions are layered onto LSM and centrifuged. The E-RFC-depleted cells are found in the interphase, while the E-RFCs are collected at the bottom of the tube. Because of the weak binding between E receptors and SRBCs, E-rosetting conditions are critical. One needs to consider the age of the SRBCs, the SRBC/lymphocyte ratio, the time and temperature of incubation, and the medium used for rosetting (Madsen and Johnsen, 1979). An SRBC pretreatment with 2-aminoethylisothiouronium bromide (AET) or with an enzyme such as neuraminidase or papain results in remarkable improvement, and it is possible to obtain stable E rosettes in a shorter time at room temperature (Madsen *et al.*, 1980).

1. 2-Aminoethylisothiouronium Bromide Treatment of SRBCs

Sheep blood is drawn in acid citrate dextrose (ACD, NIH solution A; 1.8 ml in 8.2 ml of blood) and used within 15 days, but not before 3 days after the bleeding. The SRBC suspension is centrifuged 10 min at 1000 *g*, the supernatant is discarded, and the buffy coat is carefully removed. Red cells are resuspended in saline and washed three times (1000 *g*, 5 min). Then 2 ml of packed SRBCs is resuspended in 10 ml of 140 m*M* AET solution, pH 9, and incubated at 37°C for 15 min with occasional shaking. After incubation, AET-treated SRBCs (AET-SRBCs) are washed in saline until any residual hemolysis is observed. Pasteur pipettes are used to resuspend AET-SRBCs after the first centrifugation, and thereafter AET-SRBCs are resuspended by tube inversion. Finally, packed, treated red cells are resuspended in McCoy's medium with 30% FBS to obtain a 1% suspension. The AET-SRBC suspension is distributed in aliquots of 30 ml, stored at 4°C, and used within a week.

2. Separation of E-RFCs from Nonrosetting Cells

The suspension of 3 × 10⁶ PBLs/ml McCoy's 30% FBS medium is mixed with a similar volume of 1% AET-SRBCs in McCoy's 30% FBS medium. Then 6 ml of the mixture is distributed in tubes and centrifuged at 200 g for 7 min at room temperature. The pellets are resuspended by gentle tube inversion, and 3 ml of LSM is underlayered with a Pasteur pipette. The gradient is centrifuged 15 min at 20°C with an interphase force of 1000 g.

Nonrosetting cells, i.e., B lymphocytes, are collected from the interphase, transferred to a Fisher tube, and spun for 1 min at 4000 g in a Fisher centrifuge. The supernatant is discarded, and the cells are resuspended in BSS and washed twice (1 min at 1000 g). After the last washing, the cells are resuspended in 0.5 ml of McCoy's 30% FBS medium, counted, and adjusted to 2–3 × 10⁶ cells/ml. This B lymphocyte-enriched suspension can be used for HLA-DR typing. The average yield of B lymphocytes is 12% (range 8–17%) of the PBLs used or an average of 0.1 × 10⁶ B lymphocytes/ml venous blood used.

E-rosetting cells, i.e., T lymphocytes, are collected under LSM from the bottom of the tube. The supernatant is discarded, and 3 ml of autologous plasma–BSS, previously collected and kept on ice, is added. The anti-sheep antibodies, normally present in human serum, and the preserved complement activity induce lysis of the AET-SRBCs if incubated 15 min at 37°C. The T cells, freed from SRBCs, are washed twice in BSS, resuspended in McCoy's 30% FBS medium, counted, and adjusted to 3 × 10⁶ cells/ml. This T lymphocyte-enriched suspension can be used for HLA-ABC typing.

3. Comments

The E-rosetting efficiency, when AET-SRBCs are used, is not affected by the incubation time at 4°C, after the centrifugation step, as well as not being affected by the temperature required for rosetting. For these reasons it is possible to work at room temperature, and the incubation after centrifugation of the mixture of AET-SRBCs and PBLs can be eliminated. The influence that the protein concentration in the rosetting media may have on the percentage of AET-RFCs is controversial, but in cases of a final serum concentration of more than 20% the rosettes are larger and have a compact morula appearance, and the loss of E-RFCs or non-RFCs is minimum (Bentwich et al., 1973; Madsen et al., 1980). Human AB or normal serum may be used after heat inactivation at 56°C for 30 min and after absorption with sheep and human red cells at 37° and 4°C. These sera must be checked for the presence of anti-lymphocyte alloantibodies which may inhibit formation of the rosettes. The 1% AET-SRBC suspension contains about 2×10^8 red cells/ml and, when it is mixed with a similar volume at 3×10^6 PBLs/ml, gives an SRBC/lymphocyte ratio of 70. These conditions are optimal for the rosetting procedure and permit satisfactory rosette counting.

C. Microcytotoxicity Test for B Lymphocytes

1. Test Procedure

According to NIH standard procedure, 1 μl of B-lymphocyte suspension is added to each well of the typing trays by using a 50-μl Hamilton syringe. The filled trays are incubated in a controlled-temperature incubator at 20°C. After 60 min of incubation 5 μl of complement is added to each well and the trays are incubated at 20°C in the incubator for 120 min. After complement incubation 5 μl of eosin Y dye is added, followed 5 min later by 10 μl of formaldehyde solution. After 10 min from the fixing of the reactions a cover glass is placed over each tray, and the trays are stored overnight in a cold room before reading. Trays can be read within 2 weeks.

2. Reading of the Microcytotoxicity Test

The trays are examined under an inverted phase-contrast microscope, and the percentage of stained dead cells is scored in each well (Table II). DR specificities are assigned to the studied cells, comparing the observed reactions with the declared activities of the reacting sera.

3. Complement

The main source of complement for HLA typing is rabbit serum, which is commercially available or made in the laboratory.

TABLE II

Reading Scores for Each Cytotoxic Reaction[a]

Score	Dead cells (%)	Reaction
0	—	Not tested
1	0–10	Negative
2	11–20	Doubtful negative
4	21–40	Doubtful or weak positive
6	41–80	Positive
8	81–100	Strong positive

[a] Starting from A1 and finishing at A10, the reading sequence is from A to F for the even lines and from F to A for the odd lines of the Terasaki tray. The typing protocol is according to this sequence.

Because B lymphocytes are generally more sensitive than T lymphocytes to the toxic effect of the complement, the former should be used for complement selection and titration for DR typing. A small sample of blood (3–5 ml) is taken from the ear of 2-month-old rabbits (sera from older rabbits can be easily toxic to human cells), allowed to clot at room temperature for 15 min, and then kept on ice for 2 hr. The blood samples are then spun down, at 1000 g for 20 min at 5°C, and the sera taken off and kept on ice. Dilutions of 1:1–1:16 of each complement sample are prepared using McCoy's medium with 30% FBS as diluent. For the toxicity test the dilutions of complement are simply added to the B lymphocytes with controls without complement.

For the activity test, the B lymphocytes are incubated with a well-characterized anti-B cell serum using different dilutions of serum and complement in a checkerboard. With the protocol shown in Fig. 2 both tests are performed on a plate. After a 2-hr incubation at 20°C, the killing of each sample of rabbit serum is compared with that of a control without complement, while its activity is compared with that of a standard complement.

On the basis of these tests, the rabbits whose serum produced killing and the best complement activity are selected and bled out. The new samples are kept separated and treated as in the previous tests. The sera with good activity and low cytotoxicity are pooled, dispensed in 1-ml aliquots, and stored in liquid nitrogen or in a deep freezer at −70°C. Before the new batch of pooled complement is routinely used it is further checked for activity and toxicity. The lot of the complement can be best evaluated by reaction with a standard typing tray using standard cells under standard DR-typing conditions.

Both frozen and lyophilized complement are prepared immediately before use and held on ice. For one tray the complement requirement is 0.3 ml.

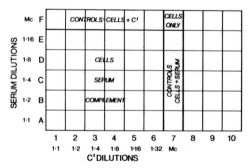

Fig. 2.   Suggested protocol for complement activity and toxicity tests.

4. Preparation of Typing Trays

Each well is filled with mineral oil by a Cornwall continuous pipetting setup to prevent evaporation of the reagent to be used in the DR typing. According to the protocol, 1 μl of each serum is seeded with a 50-μl Hamilton syringe into the tray wells in the proper sequence. Under these conditions the position of a particular antiserum is uniform for all the trays. This operation is very critical. The droplets float on the oil and stick to the sides of the well. Proper placement of the droplet in the center of the well is easier when the sera are stained with 0.001% phenol red. After the seeding each tray is examined, and missed wells are either refilled or excluded by a marker.

The filled trays are stored at $-70°C$ until use. A CO_2 atmosphere or dry ice should be avoided because the pH of the sera becomes too acid. It is most convenient to prepare a large number of trays at the same time, in a number roughly proportional to putative laboratory needs. Bubble formation or deterioration may occur when the trays are stored for more than 4–5 months. All the sera to be used in the typing trays must be clarified by centrifugation at high speed to eliminate debris and lipids. Beckman tubes are centrifuged at 15,000 rpm for 15 min at 4°C in a Beckman microfuge.

Positive and negative controls should be included. Xenogeneic anti-B lymphocyte serum is the main positive control, giving the highest cytotoxicity degree for these reactions. Allogeneic anti-DR sera will not have a greater killing effect than xenogeneic sera. If a positive control gives 50% cytotoxicity, it means that the B-cell preparation is contaminated with T cells and that the alloantisera will not give a better reaction. McCoy's medium with 30% FBS or inactivated AB serum absorbed with pooled lymphocytes is the negative control. Dilutions of 1:16 and 1:32 of the negative control with BSS can give a measure of the false positive errors. These controls measure the toxicity of complement, since the anti-complementary activity of normal serum is diluted in BSS.

5. Anti-DR Sera

The main source of anti-HLA-DR antibodies is sera obtained from planned immunization between recipients and donors compatible for HLA-ABC but different for DR antigens (Curtoni *et al.*, 1973) or sera obtained from multiparous women (Thorsby and Kissmeyer-Nielsen, 1969). When this is the case, anti-B-cell antibodies often coexist with antibodies against HLA-ABC antigens. The presence of activity not correlated with the antibodies against HLA-ABC determinant is checked by a blanketing test (Bernoco *et al.*, 1976). B lymphocytes (3 × 10⁶/ml) are incubated 120 min at 20°C with turkey anti-human β_2 microglobulin serum properly diluted (every batch of sera differs and has to be titrated). After incubation 1 μl of the cell suspension is distributed in the well of a tray containing studied sera. After 30 min at 20°C, 5 μl of complement is added and the incubation at 20°C is protracted for 60 min. Eosin Y is added, and the reaction is fixed by adding formaldehyde solution and read by dye exclusion as usual. Avian antibodies against β_2 microglobulin do not fix rabbit complement (Rice, 1948) but block lympholysis of antibodies against HLA-ABC antigens that contain β_2 microglobulins (Poulik et al., 1974). If the activity of the sera under examination is not abrogated, antibodies against DR or other surface structures not linked with β_2 microglobulin are present in the examined sera.

The specificity of the antibodies against HLA-ABC antigens is then defined against a panel of well-typed T lymphocytes, and the antibodies are removed by absorption with pooled platelets obtained from donors carrying the corresponding ABC antigens. Platelets are known to lack DR antigens. The sera are incubated with 3-week-old platelets at a concentration of 10^9/ml per antigen. After 60 min at 37°C, the incubation is extended overnight at 4°C and the sera are centrifuged 1000 g for 30 min at 4°C. The absorbed sera are tested against a panel of T lymphocytes to reveal the residual contamination of antibodies against ABC specificities and then challenged with a well-typed B-lymphocyte panel for definition of the anti-DR activity. Thereafter, activity is compared with known sera and analyzed for segregation within families.

Platelets for anti-DR sera absorption are prepared as follows. Venous blood is harvested in 5% ethylenediaminetetraacetic acid (EDTA)(2 ml EDTA solution per 10 ml of blood) and then diluted 1:20 with a 5% EDTA solution. The mixture is dispensed in 50-ml plastic tubes and centrifuged at 200 g for 10 min at 4°C. The supernatant is transferred to a new 50-ml tube and centrifuged at 800 g for 30 min at 4°C. The pellets are resuspended in cold 5% EDTA solution, pooled, and spun as before. The final pellet is resuspended in 1% ammonium oxalate by gentle manual tilting and stepwise diluted and gently shaken until 5 ml of ammonium oxalate solution for every 10 ml of drawn blood is added. The suspension is left on the bench for 10 min and then centrifuged at 800 g for 30 min at 4°C. If the $(NH_4)_2SO_4$ treatment fails to eliminate red cells, such a step is repeated. The red cell-free pellet is further washed twice in saline and finally resuspended in 0.1% NaN_3 saline. Platelets are counted, adjusted to a concentration of 10^9/ml, disposed in 10-ml round-bottomed plastic tubes, and then stored at 4°C. Platelets are used within 3 weeks.

HLA typing reagents can also be produced by xenogeneic immunization. Some sera have been produced by rabbit immunization with purified HLA antigen (Ferrone et al., 1978), but interesting results have been reported with an antibody-secreting hybridoma obtained according to Köhler and Milstein (1975). A mouse is immunized with human whole lymphoblastoid cells or with purified HLA antigens, its spleen is excised, and the splenocytes are fused with myeloma cells. The somatic hybrids grow *in vitro,* and those which produce antibodies against the immunogen are selected and cloned. This procedure secures the homogeneity of the Ig molecule directed against a single determinant. Monoclonal antibodies against β_2 microglobulin, against the common part of HLA-ABC and HLA-DR antigens (Trucco *et al.,* 1978, 1979), against HLA-A2 (Brodsky *et al.,* 1979), against MT-2 (DR3 + DR5 + DRW6 + DRW8) (Trucco *et al.,* 1979; Garotta *et al.,* 1980), and against subpopulations of T lymphocytes are available (Reinberz *et al.,* 1979).

The hybridoma approach to the production of antibodies against HLA structures is undergoing improvement and a useful reagent will be available soon (Garotta *et al.,* 1980).

D. Errors

T-lymphocyte or granulocyte contamination of B-lymphocyte preparations affect DR typing. T lymphocytes reduce the positivity of the test and false negative results occur with weak reactions, while granulocytes cause a high background of dead cells, giving false positive results. Both false positive and false negative results are also common after insufficient or excessive cell seeding.

Other errors derive from skipping wells when the cells are added or occur when lymphocyte suspension droplets are not mixed with antibody droplets in the typing tray.

Reading errors may be minimized when reactions are independently examined by two readers. To avoid typing problems, it is mandatory to use well-known sera in the typing tray or to introduce new sera on the side of well-known faithful sera.

IV. MODIFICATIONS OF THE TEST

The main modifications of the DR-typing procedure concern the method for B-lymphocyte enrichment, the microdroplet test, and the staining procedure for living or dead cells.

The B lymphocytes can be separated by depleting PBLs of T lymphocytes which form E rosettes with SRBCs pretreated with an enzyme such as papain or neuraminidase, by taking advantage of the capacity of B lymphocytes to adhere to nylon wool, or by monoclonal antibody rosetting (MAR) that allows a positive selection for cells bearing HLA-DR antigens. All these procedures are performed on PBLs after thrombin treatment.

A. Enzymatic Treatment of SRBCs

1. Papain Treatment

SRBCs are washed twice, and packed red cells are mixed with BSS to obtain a 20% suspension. Equal volumes of papain reagents and 20% washed SRBCs are mixed and incubated for 10 min at 37°C in a water bath. Papain-treated red cells (P-SRBCs) are washed three times in PBS and resuspended in McCoy's medium with 30% FBS to obtain a 2% suspension that should be used within 3 days.

Immediately before using, the papain reagent is prepared by mixing 1 vol of papain stock solution diluted 1:10 with PBS, 2 vol of L-cysteine–HCl stock solution diluted 1:500 with PBS, and 2 vol of 1 M Na$_2$HPO$_4$ solution.

2. Neuraminidase Treatment

Washed and packed SRBCs are resuspended with BSS containing 4 × 10^{-3} IU/ml of neuraminidase to obtain an 8% suspension. Usually 0.4 ml of packed SRBCs and 0.1 ml of 0.2 IU/ml neuraminidase stock solution are added to 5 ml of BSS and then incubated for 30 min at 37°C. The neuraminidase-treated red cells (N-SRBCs) are washed twice with BSS and resuspended in McCoy's medium with 30% FBS to yield a 2% suspension. N-SRBCs are used within 3 days.

3. Rosetting Procedure with Enzyme-Treated SRBCs

One volume of treated 2% SRBC suspension is mixed with 1 vol of a PBL suspension with 4 × 10^6 cells/ml. The mixture is incubated 15 min at room temperature or 15 min at 37°C in a water bath if P-SRBC or N-SRBC is used, respectively. Aliquots of 3 ml are pipetted into a 5-ml round-bottomed plastic tube and centrifuged for 7 min at 20°C with a force of 200 g; the pellets are incubated on ice for at least 30 min but no longer than 120 min. The pellets are gently resuspended by rotation; LSM is underlayered with a Pasteur pipette, and the gradients are centrifuged for 15 min at 20°C with an interphase of 1000 g.

Purified B lymphocytes are collected from the interphase and purified T lymphocytes from the pellet as reported for AET-SRBC rosetting.

B. B-Lymphocyte Isolation with Nylon Wool

Scrubbed nylon wool is divided in 0.1-gm aliquots which are soaked in BSS. Then each aliquot is uniformly packed in a 1-ml plastic syringe and further washed with 5 ml of BSS. The columns, with medium just covering the nylon wool, can be stored at 4°C overnight or frozen for a longer time when properly sealed.

Before using, the column is opened so that the medium drips out; the nylon is washed with 5 ml of BSS and then with 3 ml of McCoy's 5% FBS medium. The column filled with McCoy's 5% FBS medium is incubated horizontally at 37°C for 30 min.

For separation in T and B lymphocytes, PBLs are resuspended in 0.5 ml of McCoy's 5% FBS medium and added to the top of the preheated nylon wool column. When the cells move into the nylon wool, McCoy's 5% FBS medium is added, and the column is closed and laid flat for 30 min at 37°C. After incubation, the column is placed over a 5-ml plastic tube, and the nonadherent T lymphocytes are collected by dripping 5 ml of McCoy's 5% FBS medium, preheated to 37°C, through the column. The collecting tube is changed, and a second 5-ml volume of heated medium is dripped through the column. Purified B lymphocytes are recovered in a third tube when a volume of 1.5 ml McCoy's 5% FBS medium is added and the wool is vigorously squeezed by the syringe plunger. The squeezing operation is repeated with a second volume of 1.5 ml of medium. T lymphocytes collected in the first tube, and B lymphocytes from the third tube are washed twice with BSS, resuspended in McCoy's 30% FBS medium, counted, and adjusted to a final concentration of 2–3 × 10^6 cells/ml.

The column is designed for a maximum of 150 × 10^6 PBLs. For greater amounts, multiple columns must be used.

C. Monoclonal Antibody Rosetting

1. Principles

A monoclonal mouse antibody which reacts with cells bearing DR antigens can be helpful in separating such a population of cells. The monoclonal antibody N 5/1 is a non-complement-fixing IgG antibody with a specificity for a nonpolymorphic determinant of the DR dimer (Trucco *et al.*, 1978). This antibody, after binding to the cells, does not prevent reactivity with allogeneic, cytotoxic, anti-DR typing sera (Stocker *et al.*, 1979).

N 5/1 antibodies are raised by fusion of spleen cells from mice immunized with a human lymphoblastoid line, with mouse myeloma cells, followed by selection of hybrids. The supernatant media, from cultures of the hybrid cell line diluted 1:10 and 1:20, are the source of monoclonal antibody. To avoid E-rosette formation by T lymphocytes, the monoclonal antibody rosetting (MAR) of DR-positive cells is performed by using bovine erythrocytes (BRCs).

2. Coating of Lymphocytes with Monoclonal Antibodies N 5/1

The PBLs are adjusted to 4 × 10^6/ml in McCoy's medium containing 30% fetal calf serum and the required concentration of antibody. The mixture is held on ice for 30 min with occasional shaking. The coated cells are washed three times in BSS with centrifuging for 2 min at 1000 *g* at room temperature in a Fisher centrifuge and finally resuspended to 3×10^6/ml in McCoy's 30% FBS medium.

3. Preparation of Bovine Erythrocytes Coupled with Affinity-Purified Rabbit Anti-Mouse Ig

Bovine blood is stored in Alsever's solution and used between 1 and 4 weeks after collection. A BRC suspension is centrifuged for 10 min at 1000 g, the supernatant is discarded, and the buffy coat is carefully removed. Red cells are resuspended in saline and washed four times (1000 g, 5 min) with saline. To 0.5 ml packed BRCs, 0.5 ml 0.9% NaCl, and 1 ml affinity-purified rabbit Ig anti-mouse IgG, 800 μg/ml in 0.9% NaCl is added. The 1% stock solution of CrCl$_3$ is diluted 1:10 in saline, and 1 ml is added to the BRC–antibody mixture dropwise with constant shaking. The coupling reaction is allowed to proceed for 5 min at room temperature with occasional shaking and is terminated by the addition of an excess of PBS. The coupled BRCs are then washed three times in PBS and finally resuspended to 2% by adding 25 ml McCoy's 30% FBS medium.

4. Preparation of Affinity-Purified Rabbit Ig Anti-Mouse IgG

Rabbit anti-mouse IgG serum is inactivated at 56°C for 30 min and then passed over a column of mouse IgG coupled to Sepharose. Specific antibodies, bound to Sepharose-coupled mouse Ig, are eluted with 0.05 M glycine-HCl buffer, pH 2.5. The eluate is neutralized with 0.2 M Tris buffer, pH 8, and immediately passed over a column of Sephadex G-50 equilibrated with 0.9% NaCl. The antibody in saline is adjusted to a concentration of 800 μg/ml and frozen in aliquots.

5. Rosette Formation

Equal volumes of antibody-coated PBLs and 2% anti-mouse Ig-coupled BRCs (CBRCs) are mixed, and 0.5 ml of this mixture is added to a 10 × 75 mm plastic tube. The tube is cooled for about 5 min on ice and then centrifuged for 7 min at 400 g at 4°C. It has been found that increasing the volume of the rosetting mixture above the indicated volumes results in a severe decrease in rosette numbers.

The pellets are gently resuspended by handle tilting, 1 ml of LSM is underlayered with a Pasteur pipette, and the mixture is centrifuged at 1000 g, calculated at interphase, for 15 min at 20°C. Nonrosetting cells, i.e., DR-negative cells, are collected from the interphase, while MAR cells, i.e., DR-positive cells, are collected from the bottom of the tube. The pellet containing MAR cells is resuspended with autologous plasma–BSS and treated as reported for AET-SRBC rosetting. DR-positive and DR-negative cells are finally resuspended at 3.0×10^6/ml in McCoy's 30% FBS medium for dispensing into typing trays.

A variant of MAR for the separation of DR-positive cells has been recently reported (de Kretser *et al.*, 1980). DR-bearing cells are rosetted by monoclonal antibodies, against a common part of the DR dimer, coupled to Sepharose beads, and separated by centrifugation on LSM. The DR-positive cells bound to Sepharose beads are collected under the gradient, while the DR-negative cells are collected at the interphase. DR-positive cells are then freed by gently vortexing.

D. Modifications of the Microdroplet Test

1. The Kissmeyer–Nielsen Modification

This method utilizes glass oil chambers, and the cytotoxic reactions are performed in drops placed on the coverslip that forms the bottom of the Hamax glass oil chamber (Kissmeyer-Nielsen and Kjerbye, 1967). The optics of this type of tray are superior as compared to the plastic Terasaki tray, but such a tray requires a restricted volume of reaction mixture. For this reason 0.5 μl of serum, 0.5 μl of cell suspension, and 3 μl of complement are mixed, and the cytotoxic reaction is visualized by 0.5 μl of 1% trypan blue solution in saline. The volume of 0.5 μl is dispensed by a 25-μl Hamilton syringe. The concentration of trypan blue is critical. This vital stain is bound by serum albumin; too low a concentration will result in the failure of killed cells to stain, and too high a concentration will result in the staining of living cells. In addition, trypan blue has anti-complementary properties, and this addition to the mixture stops the cytotoxic reaction and can preserve the reaction for the next day's reading. When this method is used, it is important to remember that the amount of vital stain is calibrated for the serum content of albumin. If DR typing sera must be used diluted, the diluent must be human AB inactivated serum.

2. The Amos Modification

This method involves flicking of the plates to remove serum after serum–cell incubation and to remove complement after cell–complement incubation (Amos *et al.*, 1969). The dead cells are stained by adding 5 μl of 0.3% trypan blue in saline solution to each well, which is then filled with a drop of 1.4% EDTA solution. After 10 min the vital stain is removed by flicking the plates, a drop of medium is added to each well, and the reactions are read.

E. Fluorochromasia

Fluorochromasia is a modification of a staining procedure that involves labeling of the cells with fluorescein diacetate (FDA) (Celada and Rotman, 1966; Bodmer *et al.*, 1967).

After washings, PBLs are resuspended in McCoy's 30% FBS medium, and 3 μl of FDA reagent is added to each milliliter with a maximum cell concentration of 20 × 10^6/ml. The mixture is incubated 10 min at room temperature in the dark (the tube is wrapped in aluminium foil). After incubation the tube is filled with cold BSS and the cell suspension is centrifuged under the usual conditions. The supernatant is discarded, and the labeled cells, which appear yellow, are washed twice with BSS. For these washings BSS without serum is used. Serum contains esterases that break down free FDA, producing fluorescein. Finally the cells are resuspended in McCoy's 30% FBS medium, counted, and adjusted to 3 × 10^6 cells/ml.

One microliter of cell suspension is seeded in a Terasaki tray containing sera against DR antigens, and the test is performed according to the standard NIH technique.

After the complement incubation the plates are immediately read with an inverted microscope equipped with a source of uv light with filters for fluorescein.

Fluorescein diacetate is a nonfluorescent derivative of fluorescein that penetrates cells. Inside the cells FDA is hydrolyzed by esterases, fluorescein is produced, and living cells fluoresce brightly under blue uv light. Damage to the cell membrane caused by the action of antibodies and complement results in release of the fluorescein. Because dead cells are invisible, the positive cytotoxic reactions are indicated by the decrease in or the disappearance of fluorescent cells.

This technique allows the background of dead cells to be typed but, if such a background is too high, a damaged cell removal step is introduced. The cell suspension is layered on a Ficoll-Urovison mixture with a density of 1.094 and centrifuged at 2200 rpm for 15 min at 20°C. The cells are removed from the interphase, washed twice, and treated with FDA reagent. After the above-mentioned treatment the viability of the cell suspension is higher than 90%.

The addition of 1 μl of a 0.4 mg/ml ethidium bromide solution to each well makes dead cells evident. Under these conditions, under uv blue light dead cells appear red and living cells appear green; the test can be read, scoring the percentage of killed cells as well as in the classic NIH test.

F. Two-Color Technique

The PBLs obtained from 5 ml of venous heparinized blood are resuspended in 0.5 ml BSS 1% bovine serum albumin (BSA) and incubated with 0.05 ml of goat Ig anti-human Ig fluorescein isothiocyanate (FITC) conjugates diluted 1:3 for 5 min at 37°C (van Rood et al., 1976). After three washings with BSS and 1% BSA the PBLs are adjusted to 8 × 10^6/ml and 0.5 μl of cell suspension is dispensed in a Hamax glass oil chamber prefilled with DR-typing sera. After 60 min of incubation at 20°C, 3 μl of complement is added, and the mixture is incubated 120 min at 20°C. At the end of the incubation, dead cells are visualized in each reaction drop by adding 0.5 μl of a 1:70 dilution of ethidium bromide stock solution. A cover glass is placed on the tray, and the reading is done with an inverted microscope equipped with a monochromatic 50-W light source, a LP455 and SP490 excitation filter combination, a FT510 dichroic mirror, and a LP520 barrier filter. Under these conditions the green fluorescence of the FITC conjugates and the red fluorescence of the ethidium bromide are visible simultaneously. The two-color technique requires the optical properties of a Hamax glass oil chamber because the reactions are read in the dark by mounting on the microscope a 25× water immersion objective. B lymphocytes bear a green cap, as a result of the reaction with FITC goat anti-human Ig, if they are still alive, while they bear a green cap and are red if they have been killed by anti-DR serum. In very expert hands the two-color technique is reliable and reproducible, saves time, and allows identification of alloantisera reactions against subpopulations of mononuclear cells.

V. CRITICAL APPRAISAL

The quality of HLA-DR typing mainly depends on the purity of the B lymphocytes being studied. The purification method of choice for routine typing must give the highest yield of these cells (whose percentage in the peripheral blood is low), must be simple, rapid, and reproducible, and must fit to blood samples from normal or diseased persons, although the bleeding is performed in different places or under different conditions. Thus far our experience indicates that the AET E-rosette method gives reliable and reproducible results as compared with the other methods discussed (Table III). Such an enrichment technique is relatively simple, does not need unusual or expensive equipment and supplies, and can be performed in every laboratory without problems involving special training of a technical staff.

The nylon procedure for purifying B lymphocytes is simpler and faster than all the rosette-forming cell depletion methods. Nevertheless, in our hands, this enrichment technique is not yet fully reproducible even though it has been considerably improved.

The MAR technique requires some comment. Where monoclonal antibodies recognize antigens carried by cell subpopulations, the potentiality exists for their use in separating such populations. This method may be too elaborate for the routine purpose of HLA-DR typing but could be useful for special work in the quantitation or purification of a subset of cells.

The Kissmeyer–Nielsen and the Amos modifications of the microdroplet test, used in some laboratories, do not increase the sensitivity of the test.

TABLE III

Comparison of Different Procedures for the Separation of Human T and B Lymphocytes

Separation procedure	Total peripheral blood lymphocytes		B-enriched lymphocytes		T-enriched lymphocytes	
	E rosette (%)	SIgm + (%)	E rosettes (%)	SIgm + (%)	E rosettes (%)	SIgm + (%)
Spontaneous E rosettes[a]	62.1 ± 10.1	11.8 ± 4.2	17.0 ± 6.1	41.2 ± 5.5	85.6 ± 9.3	4.6 ± 3.2
AET E rosettes	87.9 ± 9.9	15.0 ± 6.1	5.5 ± 2.8	79.6 ± 2.3	88.1 ± 5.7	4.3 ± 1.2
Papain E rosettes	78.4 ± 7.3	12.6 ± 7.6	7.9 ± 4.3	70.5 ± 7.7	81.9 ± 6.7	3.8 ± 2.3
Neuraminidase E rosettes	67.0 ± 9.3	13.8 ± 5.4	8.2 ± 4.3	59.1 ± 3.6	85.3 ± 7.7	3.0 ± 2.2
Nylon	81.2 ± 5.6	15.3 ± 8.2	17.4 ± 9.8	66.0 ± 18.7	90.1 ± 10.7	7.3 ± 3.6
MAR	85.1 ± 4.8	16.6 ± 4.8	2.6 ± 2.1	76.4 ± 5.3	89.5 ± 9.6	5.5 ± 3.1

[a] After overnight incubation at 4°C.

When the Amos shaking-out method is used, the possibility of losing cells counterbalances the advantages of overcoming anti-complement activity of some typing sera.

Fluorochromasia could be the preferred staining procedure when leukemic, lymphoblastoid, or normal cells, differing from lymphocytes, are used as targets in the typing. These cells have a large cytoplasmic mass, and eosin Y or trypan blue stains the cytoplasm of living cells as well as the cytoplasm and nucleus of dead cells. These conditions make it difficult to score the cytotoxic reactions. Furthermore, the FDA method has the advantage that a background of 30% dead cells can be ignored. The disadvantage of fluorochromasia is that the test must be read within 12 hr.

The two-color technique is the only DR-typing technique that does not need B-lymphocyte purification and that can be performed on PBLs. It is a rapid procedure, but the reading of the cytotoxic reactions is almost critical. The reader must be very well trained to detect cell surface fluorescence and to score every killing reaction in the numerous small microscope fields observed at 250×.

VI. EQUIPMENT, SUPPLIES, AND SOLUTIONS

A. Main DR-Typing Procedure

1. Equipment and Supplies

Centrifuge capable of generating 4000 g at a controlled temperature. Fisher centrifuge Model 59 No. 4–978–100 and Fisher tubes No. 4978–145 (Fisher Scientific Co., Pittsburgh, Pennsylvania).

Beckman Model 152 microfuge and Beckman tubes No. 338802 (1.5 ml) and No. 314326 (0.4 ml) (Beckman Instruments International SA, Geneva, Switzerland).

Heraeus incubator Model KB500, temperature regulation between 5° and 40°C, not humidified (W.C. Heraeus GmbH., Hanau, West Germany).

Deep freezer, −70°C, Forma Bio-freezer Model 8200 (Forma Scientific, Marietta, Ohio).

Liquid nitrogen refrigerator Model LR-40 and drawers for storage in the liquid nitrogen refrigerator Model LR-10 (Union Carbide, United Kingdom, Ltd.).

Phase-contrast inverted microscope with 10× objective and 10× oculars.

Hamilton microsyringes, needle gauge 22, point style 3: 50 µl No. 705N (dispensed volume 1 µl per step), 250 µl No. 725N (dispensed volume

5 μl per step), 500 μl No. 750N (dispensed volume 10 μl per step); Hamilton Terasaki multiple repeating dispensers (space between needles 6.4 mm) No. 83725 for six 50-μl syringes 705N, No. 83728 for six 250-μl syringes 725N, No. 83729 for six 500-μl syringes 750N (Hamilton Co., Reno, Nevada).

Cornwall 3052F continuous pipetting outfit with 2-ml Luer lock syringe (Becton-Dickinson Co., Waltham, Massachusetts).

Multiple needle dispenser for Cornwall syringe, six needles attached to a manifold with a Luer lock inlet (made by institute workshop).

Multipurpose rotator wheel Model 150v (Scientific Industries Inc., Springfield, Massachusetts).

Neubauer hemacytometer, $\frac{1}{10}$ mm depth, $\frac{1}{400}$ mm^2, Brand pipettes for white blood cell counting (Müller and Krempel, Bülach, Switzerland).

Terasaki microtest trays No. 3034, plastic tubes No. 2051 (10 ml), plastic tubes No. 2025 (13 ml), plastic tubes No. 2070 (50 ml) (Falcon Plastics, Division of BioQuest, Los Angeles, California).

Siliconized Pasteur pipettes, long and short (WU, Mainz, West Germany).

Microscope cover glasses, 47 × 75 mm, No. 1 (Charles Berdat, Delémont, Switzerland).

Nalgene filter units, 0.45 μm (Nalge Co., Rochester, New York).

Heparin, Liquemin, 5000 U/ml (Roche, Basel, Switzerland).

Thrombin, Topostasine, 3000 NIH U/vial (Roche, Basel, Switzerland).

Mineral oil, Olio di Vaselina No. 356601 (Carlo Erba, Milano, Italy).

Hank's balanced salt solution No. 310–4060, modified McCoy's 5a medium with glutamine and 30% FBS No. 320–6630, modified McCoy's 5a powdered medium No. 430–1500, L-glutamine, 200 mM, No. 320–1140, FBS No. 200–6290, Pen-Strept solution No. 200–6290 (Grand Island Biological Co., Grand Island, New York).

Eosin Y No. 21005 (Serva, Feinbiochemica, Heidelberg, West Germany).

2-Aminoethylisothiouronium bromide No. A-5879 (Sigma, St. Louis, Missouri).

Formaldehyde, 37% acid-free, No. 3999 (Merck AG, Darmstadt, West Germany).

Ficoll 400 (Pharmacia, Uppsala, Sweden).

Urovison, 58% (Schering AG, Berlin/Bergkamen, West Germany).

2. Solutions

Heparin: Use 0.1 ml/10 ml of blood.

Thrombin: Reconstitute the vial contents with 30 ml of sterile distilled water to obtain a solution of 100 U/ml; freeze in 0.5-ml aliquots in Beckman tubes No. 338802.

Phosphate-buffered solution, 0.15 M, pH 7.2: Mix 140 ml 0.2 M

NaH_2PO_4 ($NaH_2PO_4 \cdot H_2O$, 27.6 gm/liter) with 360 ml 0.2 M Na_2HPO_4 ($NaH_2PO_4 \cdot 7H_2O$, 53.65 gm/liter); dilute to obtain 0.15 M.

Saline: Use 0.15 M NaCl (9 gm/liter NaCl).

McCoy's 5a medium: This medium is available commercially or can be prepared by dissolving McCoy's 5a powdered medium according to the directions and adding 2.2 gm/liter of $NaHCO_3$, 1% L-glutamine 200 mM, 30% heat-inactivated FBS, and Pen-Strept to a final concentration of 100 U/ml and 100 μg/ml, respectively; AB or normal human serum can be substituted for FBS (Section III,B,3).

ACD NIH solution A: Dissolve 4.8 gm citric acid, 13.3 sodium citrate, and 30 gm glucose in 1 liter of distilled water.

AET solution: Dissolve 0.79 gm AET in 20 ml of distilled water and adjust the pH to 9.0 with 10 N NaOH.

Eosin Y solution: Dissolve 25 gm eosin Y in 500 ml distilled water and filter through a 0.45 μm Nalgene filter unit; store the solution at 4°C.

Formaldehyde solution: Add 4 ml of 0.5% phenol red to 1 liter of 37% formaldehyde and add 1 M KOH dropwise to pH 7.2; filter through a 0.45-μm Nalgene filter unit and store at 4°C.

Ficoll-Urovison solution (LSM): Mix 55 gm of Ficoll 400 with 150 ml of Urovison and 800 ml of distilled water and then stir at room temperature in the dark; when the Ficoll is dissolved, adjust the density of the solution to 1.077 by the addition of water; sterilize the mixture by filtration and store in the dark at 4°C; LSM is also commercially available as Lymphodex (Litton Bionetics, Kensington, Maryland), as Lymphoprep (Nyegaard and Co., AS, Oslo, Norway), and as Ficoll-Paque (Pharmacia Fine Chemicals, Uppsala, Sweden).

B. Modifications of the DR-Typing Procedure

Papain stock solution No. P3125 with a protein content of 25 μg/ml (Sigma, St. Louis, Missouri) stored at 4°C.

L-Cysteine-HCl, 2% solution in PBS, kept frozen in small aliquots (BDH Chemicals, Ltd., Poole, England).

Neuraminidase stock solution with a protein content of 50 μg/ml and 0.2 IU/ml (Behringwerke AG, Marburg/Lahn, West Germany).

Nylon wool from Leuko-Pak leukocyte filters code 4C2400 (Fenwal Laboratories, Deerfield, Illinois) boiled in distilled water for 30 min, dried, and scrubbed.

$CrCl_3$ stock solution: $CrCl_3$ (BDH Chemicals, Poole, England) is dissolved in saline to obtain a 1% solution; twice a week for 3 weeks the pH is adjusted to 5 by dropwise addition of 1 M NaOH, and then the solution is stored at room temperature; the pH must not exceed 6, otherwise the $CrCl_3$ will precipitate as chromate.

Plastic tube, 10 × 75 mm, No. 2038 (Falcon Plastics, Division of Bio-Quest, Los Angeles, California).
Hamax plates with 60 rings for Kissmeyer–Nielsen microdroplet method or for the two-color technique, and coverslips, 66.5 × 41 mm (Hamax Industries, AS, Moss, Norway); Hamax plates require Hamilton microsyringes, 25-µl, No. 702N (dispensed volume 0.5 µl per step) and Hamilton Leiden multiple repeating dispensers (space between needles 9 mm): No. 83750 for six 25-ml syringes 702N, No. 83751 for six 50-µl syringes 705N, No. 83753 for six 250-µl syringes 725N.
Trypan blue solution: 1% trypan blue (Fluka AG, Buchs SG, Switzerland) in saline.
Fluorescein diacetate reagent: FDA No. 7378 (Sigma, St. Louis, Missouri) is dissolved at a concentration of 5 mg/ml in acetone and stored at −30°C.
Ethidium bromide solution for fluorochromasia: Ethidium bromide No. E8751 (Sigma, St. Louis, Missouri) is dissolved in PBS to obtain 0.4 mg/ml.
Ethidium bromide stock solution for the two-color technique: Ethidium bromide is dissolved in saline containing 5% EDTA to obtain 0.1 mg/ml; the solution is used diluted 1:70 in saline.
Goat Ig anti-human Ig, FITC-conjugated (Behringwerke AG, Marburg/Lahn, West Germany).
Ficoll–Urovison solution for dead cell removal: 34 gm of Ficoll 400 is mixed with 75 ml of Urovison and with 360 ml of distilled water and then stirred at room temperature in the dark; when the Ficoll is dissolved, the density is adjusted to 1.094 by the addition of water, and the mixture is sterilized by filtration and stored in the dark at 4°C.
Fluorochromasia and two-color techniques require a Zeiss or Leitz inverted microscope equipped with a monochromatic 50-W light source (HBO 50W/ac), a LP455 and SP490 excitation filter combination, a FT520 dichroic mirror, and an LP barrier filter; under these conditions the green fluorescence of the fluorescein and the red fluorescence of the ethidium bromide becomes visible simultaneously.

REFERENCES

Aiuti, F., Cerottini, J. C., Coombs, R. R. A. *et al.* (1974). *Scand. J. Immunol.* **3**, 521.
Albert, E., Amos, D. B., Bodmer, W. F., Ceppellini, R., Dausset, J., Kissmeyer-Nielsen, F., Mayr, W., Payne, R., van Rood, J. J., Terasaki, P. I., and Walford, R. L. (1980). "Histocampatibility Testing" (P. I. Terasaki, ed.), p. 18. UCLA Tissue Typing Laboratory, Los Angeles, California.
Amos, D. B., Bashir, H., Boyle, W., MacQueen, M., and Tiilikainen, A. (1969). *Transplantation* **7**, 220.
Bentwich, Z., Douglas, S. D., Siegal, F. P., and Kunkel, H. G. (1973). *Clin. Immunol. Immunopathol.* **1**, 511.

Bernoco, D., Bernoco, M., Ceppellini, R., Poulik, M. D., Van Leeuwen, A., and van Rood, J. J. (1976). *Tissue Antigens* **8**, 253.

Bodmer, W., Tripp, M., and Bodmer, J. (1967). In "Histocompatibility Testing" (E. S. Curtoni, P. L. Mattiuz, and R. M. Tosi, eds.), p. 341. Munksgaard, Copenhagen.

Bodmer, W. F., Bodmer, J. G., Batchelor, J. R., Festenstein, H., and Morris, P. J., eds. (1977) "Histocompatibility Testing." Munksgaard, Copenhagen.

Brodsky, F. M., Parham, P., Barnstable, C. J., Crumpton, M. J., and Bodmer, W. F. (1979). *Immunol. Rev.* **47**, 3

Celada, F., and Rotman, B. (1966). *Proc. Natl. Acad. Sci. U.S.A.* **57**, 630.

Curtoni, E. S., Scudeller, G., Mattiuz, P. L., Savi, M., Belvedere, M. C., and Ceppellini, R. (1973). *Symp. Ser. Immunobiol. Stand.* **18**, 39.

de Kretser, T. A., Bodmer, J. G., and Bodmer, W. F. (1980). *Tissue Antigens* **16**, 317.

Ferrone, S., Naeim, F., Indivieri, F., Walker, L. E., and Pellegrino, M. A. (1978) *Immunogenetics* **7**, 349.

Francke, U., and Pellegrino, M. A. (1977). *Proc. Natl. Acad. Sci. U.S.A.* **74**, 1147.

Garotta, G., Barbanti, M., Calabi, F., Neri, T. M., Trucco, M. M., and Ceppellini, R. (1980a). In "Histocompatibility Testing" (P. I. Terasaki, ed.), p. 864. UCLA Tissue Typing Laboratory, Los Angeles, California.

Garotta, G., Trucco, M. M., and Ceppellini, R. (1981). In preparation.

Kissmeyer-Nielsen, F., and Kjerbye, K. E. (1967). In "Histocompatibility Testing" (E. S. Curtoni, P. L. Mattiuz, and R. M. Tosi, eds.), p. 381. Munksgaard, Copenhagen.

Köhler, G., and Milstein, C. (1975). *Nature (London)* **256**, 495.

Madsen, M., and Johnsen, H. E. (1979). *J. Immunol. Methods* **27**, 61.

Madsen, M., Johnsen, H. E., Hansen, P. W., and Christiansen, S. E. (1980). *J. Immunol. Methods* **33**, 323.

Park, M. S., Terasaki, P. I., Nakata, S., and Aoki, D. (1980). In "Histocompatibility Testing" (P. I. Terasaki, ed.), p. 854. UCLA Tissue Typing Laboratory, Los Angeles, California.

Poulik, M. D., Ferrone, S., Pellegrino, M. A., Sevier, D. F., Oh, S. K., and Reisfeld, R. A. (1974). *Transplant. Rev.* **21**, 106.

Ray, J. G., Hare, D. B., Pederson, P. D., and Kayhoe, D. A., eds. (1974). "Manual of Tissue Typing Techniques," NIAID Transplants Immunol. Branch DHEW. Publ. No. (NIH) 75-545. USDHEW, Washington, D. C.

Reinherz, E. L., Kung, P. C., Goldstein, G., and Schlossman, S. F. (1979). *J. Immunol.* **123**, 1312.

Rice, C. E. (1948). *J. Immunol.* **59**, 365.

Stocker, J. W., Garotta, G., Hausmann, B., Trucco, M., and Ceppellini, R. (1979). *Tissue Antigens* **13**, 212.

Suciu-Foca, N., Godfrey, M., Rohowsky, C., Khan, R., Susinno, E., and Hardy, M. (1980). In "Histocompatibility Testing" (P. I. Terasaki, ed.), p. 881. UCLA Tissue Typing Laboratory, Los Angeles, California.

Terasaki, P. I., and McClelland, J. D. (1964). *Nature (London)* **204**, 998.

Terasaki, P. I., Bernoco, D., Park, M. S., Ozturk, G., and Iwaki, Y. (1978). *Am. J. Clin. Pathol.* **69**, 103.

Thorsby, E., and Kissmeyer-Nielsen, F. (1969). *Vox Sang.* **17**, 102.

Trucco, M. M., Stocker, J. W., and Ceppellini, R. (1978). *Nature (London)* **273**, 666.

Trucco, M. M., Garotta, G., Stocker, J. W., and Ceppellini, R. (1979). *Immunol. Rev.* **47**, 219.

van Rood, J. J., Van Leeuwen, A., Porlevliet, J., Termijtelen, A., and Keuning, J. J. (1975). In "Histocompatibility Testing" (F. Kissmeyer-Nielsen, ed.), p. 629. Munksgaard, Copenhagen.

van Rood, J. J., Van Leeuwen, A., and Ploem, J. S. (1976). *Nature (London)* **262**, 795.

9

The Protein A Plaque Assay for the Detection of Immunoglobulin-Secreting Cells

Rosa R. Bernabé, Margaretha Tuneskog,
Luciana Forni, Carlos Martinez-A.,
Dan Holmberg, Fredrick Ivars, and António Coutinho

I. INTRODUCTION

Protein A is a major component of the cell wall of *Staphylococcus aureus,* which has an affinity for the Fc region of immunoglobulin G (IgG) of some species, including humans, rabbits, and mice (Sjöquist *et al.,* 1967). This property of staphylococcal protein A (SPA) has made it a very useful tool in the purification of classes and subclasses of Ig's and as a detecting reagent when labeled with fluorochromes or radioactive iodine (Goding, 1978).

The protein A plaque assay was introduced as a simple method for

IMMUNOLOGICAL METHODS, VOL. II

enumerating Ig-secreting cells, regardless of the combining site specificity of the secreted antibodies (Gronowicz *et al.*, 1976). Protein A-coated erythrocytes were used as indicators of the reactions between secreted Ig and anti-Ig "developing antibodies," in view of the above-mentioned property of protein A to bind the Fc region of IgG in some species (Sjöquist *et al.*, 1967). The advantage of this method over the previously described "reverse plaque assay" (Molinaro *et al.*, 1974) was that affinity purification of anti-Ig antibodies, required by the latter, was not necessary in the protein A assay. As the detection of plaque depends solely upon the specificity of the developing antiserum, isotype-specific assays could be performed, and it was thought plausible that this assay would be applicable to any molecule secreted in sufficient amounts and for which a specific developing antiserum was available. Examples of these assays have now appeared in the literature.

In this chapter we shall discuss our experience in dealing with the practical details of this assay.

II. REAGENTS

A. Staphylococcal Protein A–Red Cells

Sheep erythrocytes (SRBCs) kept in Alsever's solution at 4°C for periods from 1 week to 1 month are washed three times in 10–20 vol of saline (600 gm). Chromium chloride is diluted 1:200 in saline from a 0.05 M stock solution. Ten volumes of chromium chloride are mixed first with 1 vol of a solution of SPA (Pharmacia) in saline at 0.5 mg/ml and then with 1 vol of packed red cells. The mixture is incubated for 1 hr at 30°C in a water bath with occasional mixing, then washed once in saline and twice in balanced salt solution (BSS), and finally resuspended 1:4 in BSS. Erythrocytes become slightly "sticky" after coupling, but the presence of either lysis or visible agglutinates of any size during the washings is an indication of poor coupling. The age of the red cells is the important factor in these problems. Erythrocytes from all sheep donors tried gave satisfactory results, as well as erythrocytes from other species, such as horse and donkey. The age of the stock solution of chromium chloride does not appear to influence the coupling reaction either. There is an absolute requirement for normal saline (0.15 M NaCl) in washing the erythrocytes and during the coupling, since phosphate ions abolish chromium chloride reactivity in this reaction. Coupled red cells may be kept in BSS at 4°C for periods up to 1 week without changing properties, if there is no visible lysis and if the cells are extensively washed immediately prior to the assays. Conservation of coupled red cells might be improved in 1% $MgSO_4$ solutions in saline.

B. Agar

Bacto-agar (Difco) (0.5% in BSS preferably buffered with phosphates) containing phenol red or any other pH indicator. The agar is dissolved by boiling it until it is completely clear and kept at 46°C in a water bath. The solution should be used in the next 6–8 hr after preparation, and the presence of visible precipitates makes it unsuitable. After equilibration at 46°C, a solution of DEAE–dextran (Pharmacia) at 50 μg/ml in BSS or phosphate-buffered saline (PBS) is added with simultaneous mixing to a final concentration of 0.75 μg/ml. Upon addition of DEAE–dextran, the clear agar solution becomes milky. Obviously, α-1,6-dextran-specific plaque-forming cells (PFCs) will not be detectable as Ig-secreting PFCs under these conditions because of inhibition of diffusion of the secreted Ig's. This may be a problem, particularly when testing cell lines with this specificity, and can be obviated by adapting the method in Cunningham's system (Cunningham et al., 1966).

C. Complement

Normal guinea pig serum is obtained from Gibco or Behringwerke, or prepared by pooling sera from at least 50 animals. Each batch of freshly prepared (or reconstituted) serum is frozen in small aliquots and kept at −20°C for periods up to 1 month without loss of activity. The serum is thawed and diluted with cold BSS immediately before the assays and, if kept on ice, can be used for the next 12 hr. Diluted complement cannot be saved by refreezing. The appropriate dilution of each new batch of complement must be tested in parallel with a previously tested batch in the standard assay. Of many different batches tested to date, all proved suitable for use in this assay, without any need for prior absorption, in final dilutions ranging from 1:60 to 1:150. Supraoptimal concentrations of complement may result in partial lysis of the red cell monolayer, while the plaques obtained with suboptimal concentrations are smaller and require long incubation periods. On the other hand, the titration curves are usually quite flat, allowing for a considerable variation in the final concentrations (see below).

D. Developing Antisera

Rabbit antisera or immune sera from any other species binding SPA are titrated for optimal PFC development and controlled for specificity using myeloma or Ig-secreting hybridoma cell lines. Because most of the antisera are used in isotype-specific plaque assays, the simple titration for optimal PFC numbers with normal or stimulated plasma cell-containing populations is not sufficient. If no Ig-secreting cell lines are available, anti-IgM developing antisera can be tested by using normal spleen cells stimulated by lipopolysaccharide (LPS) in culture at a concentration of 10^6 cells/ml [see Coutinho (1976) for standard culture conditions]. Over 95% of all PFCs in these populations after a 72-hr culture are IgM-secreting. The tests for IgG subclasses, however, necessarily require cell lines.

Practically all our experience concerns rabbit antisera to mouse Ig subclasses. Although all antisera will reveal PFCs at appropriate dilutions, the numbers and morphological quality of the plaques vary greatly. In assessing the efficiency of PFC development, it is advisable to perform simultaneously a test for intracytoplasmic Ig of the same isotype in the cell population used to test the antisera by immunofluorescence. Simple viable cell counts are a poor indication, since in all cell populations, including cloned cell lines, a variable proportion of all cells are not Ig secretors at any given point in time. In principle, the SPA plaque assay should reveal as many PFCs as the number of cells in the same population containing intracytoplasmic Ig's.

Another method to calculate the efficiency of isotype-specific SPA-PFC assays is to plaque antibody-secreting hybridoma cells of known specificity in parallel on antigen-coated red cells or in the SPA assay. An example is shown in Table I. Two hybridoma cell lines, secreting TNP-specific IgM molecules, gave relative efficiencies in the two tests of 68% and 98%. Such a difference in relative efficiency could be due to the affinity of the secreted antibodies and to the different amounts of Ig secreted by single cells. In fact, if the antibody has very high affinity, the plaque assay on antigen-coated red cells could be more sensitive in detecting cells secreting small amounts of Ig; thus the relative efficiency will be lower than for a cell

TABLE I

Comparison of Efficiency of PFC Detection by Conventional Antigen-Specific or SPA-Isotype Specific Plaque Assays

Antibody-secreting cells[a]	Number of cells plated	PFC/plate on:			Relative efficiency (%)
		SRBC	TNP-SRBC[b]	SPA + anti-IgM	
TNP-11	1000	0	540	368	68
SP/603	100	0	63	62	98

[a] The hybridoma lines were kindly provided by Drs P. -A. Cazenave and G. Köhler.
[b] The cells were plaqued on SRBC derivatized with various amounts of TNP, namely 3, 10, and 30 mg of TNBS per ml of packed red cells. The numbers indicated are averages of those detected on each of the three types of target cells, since both cell lines secrete antibodies lysing all three targets; however, the plaquing conditions may lead to small variations in the numbers of PFC detected on each target.

population secreting low affinity antibodies. In addition, differences in relative efficiencies will be averaged in polyclonal populations. While efficiency may vary with different isotypes, in our experience all Ig classes and subclasses are detected with efficiencies greater than 50%, IgM PFC detection often approaching 90%.

If the quality or number of PFCs obtained with a particular developing antiserum is not satisfactory, improvement can be obtained by prior purification of SPA-binding antibodies on a protein A–Sepharose immunoadsorbent (Goding, 1976). It has been recently observed that SPA-selected antibodies will develop clearer and larger PFCs and that the inhibition of PFC numbers observed at supraoptimal concentrations of antiserum is lost (Fig. 1). Neither the titer nor the optimal number of PFCs revealed is much affected by the procedure. These effects are likely to be due to inhibition of the activity of SPA-binding antibody classes by other antibodies in the antisera which do not bind SPA at the pH of the assay. The inhibition of PFC development in the region of antibody excess, described earlier as a "prozone" effect, is therefore probably not due to the requirement for a critical size of complexes for binding to SPA but rather to competition with non-SPA-binding antibodies.

The original description of the SPA plaque assay for isotype-specific PFCs involved the use of antisera made class-specific by appropriate absorption. We have found however, that in many cases unabsorbed antisera, while not isotype-specific when tested in fluorescence or even in double immune diffusion, have proved satisfactorily specific in PFC development. This is probably due to the relatively high final dilution of the antisera in

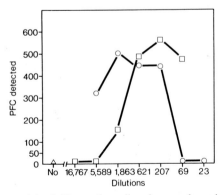

Fig. 1. Cell cultures containing IgM-secreting cells only were plaqued, using for development a rabbit anti-MOPC-104E antiserum at the indicated dilutions (circles) or rabbit IgG prepared by the same antiserum by chromatography on protein A–Sepharose (squares). The plaque morphology was very clearly improved using SPA-binding antibodies.

the PFC assay, with a consequent subthreshold dilution of contaminating antibodies (mostly anti-light chain). We routinely immunize rabbits with the mouse myeloma proteins MOPC-104E, MOPC-21, UPC-10, MOPC-195, FLOPC-21, and MOPC-315 in order to obtain developing antisera to IgM, IgG_1, IgG_{2a}, IgG_{2b}, IgG_3, and IgA, respectively. After the third or fourth boost, most antisera can be used at such high dilutions that they are operationally class-specific in the plaque assay. It should be clear, however, that at higher concentrations contaminating antibodies will also be detected. Figure 2 shows an example of these operational specificities. IgG_{2a}- and IgG_{2b}-secreting hybridomas (kindly provided by M. Trucco) were plaqued with unabsorbed anti-UPC-10 and anti-MOPC-195, both being x-bearing and showing known isotype cross-reactivity higher than that of any other pair of Ig classes. Unabsorbed anti-UPC-10 serum at optimal dilutions for IgG_{2a} PFCs shows less than 10% cross-reactivity with IgG_{2b}-secreting cells. On the other hand, anti-MOPC-195 had to be absorbed or used at concentrations suboptimal for IgG_{2b}-PFC development. Even in this case, however, at optimally developing concentrations, only 34% of the PFCs with the cross-reacting isotype are detected.

In addition to isotype-specific PFCs, it might be convenient to detect total Ig-secreting cells. This can be conveniently done by the use of rabbit anti-mouse total IgG raised by injection of commercially available IgG. These antisera always contain sufficient titer of anti-light chain antibodies to allow development of IgM-secreting PFCs in addition to all other IgG subclasses. Table II shows that an appropriate concentration of such an an-

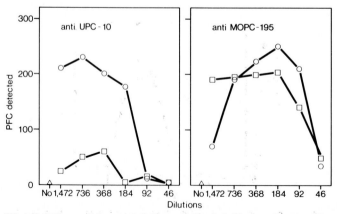

Fig. 2. (Circles) IgG_{2a}- and (squares) IgG_{2b}-secreting hybridoma cells were plaqued in the presence of the indicated concentration of *unabsorbed* rabbit antisera prepared against UPC-10 and MOPC-195 myeloma proteins, respectively.

TABLE II

Comparison of the Efficiency of Plaque-Forming Cell Detection by Anti-Class Antisera and of an Antiserum to Mouse IgG

Specificity of the antiserum	Antigen used for immunization		PFCs per spleen[a]
Anti-μ	MOPC-104E		106,000
Anti-γ1	MOPC-21		6,325
Anti-γ2a[b]	UPC-10		62,350
Anti-γ2b[b]	MOPC-195		12,825
Anti-γ3	FLOPC-21		1,210
Anti-α	MOPC—315		27,300
		Total PFCs	216,010
Anti-total Ig's	Mouse IgG		229,000

[a] CBA/J, 3 months old.

[b] An antiserum raised against a mixture of UPC-10 and MOPC-195 detected 72,200 PFCs per spleen, compared to the 75,175 detected separately by anti-UPC-10 and anti-MOPC-195.

tiserum does in fact develop all PFCs that can be detected in a mixture of secretors of all isotypes with individual class-specific reagents. As also shown in the table, an antiserum prepared by immunizing with a mixture of UPC-10 and MOPC-195 detects all $IgG_{2(a + b)}$-secreting PFCs. It is also possible to perform assays for total IgG-secreting PFCs, but this has to be done by mixing appropriate dilutions of the different class-specific antisera rather than by absorbing anti-total IgG antisera to decrease the number of anti-light chain antibodies. Whenever mixing antisera that have been titrated and controlled for operational specificity in separate, it should be considered that anti-light chain or other contaminating antibodies present in the sera might reach effective concentrations and develop PFCs of undesired specificities. It is mandatory, therefore, to control for operational specificities also in mixtures of antisera. Out of a number of anti-$\varkappa$ antisera tested while developing PFCs with variable efficiencies, none has been found to reveal satisfactorily all $\varkappa$-secreting cells (that is at least 90–95% of all Ig secretors in the mouse). Developing antisera, after testing for titer and specificity, are frozen in small aliquots, kept at 20°C for indefinite periods of time, and appropriately diluted before use. Antisera prepared in species whose IgG does not bind SPA at physiological pH are obviously unsuitable for use as developing antisera. These include goat and sheep antisera very often used to prepare anti-mouse and anti-human antibodies.

III. CELL SUSPENSIONS

In vitro cultured cells or cell suspensions obtained from lymphoid tissues are washed in cold BSS (200 gm) and suspended to appropriate concentrations resulting in between 50 and 200 PFCs per plate. This might be difficult to achieve for those not acquainted with the method. As a rough estimate, a spleen from a normal unprimed adult mouse contains between 80,000 and 500,000 IgM-secreting PFCs (depending on the environmental conditions of the animal colony, on bacterial flora, in particular, and on the age and strain), 3000–15,000 IgG_1-, 20,000–80,000 IgG_2-, 1000–5000 IgG_3-, and 10,000–80,000 IgA-secreting cells.

A culture of 6×10^4 normal spleen cells stimulated by LPS in 0.2-ml volumes (Coutinho, 1976) contains roughly 30,000–50,000 IgM-secreting PFCs by day 4 or 5 of culture. While 50–200 PFCs per plate are optimal numbers for detection and counting, up to 500 PFCs per plate can still be easily counted and reveal correct numbers of secreting cells. Numbers higher than these, however, cannot be accepted, as there will be inhibition of both the size and number of PFCs detected.

Washed cell suspensions are kept in BSS on ice until tested. The PFCs detected in concentrated cell suspensions (3×10^6/ml) will be reasonably stable on ice up to 3–4 hr (maximum decrease 10–15%), while PFCs in diluted cell suspensions, for example, cells harvested from cultures, will rapidly "disappear," even if kept on ice. Cultures have to be appropriately washed, particularly if large numbers of Ig-secreting cells are present in the culture or if anti-mouse Ig reagents have been included in the culture. This is because soluble mouse Ig will obviously inhibit the development of PFCs in the SPA assay.

IV. PLAQUING PROCEDURE

The test is performed under nonsterile conditions, but all the stock reagents—in particular BSS, DEAE–dextran, SRBCs, and developing antisera—should be kept sterile, otherwise bacterial hemolytic plaques will develop upon incubation and these might be difficult to distinguish from true PFCs. In a standard test, the following reagents are added to hemolysis tubes kept on ice: (1) 100 μl of the cell suspension to be tested; for convenience this can be varied from 20 to 120 μl without affecting the efficiency of the method; (2) 20–25 μl SPA-coated SRBCs; (3) 20–25 μl complement; (4) 20–25 μl developing antisera.

After a few minutes on the bench, the mixture is vortexed in the tube and 0.3 ml of agar (kept at 46°C) is added. The tube is then quickly shaken by hand, and its contents poured into a 9-cm-diameter plastic petri dish and spread in a spot of 6–7 cm diameter using the edge of the same hemolysis tube. Both the "top" and "bottom" of the petri dishes should be used to spread a spot, as these provide by themselves necessary humidification during the incubation period. For this purpose, it is recommended to use petri dishes that close tightly and are designed not to permit ventilation. After a few minutes in an undisturbed position, the petri dishes are closed and should be brought within 5–10 min into a humidified bacteriological incubator kept at 37°C. The plates are incubated for a minimum of 3 hr to a maximum of 6 hr, depending on the efficiency of PFC development for each isotype. Periods of incubation longer than 6 hr are unsuitable, as bacterial growth might interfere with the test. The plates should be spread inside the incubator to allow uniform and rapid equilibration at 37°C of all the plates. Under suboptimal conditions (of complement in particular) it might be observed that top and bottom duplicates show considerable differences in the number and size of PFCs. This may be corrected by turning over the plates after a 30-min incubation on one side and by piling them up thereafter. It is critical that a humidified atmosphere be maintained in the incubator.

For plaquing large numbers of samples the following procedure may be followed: The aliquots of cell suspension and red cells are added to the tubes which are kept on ice up to 30–60 min. Racks with 36–50 tubes are taken from the ice one by one, and a mixture of complement and developing antisera (that may be kept for several hours) is distributed to all tubes with automatic dispensers. All the tubes in one rack are then plaqued. Mixtures of indicator red cells and developing antiserum, however, cannot be kept for longer than 10–15 min.

Problems that might arise include:

1. Visible agglutinates in the red cell suspensions; these may be checked by spreading agar containing erythrocytes on a plate before starting the test, which also allows one to assess whether the red cell concentration and the color of the monolayer are suitable.

2. "Clumps" in the agar, in spite of the fact that the agar solution was clear; this is due to a slightly low temperature of the water bath, to slowness in the spreading on the plates, or to the fact that the glass tubes were kept for too long on ice and were not equilibrated at room temperature before addition of the agar. Hemolysis tubes more than 4–5 cm long should not be used for this reason. Nonhomogeneous solidification of the agar should be avoided, as small "precipitates" could be confused with PFCs.

3. "Bubbles" in the monolayer; large bubbles, formed during the spread of the agar are not particularly disturbing. Small bubbles, however, which are formed during the vortexing of the tubes before spreading can also be

difficult to distinguish from PFCs, and therefore protein supplementation of the plaquing medium should be avoided and the tubes vortexed before addition of the agar.

V. COUNTING OF PLAQUE-FORMING CELLS

After incubation, the plaques are counted in a plaque counter under low (2–4×) magnification and indirect light. SPA-PFCs in general are morphologically more homogeneous than antigen-specific PFCs. Their size shows little variation and, primarily, they are never totally clear; that is, lysis of the red cell monolayer is never complete and the plaques appear slightly "foggy." Fully transparent, clear plaques in the monolayer are almost always either air bubbles or the result of bacterial activity. After incubation at 37°C the plates may be kept at 4°C for periods of up to 3–4 days.

VI. GENERAL COMMENTS

The same reagents, at appropriate concentrations, reveal very similar numbers of PFCs when used in the Cunningham liquid layer plaque assay (R. Benner, personal communication). These, however, must be read immediately after incubation.

Most commercially available rabbit antisera have proved appropriate for use in the SPA plaque assay with human as well as mouse Ig-secreting cells. Rabbit antiallotype antisera have also been used successfully in detecting rabbit Ig-secreting PFCs.

It is obvious that, in so far as the efficiencies of PFC detection are not 100%, this method requires improvement and it cannot be taken *a priori* as detecting *all* Ig-secreting cells.

VII. APPENDIX

Myeloma cell lines, secreting Ig's of different classes, can be obtained from the Cell Distribution Center of the Salk Institute, San Diego, California.

Myelomas carried *in vivo* as subcutaneous tumors can be obtained from Litton Bionetics, Kensington, Maryland.

Myeloma proteins, either purified or in serum or ascites fluid are available from Litton Bionetics, Kensington, Maryland.

Anti-Ig antisera: We use the following schedule of immunization for preparation of rabbit antisera to mouse IgG or to mouse myeloma proteins:

1. One milligram antigen in 1 ml saline, emulsified with 1 ml complete Freund's adjuvant, injected subcutaneously and intramuscularly into at least four sites.
2. After 1 month, 500 μg antigen emulsified in incomplete Freund's adjuvant.
3. After another month, 100 μg alum precipitate.
4. First bleed (50 ml blood); the rabbits are then boosted every month with 100 μg alum-precipitated antigen and bled (50 ml) 1 and 2 weeks thereafter.

Since a careful titration is quite laborious, it is advisable to collect three or four bleeds (about 100 ml) of antiserum before performing it, in order to have a batch of titrated serum that can be used over many months.

The titrated sera are divided into small aliquots and kept frozen at $-20°C$. The serum is diluted in BSS when needed and Millipore-filtered before use. Diluted antisera can be kept at 4°C for a maximum of 2 weeks.

ACKNOWLEDGMENT

Part of this work has been supported by the Swedish Medical Research Council.

REFERENCES

Coutinho, A. (1976). *Scand. J. Immunol.* **5,** 129.
Cunningham, A. J., Smith, J. B., and Mercer, E. N. (1966). *J. Exp. Med.* **124,** 701.
Goding, J. (1976). *J. Immunol. Methods* **13,** 215.
Goding, J. (1978). *J. Immunol. Methods* **20,** 241.
Gronowicz, E., Coutinho, A., and Melchers, F. (1976). *Eur. J. Immunol.* **6,** 558.
Molinaro, G. A., Maron, A., and Dray, S. (1974). *Proc. Natl. Acad. Sci. U.S.A.* **71,** 1229.
Sjöquist, J., Forsgren, A., Gustafson, G. T., and Stalenheim, G. (1967). *Cold Spring Harbor Symp. Quant. Biol.* **32,** 577.

10

In Vitro Production and Testing of Antigen-Induced Mediators of Helper T-Cell Function

Sarah Howie

I. INTRODUCTION

Three classes of cell-free supernatants derived from murine lymphocytes which can replace helper T cells in the antibody response have been described: (1) those from allogeneically stimulated lymphocytes, (2) those from mitogen-stimulated lymphocytes, and (3) those from antigen-stimulated lymphocytes. Some of the characteristics of these helper supernatants are compared in Table I.

The use of such supernatants allows the activation of B cells to be studied *in vitro* in the absence of helper T cells and allows aspects of T- and B-cell interaction to be studied in detail.

This chapter deals with an *in vitro* method for inducing from unprimed lymphocytes a helper factor which is antigen-specific and non-H-2-restricted.

IMMUNOLOGICAL METHODS, VOL. II

TABLE I

Comparison of Some Characteristics of Helper Supernatants

Type of stimulus	Functional characteristics of help	Reference
Allogeneic cells	Antigen nonspecific, non-H-2-restricted	Dutton *et al.*, 1971; Schimpl and Wecker, 1972
Allogeneic cells	Antigen nonspecific, H-2-restricted	Armerding and Katz, 1974
T-cell mitogens	Antigen nonspecific, non-H-2-restricted	
Antigen	Antigen-nonspecific, non-H-2-restricted	Waldmann and Munro, 1973
Antigen	Antigen-specific, non-H-2-restricted	Taussig, 1974; McDougall and Gordon, 1977; Howie and Feldmann, 1977

II. MATERIALS

Culture medium: RPMI 1640 or Eagle's minimal essential medium, penicillin, streptomycin, L-glutamine, and fetal calf serum (FCS) available from Gibco Biochemicals, Ltd., and 2-mercaptoethanol, from BDH Chemicals Ltd., Poole, England
Tissue cultures:
Humidified CO_2 incubator
Dry incubator with rocking platform
Marbrook cultures:
Dialysis membrane (Union Carbide Corp., Chicago, Illinois) or Nucleopore membrane (Millipore SA, Molsheim, France)
Silicon rubber tubing
Large Marbrook cultures
10-cm-diameter Pyrex crystallization dishes
15-cm-diameter Pyrex ramekin dishes
Specially made glass inserts
Medium-sized Marbrook cultures:
30-ml sterile plastic Universal bottles (No. 128A, Sterilin United Kingdom, Ltd.)
Silicon rubber corks
Cotton wool
Specially made glass inserts
A ready-made culture apparatus of this type is also available from Corning.

Small Marbrook cultures:
  24-well Costar tissue culture plates (No. 3524)
  Selectapette pipette tips (No. 4696, Becton Dickinson, Ltd.)
  Specially made autoclaveable plastic plates
Mini-Mishell–Dutton cultures:
  Flat-bottomed microtiter plates (No. 3040F, Falcon)
Mice and antigens: The choice of these is left to the investigator. I have
  had experience with the following antigens: keyhole limpet hemocyanin
  (KLH) (Calbiochem) as a slurry (the lyophilized antigen is not ap-
  propriate for these purposes); the synthetic polymers (T,G)-A—L and
  GAT[10] (Miles Yeda Products, Ltd., Rehovot, Israel.)
Plaque assay:
  Cunningham assay chambers each consisting of two glass slides held
  together with double-sided adhesive tape
  Sheep red blood cells
  Picrylsulfonic acid (TNBS)
  Cacodylate buffer, pH 6.9
  Glycylglycine
  Guinea pig complement

III. USE OF THE MARBROOK CULTURE SYSTEM FOR INDUCING ANTIGEN-SPECIFIC HELPER SUPERNATANTS

Two basic technologies for growing lymphocytes *in vitro* have been described, the Mishell–Dutton culture system and the Marbrook culture system. For reasons which remain unclear, the Mishell–Dutton culture system does not allow the induction of antigen-specific helper supernatants and the Marbrook system must be employed.

The Marbrook culture system was first described in 1967. Basically it consists of two chambers, an inner and an outer, separated by a semipermeable membrane (Fig. 1). A dialysis membrane is routinely used, but Nucleopore membranes may also be used. Cells are grown in a small volume of medium in the inner chamber which is immersed in a larger volume of fluid in the outer chamber. The volumes naturally depend on the size of the culture system employed, but the ratio of inner to outer fluid should not exceed 1:5 for optimal results, and a ratio of 1:10 is routinely used.

A. Production of Antigen-Specific Helper Factor

These conditions were originally developed using a medium-sized Marbrook apparatus (Fig. 2). This consists of a sterile plastic Universal bottle or

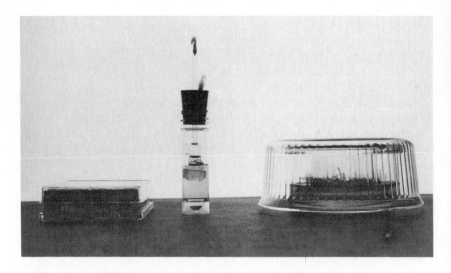

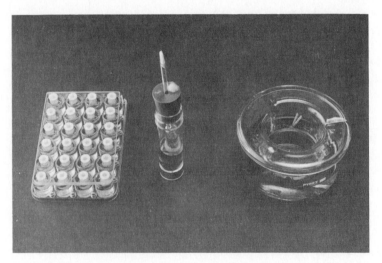

Fig. 1.   Small, medium-sized, and large Marbrook tissue culture apparatus.

a similar sterilizeable glass bottle, a specially made glass insert (which may be replaced by 1-cm-diameter glass tubing of Pyrex quality), and a silicon rubber cork specially bored to hold the insert and having a second hole for ease of gas exchange in the incubator. Silicon rubber is chosen because it is nontoxic to the cells, however, other types of corks may be used but should be tested for toxicity by incubating small pieces with the cells and checking

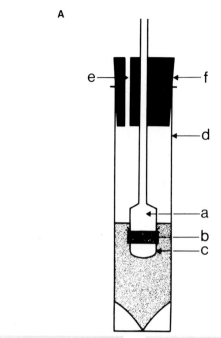

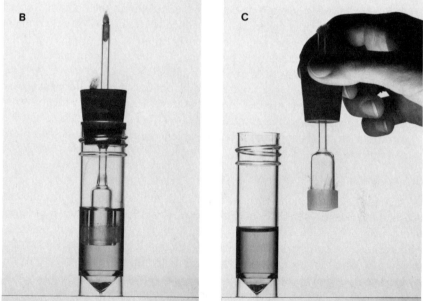

Fig. 2. Medium-sized Marbrook culture apparatus. (A) Diagrammatic representation: a, glass insert containing cell suspension; b, silicon rubber ring; c, dialysis membrane; d, Sterilin Universal bottle containing medium; e, air outlet; f, silicon rubber cork. (B and C) Photographs of actual apparatus used; see text for details.

for cell viability. After 4 days the expected viable cell recovery is 20–40% of the original number of cells cultured.

1. Preparation of the Culture Flasks

A dialysis membrane is cut to fit over the end of the insert and boiled in distilled water four or five times or until it no longer has an odor. The boiled dialysis membrane is fitted over the end of the insert and held tightly in place, either by a rubber ring or by a piece of 1-cm-diameter silicon rubber tubing. Tubing is preferred because it can be cut to make thicker rings than are commercially available and it is advisable to have the dialysis membrane as closely bound to the insert as possible to avoid nondialysis transfer of material into and out of the inner chamber. The tubing should also be boiled before use. It is convenient to boil it with the dialysis membrane. The open end of the insert and the air exchange outlet in the cork are plugged with cotton wool, and the entire apparatus is sterilized by autoclaving.

2. Use of the Culture Flasks

Culture medium (10 ml) is pipetted into a sterile plastic Universal bottle. The lid of the bottle is discarded and replaced by the sterile insert so that the dialysis membrane is beneath the level of the medium in the outer chamber. At this stage the inner chamber can be checked for leaks, as it should remain fluid-free if the membrane is intact. Then 1–1.5 ml of cell suspension is introduced into the inner chamber by means of a sterile Pasteur pipette. It is convenient to use tubing to attach a 2-ml plastic syringe to the end of the Pasteur pipette instead of a pipette bulb to obtain an accurate measure of the volume introduced into the inner chamber. The insert is plugged with sterile cotton wool, and the culture is ready to be incubated. These culture flasks are a bit top-heavy, and it is advisable to support them in a test tube rack at all stages.

3. Induction of Antigen-Specific Helper Factor

A single-cell suspension is made from fresh mouse spleens. The cells are washed by centrifugation at 1100 rpm for 10 min either at room temperature or in a refrigerated centrifuge at 4°C. The cell pellet is resuspended in culture medium (RPMI 1640 or Eagle's minimal essential medium) containing supplementary penicillin (200 U/ml), streptomycin (100 μg/ml), 20 mM L-glutamine, 10^{-5} M 2-mercaptoethanol, and FCS. The optimal amount of FCS depends on the batch but is normally between 2 and 10%. The cells are counted using a viable cell stain and made up to 10^7 viable cells/ml (the cell density can be within the range 5×10^6 to 1.5×10^7 cells/ml without seriously affecting the culture conditions). Antigen is added to the cell suspension, the amount varying with the antigen; e.g., for KLH 0.1 μg/ml is used, whereas for the synthetic polymers (T,G)-A—L and GAT[10] 1 μg/ml is used. The cell suspension is then introduced into the Marbrook flasks as described above.

The induction of helper factor is accomplished in two stages. In the first stage helper cells are induced; this requires 4 days' incubation at 37°C in a humidified incubator with 5% CO_2. At the end of the 4 days the cells are

TABLE II

Comparison of Helper Cells Generated in Large, Medium, and Small Marbrook Flasks

Cell type	IgM anti-DNP PFCs/10⁶ cells		
Spleen cells with no antigen	4		
Spleen cells plus DNP–KLH	20		

	IgM anti-DNP PFCs/10⁶ cells		
	Large	Medium	Small
Spleen cells plus DNP–KLH			
Plus helper cells, 2.5 × 10⁵/ml	188	240	256
Plus helper cells, 1.25 × 10⁵/ml	240	232	292
Plus helper cells, 3 × 10⁴/ml	0	96	32

TABLE III

Comparison of Helper Factors Generated in Large, Medium, and Small Marbrook Flasks [a]

Cell type	IgM anti-DNP PFCs/10⁶ cells		
Spleen cells with no antigen	4		
Spleen cells plus DNP–KLH	16		

	IgM anti-DNP PFCs/10⁶ cells		
	Large	Medium	Small
Spleen cells plus DNP–KLH			
Plus helper factor, 1:30	300	224	300
Plus helper factor, 1:300	272	240	236
Plus helper factor, 1:3000	88	78	20

[a] Helper factors assayed in 200-μl mini-Mishell–Dutton cultures (2.5 × 10⁶ spleen cells/ml plus 0.3 μg DNP-KLH/ml) harvested on day 4.

harvested and can be used either directly as helper cells or to produce helper factor (Tables II and III). To produce helper factor the cells are extensively washed in serum-free medium and resuspended in culture medium containing *no* FCS. The cells are counted and again made up to 10^7 viable cells/ml with the same amount of antigen as used in the original culture. The cells are then placed in Marbrook flasks such that the medium in the outer chamber contains FCS and the medium in the inner chamber contains cells and antigen but no serum. The cells are then recultured for 18–30 hr. After 30 hr the activity in the supernatant declines, possibly because of a build-up of dead cell products or degradation of the factor. At the end of the second culture period the contents of the inner chamber are harvested, spun for 10 min at 1100 rpm to remove the cells, and then respun at 3000 rpm for 15 min to remove any remaining cell debris. The supernatant is then aliquoted and stored at − 20°C. The cells can be restimulated for 24 hr with fresh antigen to produce a second batch of helper factor.

B. Production of Large Volumes of Supernatant for Biochemical Analysis

The volumes of supernatant obtained from the 1-ml Marbrook cultures described above are necessarily rather small. In order to characterize biochemically and purify the active molecules, large volumes are required. With this in mind, culture flasks capable of holding 3×10^8 cells rather than 10^7 were designed (Fig. 3). The factor limiting the size of these flasks was that the widest commercially available dialysis tubing had a maximum width of approximately 43 mm; slit up one side, it unfolded to give a width of approximately 85 mm so that the largest practical inner chamber diameter was 60 mm. The inner chambers were made from Pyrex-quality glass and designed to fit over 10-cm-diameter Pyrex crystallization dishes.

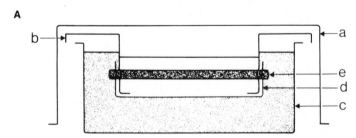

Fig. 3. Large Marbrook apparatus. (A) Diagrammatic representation: a, glass ramekin dish; b, glass insert containing cell suspension; c, crystallization dish containing medium; d, dialysis membrane; e, silicon rubber tubing. (B–D) Photographs of apparatus in use; see text for details.

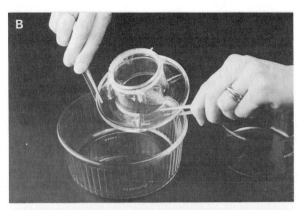

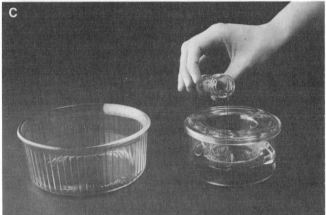

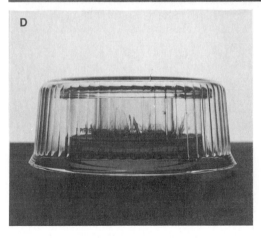

Fig. 3. *(continued)*

The lids of the chambers had to be shorter than the crystallization dishes when in place to avoid contamination by air currents in the incubator, and the most suitable were Pyrex ramekin dishes 15 cm in diameter. These culture flasks hold 30 ml of cell suspension suspended in 150 ml of medium and allow the convenient collection of relatively large volumes of helper factor.

IV. TESTING THE ACTIVITY OF ANTIGEN-SPECIFIC FACTORS

Antigen-specific factors can be tested for their *in vitro* antibody-inducing capacity in either Marbrook or Mishell–Dutton cultures.

If a Marbrook culture system is employed, the most convenient type is the mini-Marbrook system (Fig. 4). This consists of an autoclaveable plastic

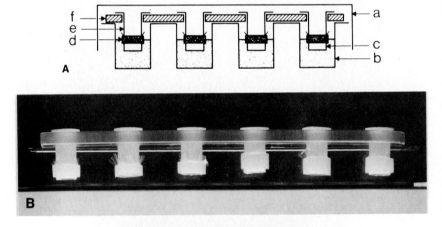

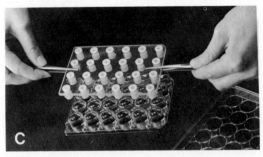

Fig. 4. Small Marbrook tissue culture apparatus. (A) Diagrammatic representation: a, Costar tray lid; b, Costar well containing medium; c, dialysis membrane; d, silicon rubber tubing; e, insert; f, plastic plate supporting inserts. (B and C) Photographs of actual apparatus; see text for details.

plate cut to fit over a 24-well Costar tissue culture plate. Twenty-four holes are drilled in the plate to hold the inserts, which are made from cut-off Selectapette pipette tips. These particular tips are chosen because of the rim around their tops. Dialysis or Nucleopore membranes are fixed to the ends of the pipette tips by silicon rubber tubing. [*Note:* The use of Nucleopore membranes in this culture system affords a quick way of testing whether cells (helpers, suppressors, T-cell hybridomas, etc.) are secreting mediators.] The cells to be tested are grown in the bottom of Costar wells, and the assay cells in the inserts.

The Costar wells are filled with 2.5 ml of medium, and the sterile plate with inserts is placed in position. Then 200 μl of a suspension of 1.5×10^7 viable spleen cells per milliliter plus an appropriate amount of antigen and helper supernatant is placed in each insert. The tray is covered with the lid, and the cultures are incubated for 4 days in a humidified CO_2 incubator. At the end of the culture period the cells in the inserts are harvested and the number of antigen-specific plaques determined by the Cunningham plaque-forming cell assay.

The amounts of antigen, etc., vary with the antigen; to test KLH-specific factors 0.3 μg/ml dinitrophenyl (DNP)-KLH with approximately 36 mol DNP/mol of KLH and dilutions of helper supernatant in the range 10–0.01% by volume are used.

One-milliliter Marbrook cultures can also be used to assay the effect of helper cell supernatants. In this case a cell suspension containing 10^7 viable spleen cells and appropriate amounts of antigen and helper factor is introduced into the inner chamber of the culture flask. The flasks are incubated for 4 days, and the number of plaque-forming cells (PFCs) determined. It should be stressed that the number of plaques per culture obtained in 200-μl and 1-ml Marbrook cultures is approximately the same, so that the smaller culture system, apart from being more economical, is three to five times more efficient for inducing antibody formation. The reason(s) for this discrepancy remain(s) unclear.

However, for the B-cell assay the culture system of choice, both for reasons of economy and culture efficiency, is the mini-Mishell–Dutton type of culture on microtiter plates. This is technically far simpler to work with than the Marbrook system and in terms of the number of plaque-forming cells generated is 5–10 times more efficient than the mini-Marbrook system.

To test KLH helper factor in this system, quadruplicate cultures consisting of 200 μl of a cell suspension of 2.5×10^6 viable spleen cells per milliliter, 0.3 μg DNP-KLH/ml, and an appropriate amount of helper factor in RPMI 1640 medium-containing FCS are incubated for 4 days on flat-bottomed microtiter plates in sealed boxes containing 5% CO_2 on a rocking platform. After 4 days the cultures are harvested and the number of PFCs determined.

The specificity of the helper factors generated in the Marbrook system is tested by incubating cells, helper factor, and inappropriate antigens. It should be noted that these factors do not help nude mouse spleen cells produce a sheep cell response, although they will help them produce a response to the appropriate antigen.

Tables II and III show a comparison of the helper cells and factors produced in all three Marbrook systems described and tested in the mini-Mishell–Dutton system. It can be seen that they are all comparable, and the choice of system used depends on the availability of particular mice and whether the functional or the biochemical properties of the helper factors are to be studied.

In previous studies (Howie and Feldmann, 1977, 1978; Howie *et al.*, 1979) such helper factors were demonstrated to be derived from T cells and to exert their function on B cells indirectly via macrophage accessory cells. By the use of appropriate immunoadsorbent columns they were also demonstrated to have antigen-binding capacity and to carry immune-associated (Ia) antigens belonging to the carbohydrate rather than the protein series of polymorphic Ia antigens.

V. PLAQUE ASSAY

To determine the number of DNP-specific immunoglobulin M (IgM) antibody-secreting cells in the assay cultures the Cunningham plaque assay is used.

The cultures are harvested and resuspended to an appropriate volume (it is convenient to count between 50 and 150 plaques per chamber). In most cases the cultures are resuspended in their original volume of balanced salt solution (BSS). For every culture both the number of plaques with uncoupled sheep erythrocytes (background plaques) and the number of plaques with trinitrophenyl (TNP)-conjugated sheep erythrocytes (TNP-SRBCs) are determined. The number of hapten-specific plaques is calculated by subtracting the number of background plaques from the number of plaques to TNP-SRBCs.

In this assay the following procedure is used to couple TNP to SRBCs. The SRBCs are washed three times with BSS or phosphate-buffered saline (PBS). An appropriate amount of SRBCs is made up to 20% in cacodylate buffer, pH 6.8, and mixed with an equal volume of a 2 mg/ml solution of picrylsulfonic acid in cacodylate buffer for 10 min at room temperature. The cells are then washed once with glycylglycine (2 mg/ml in BSS) and then three times with BSS or PBS.

VI. SUMMARY

In summary, antigen-specific helper supernatants (or helper factors) capable of replacing helper T cells *in vitro* can be induced *in vitro* in the Marbrook tissue culture system. However, it should be stressed that the relative technical complexity of the system requires that a great deal of care be applied to details, e.g., a dialysis membrane which is not sufficiently washed, the wrong type of rubber cork, the wrong type of tubing for holding the dialysis membrane can be toxic to the cells in culture and lead to disappointing results.

REFERENCES

Armerding, D., and Katz, D. H. (1974). Activation of T and B lymphocytes *in vitro*. II. Biological and biochemical properties of an allogeneic effect factor (AEF) active in triggering specific B lymphocytes. *J. Exp. Med.* **140**, 19–37.

Dutton, R. W., Falkoff, R., Hirst, J. A., Hoffman, M., Kappler, J. W., Kettman, J. R., Lesley, J. F., and Vann, D. (1971). Is there evidence for a non-antigen specific diffusible chemical mediator from the thymus derived cell in the initiation of the immune response? *In* "Progress in Immunology" (B. Amos, ed.), p. 355. Academic Press, New York.

Howie, S., and Feldmann, M. (1977). *In vitro* studies on H-2 linked unresponsiveness to synthetic polypeptides. III. Production of an antigen specific T helper cell factor to (T,G)-A—L. *Eur. J. Immunol.* **7**, 417–421.

Howie, S., and Feldmann, M. (1978). Immune response (Ir) genes expressed at macrophage-B cell interactions. *Nature (London)* **273**, 664–666.

Howie, S., Parish, C. R., David, C. S., McKenzie, I. F. C., Maurer, P. H., and Feldmann, M. (1979). Serological analysis of antigen specific helper factors specific for (T,G)-A—L and GAT. *Eur. J. Immunol.* **9**, 501–506.

McDougall, J. S., and Gordon, D. S. (1977). Generation of T helper cells *in vitro*. II. Analysis of supernates derived from T helper cell cultures. *J. Exp. Med.* **145**, 693–708.

Marbrook, J. (1967). Primary immune response in cultures of spleen cells. *Lancet* **2**, 1279–1281.

Schimpl, A., and Wecker, E. (1972). Replacement of T cell function by a T cell product. *Nature (London) New Biol.* **237**, 15.

Waldmann, H., and Munro, A. (1973). T cell dependent mediator in the immune response. II. Physical and biological properties. *Immunology* , 27–53.

11

A Helper Cell Assay of Cellular Antigens and Its Applications to Hapten-Specific T Cells

Carlos Martinez-A., Andrei A. Augustin, and
António Coutinho

I. INTRODUCTION

The cellular and molecular mechanisms underlying helper T-cell-dependent B-cell induction remain one of the most controversial subjects in immunology. In addition, our knowledge of the structural aspects of helper T cells and their mode of activation is very limited. Undoubtedly, the complexity of this process, involving several cell types, contributes to the present difficulties. The requirement for cooperation between at least two types of specific clonally distributed cells results in a very low frequency of relevant interactions in cultures of normal cell populations stimulated *in vitro*

IMMUNOLOGICAL METHODS, VOL. II

with antigens. The technical possibilities for inducing primary *in vitro* thymus-dependent (TD) antibody responses have thus been limited to those against heterologous erythrocyte antigens, as reports on the successful induction of primary *in vitro* reponses to soluble TD antigens have remained controversial.

Prior specific *in vivo* priming of either carrier-specific helper cells or hapten-specific B cells is currently used as a method for partially overcoming the very low frequency of relevant interactions *in vitro*. Long-term *in vitro* culture of helper T lymphocytes (Augustin *et al.*, 1979; Schrier *et al.*, 1979; Schreier *et al.*, 1980), which selects populations of helper cells containing T lymphocytes displaying the desired specificity in a high frequency, has provided further progress in this area.

On the other hand, the available techniques for enrichment of specific B cells by antigen binding (Haas, 1979) are quite elaborate and involve extensive handling of cells with consequent negative effects upon the cloning efficiency of treated cell populations. A helper assay has been recently devised (Augustin and Coutinho, 1980; Martinez-A. *et al.*, 1980a) in which all B cells seeded in culture are *potentially* capable of undergoing specific interactions with helper cells. This was done by preparing helper T cells with a specificity for naturally occurring or artificially coupled determinants on the surfaces of most (or all) B cells. Long-term *in vitro* selection of specific helper T cells adds to the increase in specific cooperative interactions obtained in this system. The responses are assayed either by measuring proliferative responses of primed and enriched T cells to the cellular antigens upon culture with *irradiated* stimulator cells, or by measuring their helper activity as reflected in the activation of nonirradiated, "antigenic" B cells to exponential growth and secretion of immunoglobulin (Ig) as revealed in a polyclonal plaque assay (Gronowicz *et al.*, 1976; see also Chapter 9).

II. PRINCIPLES OF THE METHOD AND ITS MODIFICATIONS

With the work of Cammisuli *et al.* (1978), it has become clear that helper T-cell-dependent B-cell induction, while requiring specific helper cell recognition, occurs in the absence of antigen recognition by the responding B lymphocytes. It is then possible to assess helper activity by measuring B-cell responses irrespective of antibody specificities, once specific antigen recognition by helper cells on the responding B-cell membranes is ensured.

Large enrichments of specific helper T cells have been recently achieved for soluble antigens by Corradin *et al.* (1977) by using appropriate *in vivo* priming protocols, and further extended by Augustin *et al.* (1979) by long-term *in vitro* selection. These culture conditions allow a manifold positive selection of specific cells and the concomitant negative selection of cells with other specificities, particularly those that are alloreactive.

We (Augustin and Coutinho, 1980) have used the same methods for cellular antigens expressed on B-cell (and macrophage) membranes to prepare enriched helper cells. These cells, upon coculture with antigenic functionally competent spleen cells initiate proliferation and the cooperative interactions leading to "target" B-cell triggering, proliferation, and differentiation. The system can in principle be applied to any naturally occurring antigen and, in view of the very high frequency of specific interactions, appears suitable for the study of mechanisms of collaboration, B-cell activation, and regulation. In particular, it allows study of the precise roles of antigen recognition by B cells.

On the other hand, the study of antigen recognition by helper T cells, their activation and growth requirements, and the structural aspects of effector functions requires defined antigenic determinants rather than natural antigens, the structure and cellular representation of which are in most cases poorly defined. To this end, we (Martinez-A. *et al.,* 1980a) have introduced further modifications in these systems for preparing and testing helper T cells with a specificity for haptens that can be directly coupled to lymphoid cell populations without impairing their functional capabilities. The present methods therefore also allow the study of functional fine specificity and the avidity of helper T cells.

It has not been possible so far to clone either helper cells or responding B cells in these systems, and this limits the use of this method in precise quantitative experiments. We do not know, for example, the exact number of normal B lymphocytes that can be activated by cooperative interaction of this type, regardless of their antigenicity for helper cells. The role of nonlymphoid accessory cells in the system, in regard to both T-cell activation and B-cell response, is also unclear. These limitations are likely to be removed by further experimentation, but at present they restrict the use of this method.

III. MATERIALS

Phosphate-buffered saline (PBS), pH 7.2 and 8.7
Balanced salt solution (BSS), pH 7.2
Borate buffer: 0.035 M borate and 0.08 M NaCl, pH 9.1–9.2
PBS–Borate buffer: 1 part borate buffer plus 50 parts PBS, pH $\simeq$ 8.2
Dimethyl formamide (DMF)
3-(p-Sulfophenyldiazo)-4-hydroxyphenyl (SP) (gift of H. Pohlit)
2,4,6-Trinitrobenzenesulfonic acid (TNBS) (Sigma)

Fluorescein isothiocyanate (FITC) (Nordic)
Protein A (Pharmacia)
DEAE-dextran (Pharmacia)
Sheep red cells (SRBCs)
Complete Freund's adjuvant (CFA) (Difco)
Developing antisera: Rabbit anti-mouse Ig specific for the various Ig isotypes, as described (Gronowicz et al., 1976; see also Chapter 9)
Culture media and supplements: RPMI 1640 (Gibco), HEPES (Flow Laboratories), fetal calf serum (FCS) (Gibco), antibiotics (penicillin and streptomycin) (Gibco)

IV. PROCEDURES

A. Hapten-Derivatized Spleen Cells

Mice are killed by cervical dislocation, and the spleen removed and placed in cold BSS. Cell suspensions are prepared by pressing the spleen against a stainless steel sieve immersed in a BSS solution. Large cell aggregates are removed by a 3-min 1-g sedimentation and the cells washed once. Red cells are removed using Gey's solution (Gey and Gey, 1936) (approximately one spleen per 3 ml for 5 min on ice). Thereafter the cells are extensively washed in PBS, irradiated (3.300 rads), and haptenated. The hapten concentrations given here are those used for *in vivo* and *in vitro* immunization.

1. Trinitrophenyl (TNP_{10})–spleen cells: 10^8 spleen cells/ml are incubated for 10 min at 37°C in a solution of PBS (pH 7.2) containing 10 mM TNBS.
2. $FITC_{100}$–spleen cells: 10^8 spleen cells/ml are incubated for 15 min at 37°C in a PBS solution (pH 8.7) containing 100 μg/ml of FITC.
3. SP_{50}–spleen cells: 1–2 × 10^7 cells/ml in a PBS–borate buffer (pH 8.2) are incubated for 20 min on ice with 50 μl of a 1 mM solution of SP in DMF.

After coupling, the cells are extensively washed in BSS.

B. *In Vivo* Immunization

Irradiated hapten-derivatized spleen cells are suspended in CFA at a final concentration of 10^9 cells/ml; a homogeneous suspension is obtained by mixing. Mice are injected with 50 μl of this suspension at the base of the tail.

C. Preparation of Helper Cell Cultures

Four days after *in vivo* immunization, the inguinal and paraaortic lymph nodes are removed from the immunized mice and teased through 50-gauge steel mesh. Then 15×10^6 lymph node cells are cultured with 30×10^6 irradiated hapten-derivatized spleen cells in a volume of 5 ml of medium in a Falcon culture flask (No. 3033).

The culture medium is RPMI 1640 (Microbiological Associates) supplemented with 25×10^{-3} M HEPES, glutamine (2 mM), asparagine (36 mg/ml), arginine (116 mg/ml), penicillin and streptomycin (2000 U/ml), and human sera (5%) previously tested for T-cell growth-supporting activity (Con A stimulation on normal spleen cells). Every 7 days, cultures are fed with 3 ml of fresh medium containing 2×10^7 irradiated, hapten-coupled spleen cells.

D. Testing for Helper Activity

Putative helper cells obtained either directly from the lymph nodes or from the preparative cultures are tested for specificity and functional activity in two different ways: (1) ability to proliferate in response to homologous and control antigens (i.e., normal or haptenated, *irradiated* spleen cells); (2) ability to stimulate polyclonal B cell responses upon coculture with nonirradiated, normal or derivatized spleen cells.

1. Proliferation of Primed T Cells in Response to Hapten-Derivatized (or Normal) Syngeneic Spleen Cells

Primed cells (2×10^5 per culture) are stimulated *in vitro* with irradiated syngeneic spleen cells (6×10^5 per culture) derivatized with the homologous hapten in a total volume of 0.2 ml on microtiter plates (No. 3040, Falcon) using the medium described for the preparative cultures. Lymphocyte proliferation is assayed daily from 24 hr onward by incubating the cultures for 3 hr with 5 μCi of [*methyl-*^{3}H]thymidine ([^{3}H]Tdr, Amershan, specific activity 2 Ci/mmol) before harvesting and counting radioactive thymidine uptake.

2. Helper Activity of Primed T cells

The helper activity is assayed by mixing the same culture test cells, containing the putative helpers, with hapten-derivatized, nonirradiated spleen cells and monitoring daily the appearance of IgM- and IgG-secreting plaque-forming cells (PFCs) in these cultures, using the protein A plaque assay. The number of hapten-coupled spleen cells is kept constant, at 5×10^4 per culture, while a range (5×10^2 to 5×10^4) of helper cell concentrations are systematically tested in each experiment. Necessary controls include separate cultures of each cell population, as well as observation of the response of normal and haptenated spleen cells to a direct mitogen such as lipopolysaccharide (LPS).

In addition, a 100-fold range of hapten densities should be used to derivatize the stimulator–responder spleen cells in order to assess the functional avidity of helper cells. These test cultures are performed in 0.2-ml volumes on microtiter plates. The culture medium is RPMI 1640 supplemented with 5×10^{-5} M 2-mercaptoethanol, 10^{-3} M HEPES, penicillin and streptomycin (2000 U/ml), and FCS (10%) (Gibco).

V. COMMENTS

A. Priming

The use of CFA is mandatory, and appropriate mixing of immunizing cells and CFA appears to be the most critical parameter in priming. Successful immunization is reflected in the increase in size of the draining lymph nodes. Inguinal and paraaortic nodes from a single mouse may contain up to $30–40 \times 10^6$ cells 4 days after priming. This cell population contains 70–80 Thy-1-positive cells which respond specifically to stimulating cells by proliferation, although they do not mediate helper effects if tested directly on day 4 before *in vitro* restimulation. Intravenous or intraperitoneal priming leads to the recovery of helper cells from the spleen under conditions parallel to those described here, although at a much lower frequency.

B. *In Vitro* Enrichment

It is fundamental that helper cells in preparative cultures not be exposed to the same type of heterologous serum used to supplement test cultures. Under such conditions, in particular with FCS supplementation, only anti-FCS, self-MHC-restricted helper cells can be detected. These give rise to what will appear as "background" nonspecific activation of nonantigenic target cells. Human serum supplementation avoids this problem nearly completely, and preliminary results indicate that enrichment cultures grown in media supplemented with syngeneic mouse serum, in addition to albumin and transferrin (Iscove and Melchers, 1978; Dillner-Centerlind et al., 1979), provide suitable conditions as well. Three weeks after *in vitro* selection, 99% of all cells are Thy-1-positive, while 93 and 10% are positively stained with monoclonal antibodies to Lyt-1 and Lyt-2, respectively. Only 95% of all cells can be stained by a mixture of these two antibodies.

The timing of restimulation and feeding does not appear to be very critical. The appropriate number of days varies from experiment to experiment and should be determined by microscopic examination of the cultures.

The recoveries from preparative cultures also vary considerably with the antigenic system and the T-cell donor. After 4 weeks of culture the number of recovered cells may vary from 5 to 40% of the input.

After 4–6 weeks' selection, helper cells can be further maintained by consecutively harvesting and restimulating them with appropriate irradiated antigenic spleen cells. Helper cell lines have been maintained under this protocol for over 6 months without detectable loss of specificity or functional activity.

Preparative cultures result in functional enrichment of specific helper cells, both in terms of the average ability of the helper cell population to recognize very low hapten densities on the target responder cell (functional avidity) and of helper activity on a per T-cell basis.

C. Test of Helper Activity

Although enriched helper cells are specific for immunizing hapten-coupled cells, it is important to note that at high effector/target responder cell ratios (3:1 or 1:1), we consistently observe "nonspecific" effects in mixed cultures of helper cells and normal nonhaptenated spleen cells, primarily after short-term selection (2–3 weeks). These effects do not occur, however, at lower ratios and after longer periods of *in vitro* enrichment. This background effect makes it absolutely necessary to titrate in each experiment the number of helper cells in culture. Nonspecific effects disappear with time in selective cultures, but careful titration of helper cells is nonetheless strictly necessary whenever comparisons in activity of either helper or responder B cells are to be made. The functional ability of target spleen cells after haptenation has to be controlled in each experiment by stimulation with a polyclonal mitogen, e.g., LPS.

The B-cell responses, as measured in the plaque assay, should be determined on consecutive days, since only a complete kinetic profile can give correct indications as to the number of responding cells and their increase in culture.

Both IgM and IgG PFCs should be assayed, as a large fraction of all activated B-cell clones in these cultures switch to the production of IgG_1, IgG_2, and IgG_{2b}. No IgG_3 PFCs are induced by helper T cells.

The T- and B-cell collaboration in such a system requires helper cell recognition of antigen in association with the appropriate MHC determinants on the surface of the responding B cells. The genes responsible for such a restriction map in the *I-A* subregion (Martinez-A. *et al.*, 1980b) but also a minor fraction of the helper cells (10–20%) map in the *I-E* subregions (Martinez-A. *et al.*, 1980b,c). It follows that no "bystander" effects are observed in this system.

D. General

The cellular antigens detected in these systems are likely to be highly complex. In addition, helper cell enrichment results in the appearance of responses that are not detected in a primary mixed lymphocyte reaction. It follows that conclusions about the antigenic specificities of helper cells must be reached through appropriate genetic analysis rather than by referring to available typing results obtained under less sensitive conditions. Also, as a result of the enrichment protocol, "low-responder" cells may be detected as "high-responder" cells after long-term selection (Martinez-A. *et al.,* 1980b).

In spite of these limitations these methods appear convenient for the study of helper cells (and not just proliferating cells) with a specificity for cellular antigens and for determinants that can be coupled to lymphoid cell membranes.

ACKNOWLEDGEMENT

This work was supported in part by the Swedish Medical Research Council. Ms. Pat Young, Carina Olsson, and Margaret Tuneskog provided expert technical assistance.

REFERENCES

Augustin, A. A., and Coutinho, A. (1980). *J. Exp. Med.* **151,** 587.
Augustin, A. A., Julius, M. H., and Cosenza, H. (1979). *Eur. J. Immunol.* **9,** 665.
Cammisuli, S., Henry, C., and Wofsy, C. (1978). *Eur. J. Immunol.* **8,** 656.
Corradin, G., Etlinger, H. M., and Chiller, J. M. (1977). *J. Immunol.* **119,** 1048.
Dillner-Centerlind, M.-L., Hammarström, S., and Perlman, P. (1979). *Eur. J. Immunol.* **9,** 942.
Gey, G. O., and Gey, M. K. (1936). *Am. J. Cancer* **27,** 45.
Gronowicz, E., Coutinho, A., and Melchers, F. (1976). *Eur. J. Immunol.* **6,** 558.
Haas, W. (1979). *In* "Immunological Methods" (I. Lefkovits and B. Pernis, eds.), p. 269. Academic Press, New York.
Iscove, N. N., and Melchers, F. (1978). *J. Exp. Med.* **147,** 923.
Martinez-A., C., Coutinho, A., Bernabé, R. R., Augustin, A. A., Haas, W., and Pohlit, H. (1980a). *Eur. J. Immunol.* **10,** 403.
Martinez-A., C., Coutinho, A., Bernabé, R. R., Haas, W., and Pohlit, H. (1980b). *Eur. J. Immunol.* **10,** 411.
Martinez-A., C., Coutinho, A., and Bernabé, R. R. (1980c). *Immunogenetics* **10,** 299.
Schreier, M., Andersson, J., Lernhardt, W., and Melchers, F. (1980). *J. Exp. Med.* **151,** 194.
Schrier, R. D., Skidmore, B. J., Kurnide, J. T., Goldstein, S. N., and Chiller, J. M. (1979). *J. Immunol.* **123,** 2525.

12

Limiting Dilution Analysis of Precursors of Cytotoxic T Lymphocytes

Jean Langhorne and Kirsten Fischer Lindahl

221

IMMUNOLOGICAL METHODS, VOL. II

I. PRINCIPLE OF THE METHOD

Until recently the study of cytotoxic T lymphocytes (CTL) was based on cytotoxicity assays performed with effector cells stimulated in bulk cultures. Although assays of this type provide much information on the nature and development of cytotoxic T cells, it is not possible to determine the frequency of these cells or their precursors by direct means or to examine the specificity of large numbers of clones.

A mixed lymphocyte culture (MLC) grown with a limiting number of responding cells allows direct estimation of CTL precursor cell (CTL-P) frequency in response to a variety of cell surface antigens: major and minor histocompatibility antigens, tumor antigens, and the antigens of hapten-conjugated and virus-infected cells. With this knowledge it is possible to manipulate the responding cell input so that there is at most a single CTL-P per culture. The clonal progeny derived after cocultivation with stimulating cells can then be used to investigate the cross-reactivity and specificity of CTL derived from single precursor cells.

The basis of the assay is the culture of many replicates of a range of responder cell doses in the presence of an excess of stimulating cells. The doses of responder cells are chosen such that, for each, a fraction of the cultures will contain no CTL-P. It is essential that the only limiting component in the assay be the CTL-P; accessory cells and T-cell helper factors must be present in excess. After 6–8 days' incubation the microwells are assessed for cytotoxic activity using a ^{51}Cr release assay. The fraction of nonresponding cultures (i.e., those containing no CTL-P) for each responding cell dose is scored. From this it is possible to calculate the frequency of CTL-P using the zero-order term of the Poisson distribution (Section V).

The methods described in this chapter will be confined to determination of the number of CTL-P responsive to major alloantigens of the mouse, but the principles discussed are applicable to other antigens and species.

II. MATERIALS

A. Media

Preparation medium, Hanks' phosphate-buffered saline (HPBS): 100 ml 10 × Hanks' balanced salt solution without bicarbonate (Gibco, Glasgow, Scotland), 10 ml penicillin–streptomycin, 10,000 U/ml (Gibco), and 10 ml 1 *M* phosphate buffer, pH 7.2, made up to 1 liter with sterile, triple-distilled water.

Culture medium, RPMI 1640: 500 ml RPMI 1640 with L-glutamine and

NaHCO₃ (Gibco), 6 ml 1 M HEPES buffer (Flow, Ayrshire, Scotland, 5 ml 200 mM L-glutamine, and 0. 5 ml gentamicin, 10 mg/ml (Schering Corp., Kenilworth, New Jersey).
Culture medium for target cell blasts, Iscove's medium (Iscove and Melchers, 1978) (as an alternative, RPMI 1640 can be used): 9 gm powdered Iscove's medium (Gibco), 3.024 gm NaHCO₃, and 1 ml gentamicin, 10 mg/ml (Schering) made up to 1 liter with triple-distilled water and sterilized by filtration. The pH should not be adjusted.

B. Miscellaneous Chemical and Biological Reagents

Concanavalin A (Con A) (Sigma, Surrey, England, or Pharmacia, Uppsala, Sweden)
Ficoll–sodium metatrizoate: 72 ml 14% (w/v) Ficoll 400 (Pharmacia) and 30 ml sodium metatrizoate (32.8% solution, Nyegaard, Oslo, Norway)
Fetal calf serum (FCS) (we have obtained satisfactory batches from Flow, Gibco, and Microbiological Associates, Maryland)
Lipopolysaccharide (from *Escherichia coli,* Westphal's method of extraction, Difco or Sigma)
2-Mercaptoethanol (Merck, Darmstadt, West Germany)
α-methyl-D-mannoside (Sigma)
⁵¹Cr as Na₂CrO₄ · 1OH₂O (ca. 1 ci/mg, IRE, Zoning Industriel, Fleurus, Belgium)
Zaponin (Coulter Electronics, Harpenden, England)

C. Plastics

Tissue culture flasks: 25 cm² (No. 3013, Falcon, Oxnard, California), 75 cm² (No. 3024, Falcon), and 174 cm² (Nunclon, Roskilde, Denmark)
Sterile, V-bottom, tissue culture-treated microtiter trays with lids (Linbro IS-MVC-96-TC, Instrumentengesellschaft, Zürich, Switzerland)
Cells can be prepared in any sterile glassware (washed for tissue culture use) or plastic ware. We routinely use the following: conical centrifuge tubes, 15 ml (No. 2095, Falcon) and 50 ml (No. 2070, Falcon); petri dishes, 60 mm (No. 1007, Falcon). We use 7 × 38 mm round-bottom plastic tubes (Milian Instruments SA, Geneva, Switzerland), which fit into a microtiter tray, for harvesting ⁵¹Cr supernatants.

D. Multidispensers

Repeating dispenser with 5 ml total volume, dispensing 100 µl in each step (Hamilton, Bonaduz, Switzerland)

Adjustable 12-fold Finn pipette dispensing up to 200 µl ("Paintbrush," Titertek, Flow)

Leiden dispenser, six syringes with a capacity of 100 µl each (Hamilton)

E. Animals and Cell Lines

Mice of both sexes, specific pathogen-free or conventionally bred, can be used. We prefer them between 6 and 12 weeks of age but have used mice up to 1 year old. The choice of strain is dictated only by the purpose of the experiment.

Lewis rats are preferred for the production of Con A supernatant (Section III,A,2).

Tumor cell lines can be obtained from the Cell Distribution Center, Salk Institute, La Jolla, California).

III. METHODS (FIG. 1)

A. Addition of Helper Factors

1. Source

In limiting dilution assays it is essential that every component that facilitates the generation of CTL be present in excess. If no precautions are taken, because of the low number of responder cells used to ensure proper dilution of CTL-P, the necessary T-cell helper factors will also be limiting. Accessory cells or soluble T-cell helper factors must therefore be added.

It has been demonstrated that spleen cells from athymic *nu/nu* mice substantially enhance the CTL response, particularly at very low concentrations of responder cells (Schilling *et al.*, 1976). Since *nu/nu* mice are available in only a few strains, the number of strain combinations that can be studied is limited (Miller *et al.*, 1977; Miller, 1979).

Irradiated spleen cells syngeneic with the responder cells have also been used as a source of help (Pilarski, 1977). The addition of large numbers of cells to microcultures might, however, lead to deterioration of culture conditions such that optimum generation of CTL is not achieved. The numbers of CTL-P determined by this method are generally lower than those obtained with soluble T-cell helper factors. In addition it is difficult to know what cell interactions take place under such conditions.

Soluble growth-promoting factors derived from secondary MLC supernatants (Ryser *et al.*, 1978) and from supernatants of Con A-activated spleen cells (Con A supernatants) have been shown to be potent sources of helper factors required for cytotoxic T-cell growth and development (Gillis and Smith, 1977). Supernatants offer several advantages over the addition of accessory cells in limiting dilution assays: (1) The supernatants provide

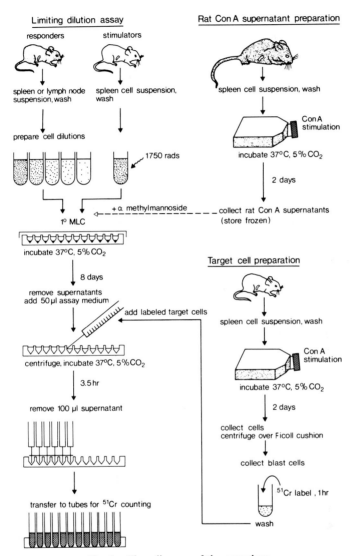

Fig. 1. Flow diagram of the procedure.

helper factors regardless of the strain combinations studied. (2) Since supernatants can be easily prepared in bulk and stored, the same preparations can be used for a series of experiments. (3) Partially purified fractions containing the active components of these supernatants can also be used, allowing a better defined assay system. For these reasons we will describe only the use of soluble growth factors.

We have found that media supplemented with secondary MLC supernatants, Con A-activated spleen cell supernatant, or partially purified T-cell growth factors (TCGF) are equally satisfactory in providing help in limiting dilution assays for CTL-P.

2. Preparation of Supernatants from Concanavalin A-Activated Rat Spleen Cells and of Partially Purified T-Cell Growth Factors

The preparation of Con A supernatant, the partial purification of TCGF, and the assessment of their activity are described by Schreier and Tees (Chapter 15, this volume). The Con A supernatants are routinely used at a final concentration of 50% (v/v), and the pooled active fractions of TCGF at a final concentration of 5% (v/v) in the primary MLC of limiting dilution assays. To prevent possible nonspecific stimulation of CTL by the remaining Con A, α-methyl mannoside to a final concentration of 0.1 M is added to the Con A supernatant before use.

3. Preparation of Secondary Mixed Lymphocyte Culture Supernatant

The preparation and use of supernatants derived from secondary MLC have been extensively described (Ryser *et al.*, 1978; reviewed in MacDonald *et al.*, 1980). The method (from H. R. MacDonald, personal communication) is briefly outlined below.

Spleen cell suspensions are prepared as described in Section III,B from 10 C57BL/6 and 20 DBA/2 mice. The primary MLC is set up by mixing 50 × 10⁶ viable C57BL/6 spleen cells with 100 × 10⁶ irradiated DBA/2 spleen cells (1750 rads) in 40 ml of RPMI containing 2% FCS in tissue culture flasks (75 cm², Falcon). Approximately 20 cultures can be initiated from this number of mice. The cultures are incubated for 12–14 days at 37°C in 5% CO_2 in air. The cells are then recovered from the primary MLC by centrifugation, and viable cells are counted. In the same flasks, 30 × 10⁶ surviving cells are then mixed with 120 × 10⁶ freshly prepared irradiated DBA/2 spleen cells in 30 ml of new medium, and the flasks incubated at 37°C. After 24 hr the supernatants are collected, pooled, and stored at −20°C in convenient volumes. A total volume of 500–600 ml can be recovered from a preparation of this size.

The activity of the supernatant can be tested in a limiting dilution assay at various concentrations. Routinely, secondary MLC supernatants are used in our laboratory at a final concentration of 50% (v/v) in the microcultures.

B. Preparation of Stimulating Cells

A single-cell suspension is prepared from spleens by gentle teasing of the tissue with forceps or by disruption of tissue fragments with a Teflon pestle. The cells are collected in HPBS containing 2% FCS (HPBS–2% FCS), passed through sterile cotton wool to remove clumps, pelleted, and washed once.

The cells are resuspended at approximately 5×10^7 viable cells/ml, irradiated (1750 rads), and made up to a concentration of 10^7 viable cells/ml in 100% rat Con A supernatant, secondary MLC supernatant, or 10% TCGF (twice the final optimum concentration). All cell handling is carried out at room temperature.

C. Preparation of Responder Cells

Responder cells are prepared from lymph nodes or spleens as described in Section III,B, pelleted, washed once in HPBS-2% FCS, and resuspended at a known concentration of viable cells. The responder cells are then serially diluted in RPMI-50% FCS with 5×10^{-5} M 2-mercaptoethanol (to give a final concentration of 25% FCS in the microcultures) so that the desired dose of cells to be added to each microwell is contained in 100 μl. The batches of FCS are selected for their ability to promote killer cell generation in bulk cultures (Fischer Lindahl and Wilson, 1977a).

D. Mixed Lymphocyte Cultures

Mixed lymphocyte cultures are grown in V-bottom wells of microtiter plates. To each well is first added 10^6 irradiated stimulator cells in 100 μl and then 100 μl of responder cells, using a Hamilton repeating dispenser. For each dose of responder cells, 24–48 replicate cultures are set up (two to four rows on a microtiter plate). An additional set of 24–48 cultures containing only stimulator cells and medium (instead of responder cells) is also included.

The microcultures are incubated at 37°C in a humidified atmosphere of 5% CO_2 in air. Cytotoxic activity reaches its maximum between days 6 and 9. We have found that an incubation time of 8 days rather than 6 days results in a clearer differentiation between positive and negative cultures and a higher CTL-P frequency.

E. ^{51}Cr Release Assay

1. Introduction

The microwells are assessed for cytotoxic activity against ^{51}Cr-labeled target cells after 8 days of incubation. Target cells are prepared either from mitogen-stimulated [Con A or lipopolysaccharide (LPS)] spleen cells or from certain mouse tumor cell lines. The most commonly used cell lines are P815, a mastocytoma of DBA/2 (H-2^d) origin, and EL4, a leukemia line of C57BL/6 (H-2^b) origin. They are particularly useful in preliminary experiments designed to determine optimum conditions for CTL generation, since the spontaneous release of ^{51}Cr is low, the amount of ^{51}Cr incorporated per cell is high, and they are easily killed.

2. Preparation of Target Cells

Spleen cells (30 × 10^6), prepared as described in Section III,B, are placed in tissue culture flasks (No. 3024, Falcon) in 30 ml of Iscove's medium containing 10% FCS, 5 × 10^{-5} M 2-mercaptoethanol, and 2 µg/ml Con A or 30 µg/ml LPS. The flasks are incubated for 2 days at 37°C in a humidified atmosphere of 5% CO_2 in air. The cells are then harvested by centrifugation (200 g), resuspended in approximately 2.5 ml of HPBS containing 5% heat-inactivated FCS (FCS$_\Delta$), and centrifuged onto a Ficoll–metatrizoate cushion (2 ml in a 15-ml tube) for 15 min at 700 g. The blast cells are collected from the interface, washed once in HPBS–5% FCS$_\Delta$, and resuspended at 10^7 viable cells/ml. The required numbers of target cells are mixed with 500 µCi ^{51}Cr/10^7 cells and incubated for 1 hr at 37°C. The labeled target cells are washed twice in HPBS–5% FCS$_\Delta$ and finally resuspended at 10^5 cells/ml in RPMI–10% FCS$_\Delta$.

Tumor cells from continuously growing cell lines are collected, centrifuged, and resuspended at 10^7 viable cells/ml. The Ficoll purification step can be omitted. Labeling with ^{51}Cr is carried out as described above.

3. ^{51}Cr Release Assay

The microtiter plates containing the primary MLC are centrifuged at 500 g for 5 min, and the culture supernatants flicked off. The cell pellets are resuspended on a vortex mixer and 50 µl of RPMI–10% FCS$_\Delta$ added to each well using a Paintbrush multidispenser. Replicate wells, usually 24 of each, are prepared on a separate plate with 50 µl RPMI–10% FCS$_\Delta$ for spontaneous release controls and 50 µl Zaponin (diluted 1:5 in water) for maximum release controls. To each well 10^4 ^{51}Cr-labeled target cells in 100 µl are added with a Hamilton repeating dispenser.

In experiments of this type, large volumes of target cells are prepared to be distributed into a large number of wells. It is therefore essential that the target cell suspension be kept well mixed to ensure proper sampling. In our hands, the addition of fewer target cells to each well results in the same percentage of ^{51}Cr released; reducing the number of target cells therefore would not increase the sensitivity of the assay.

The plates are centrifuged at 20 g for 5 min and incubated at 37°C in a humidified atmosphere of 5% CO_2 in air. We have compared the results obtained after 3, 5, 7 hr incubation and found no significant differences in the number of CTL-P obtained. Routinely, an incubation time of $3\frac{1}{2}$ hr is used, since shorter incubation times result in lower spontaneous release values and are more convenient.

After incubation, 100 µl of supernatant is removed from each well with a Leiden dispenser and transferred to counting tubes set up in a microtiter tray in the same pattern. To prevent carryover of ^{51}Cr from well to well, the syringes are then filled with saline, and this wash is added to the appropriate tubes. The amount of ^{51}Cr released into the supernatant is measured with a gamma counter. Supernatants can also be harvested with a Paintbrush multidispenser, but we feel that it may be less accurate, since it is prone to accumulate air bubbles in the tips. Accuracy is essential, since the precise amount of ^{51}Cr released in each individual well is critical for evaluation of the assay.

IV. EXPERIMENTAL DESIGN

For each combination of responders and stimulators studied it is necessary to determine the range of informative responder cell doses, i.e., cell doses at which a fraction of the wells contain no CTL-P and remain nonresponding. In a preliminary experiment a wide range of responder cell doses is used. From the results the informative range can be selected, and in the final experiment these will provide the information for calculating the CTL-P frequencies. An example is shown in Table 1. The experiment was designed to determine the frequency of CTL-P to DBA/2 ($H-2^d$) alloantigens in C57BL/6 ($H-2^b$) lymph node cells. The preliminary experiment indicates that only wells with less than 1000 cells provide useful information for the frequency estimation. In the final experiment cell doses ranging from 50 to 1000 cells per well were chosen. In order to statistically analyze the goodness of fit of the data to the zero-order term of the Poisson distribution (discussed in Section V,B) at least four responder cell doses are required, where some but not all of the individual wells respond. It is more important to have a range of different responder cell doses than a very large number of replicates of a single or a few cell doses.

Within each experiment it is necessary to include appropriate controls to establish that the response is specific. For this, responder cells can be cultured in the MLC with irradiated syngeneic stimulator cells at three or four representative cell doses.

V. ANALYSIS OF THE RESULTS

A. Definition of a Responding Microwell

The major problem in calculating the CTL-P frequency from a limiting lilution assay is the definition of a responding microwell. A convenient

TABLE I

Number of Responding and Nonresponding Cultures Obtained with Various Doses of Responder Cells[a]

Assay	No. of responder cells per well	No. of responding wells out of 24[b]	Fraction of nonresponding wells
Preliminary	—	0	(1.00)
	100	1	0.96
	500	17	0.29
	1,000	23	0.04
	3,000	24	(0.00)
	10,000	24	(0.00)
Main[c]	—	0	(1.00)
	50	1	0.96
	75	2	0.92
	100	4	0.83
	150	5	0.79
	200	9	0.62
	250	12	0.50
	500	17	0.29
	1,000	20	0.17

[a] Limiting dilution of C57BL/6 lymph node cells. Groups of 24 microcultures containing different doses of C57BL/6 LN cells were cultured with 10^6 irradiated DBA/2 spleen cells for 8 days in the presence of 50% secondary MLC supernatant. Each microwell was assessed for cytotoxic activity on ^{51}Cr-labeled P815 target cells.

[b] The determination of a responding well is described in Section V.

[c] In this assay the CTL-P frequency was 1 in 513 (calculated as described in Section V).

method for initial presentation of the data is to plot the ^{51}Cr counts in each individual microwell for each responder cell dose (Fig. 2). It can be seen from a plot of this nature that there is no clear demarcation between a non-responding and a responding well. Selection of the threshold value above which a well is considered positive is made empirically. Conventionally, if the amount of ^{51}Cr released in a well exceeds the mean spontaneous release by either 2 or 3 standard deviations (SDs), then the well is considered positive. Alternatively, others have used 10% specific ^{51}Cr release as the lower limit.

The spontaneous release is taken as the mean amount of ^{51}Cr released from target cells in the presence of stimulator cells. This value is often lower than the release from target cells incubated alone in medium and is more representative of the experimental conditions.

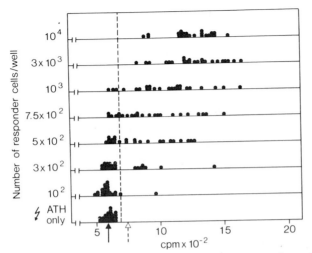

Fig. 2. Induction of cytotoxic activity by small numbers of responding cells primed in MLC. Groups of 24 microcultures containing 10^6 irradiated A.TH ($H\text{-}2^{t2}$) spleen cells and 100–1000 normal A.CA ($H\text{-}2^f$) lymph node cells were cultured for 8 days in the presence of rat Con A supernatants (50% v/v). Each microwell was assayed for cytotoxicity against ^{51}Cr-labeled A.TH Con A blasts. Each circle represents the amount of ^{51}Cr released in a single microwell. The solid arrow represents mean spontaneous ^{51}Cr release in the presence of stimulator cells alone, the dashed line the mean spontaneous release value plus 2 SDs, and the dashed arrow the mean plus 3 SDs. In this experiment ^{51}Cr release values that exceed the mean spontaneous release plus 2 SDs are considered positive (discussed in Section V,A).

B. Frequency Analysis

A detailed analysis of application of the Poisson distribution to limiting dilution assays has been given elsewhere (Miller *et al.,* 1977; Lefkovits and Waldmann, 1979). The general form of the Poisson formula gives the probability F_n that a culture contains n CTL-P:

$$F_n = \mu^n e^{-\mu}/n! \tag{1}$$

where e is the base of natural logarithms and μ is the *average* number of CTL-P per well at a given responder cell dose x; i.e.,

$$\mu = fx \tag{2}$$

where f is the CTL-P frequency to be determined in the population of responder cells studied.

With the ^{51}Cr release assay, it is only possible to distinguish cultures that do not respond, i.e., have no CTL-P ($n = 0$), from cultures that respond.

The frequency of CTL-P is calculated from the zero-order term:

$$F_0 = e^{-\mu} \tag{3}$$

or

$$-\ln F_0 = \mu \tag{4}$$

Thus there is a linear relationship between the logarithm of the fraction of nonresponding wells and the average number of CTL-P per well. For each experiment the logarithm of the fraction of nonresponding wells is therefore plotted against the responder cell dose. From Eq. (4) it can be calculated that the dose which on the average contains one precursor cell (μ = 1) is the x value determined from this plot corresponding to a y value of -1 (37% nonresponding wells).

This calculation can only be made if the experimental data conform to the straight-line relationship expressed by Eq. (4); i.e., the CTL-P must be the only limiting factor in the experiment. Before the CTL-P frequency can be estimated, the data must therefore be analyzed to determine whether they fit this relationship. As an example, the data shown in Table II are plotted in Fig. 3. The best fitting line through these experimental points (indicated by the dashed line on the graph) is calculated by the least squares method (Piazza, 1979). It can be seen that in this experiment the intercept with the y axis (a) is not zero but 0.298 $\pm$ 0.152 (the error of a). We generally assume that, if the intercept value plus or minus twice its error overlaps with zero, the (a) is not significantly different from zero and the line can be refitted to go through zero (by the least squares method as described by Lefkovits and Waldmann, 1979). This is indicated by the solid line in Fig. 3.

TABLE II

The Cytotoxic Activity of A.CA Lymph Node Cells Stimulated with A.TH Spleen Cells[a]

No. of responder A.CA cells added	No. of responding cultures out of 24	Fraction of nonresponding cultures
0	0	(1.000)
100	2	0.917
300	8	0.667
500	15	0.375
750	21	0.125
1000	22	0.083
3000	24	(0.000)

[a] Taken from the data shown in Fig. 1

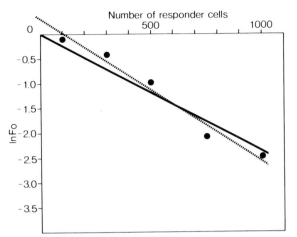

Fig. 3. Estimate of CTL-P frequency in normal A.CA (*H-2ᶠ*) lymph node cells responding to A.TH (*H-2ᵗ²*) alloantigens. Data were taken from Fig. 2 and Table II. The dashed line represents the best fitting regression line to the experimental points (o). The intercept on the *y* axis (*a*) of the best fitting line is 0.298 ± 0.152 with a slope (*b*) of 0.00287 and a correlation coefficient (*r²*) of 0.974. The solid line represents the best fitting line which intercepts the ordinate at zero. The CTL-P frequency is estimated from the value of *x* corresponding to a *y* value of −1.

The goodness of fit of the data to this regression line can be tested either by using the correlation coefficient or by carrying out an analysis of variance on the regression line (shown in Table III) (Piazza, 1979). As can be seen from the results of the analysis of variance, the variance ratio (for 1 and 2 degrees of freedom) is highly significant. Therefore most of the variation in *y* can be accounted for by variation in *x*, i.e., by a linear relationship. This suggests that the data conform to single-hit kinetics, and the zero-order

TABLE III

Analysis of Variance on the Regression Line Plotted in Fig. 2[a]

Source of variation	Degrees of freedom	Sum of squares	Variance	Variance ratio
Linear	1	11.38	11.38	179.15
Nonlinear	1	0.13	0.13	1.98
Regression	1	11.51	11.51	181.12
Error	2	0.13	0.06	
Total	4	11.63		

[a] The values are corrected to two decimal places.

term of the Poisson distribution can be used to calculate the CTL-P frequency.

The frequency can be determined either from the reciprocal of the slope of the line or as the x value corresponding to a y value of -1. In this experiment the frequency of CTL-P among A.CA lymph node cells responsive to A.TH alloantigens is 1 in 409. Testing the goodness of fit of the data to the regression line uses 4 degrees of freedom. The assay must therefore include more than four informative responder cell doses.

If the intercept is significantly different from zero, then the data do not conform to single-hit kinetics and the CTL-P frequency cannot be estimated on the basis of this hypothesis. An intercept significantly higher than zero may indicate that the threshold is set too high or that something other than the CTL-P is limiting. Conversely, an intercept significantly below zero indicates that an incorrect definition of a responding well has been made, since there are positive wells in the absence of responder cells. This reemphasizes the importance of the choice of a threshold value in distinguishing positive from negative wells. Since it is arbitrarily defined, the threshold value can be chosen in each experiment (e.g., either 2 or 3 SDs above the mean spontaneous release) such that the data conform to the zero-order term of the Poisson distribution.

VI. DEVELOPMENTS OF THE LIMITING DILUTION ASSAY

A. Introduction

The limiting dilution assay described so far has been used to study the CTL response to a single target cell preparation. The assay can be extended to determine CTL specificity and cross-reactivity with different target cell preparations, to assay CTL activity under different conditions, to compare the frequencies of proliferating and cytotoxic precursor cells, or to determine the relationships between the generation of active CTL and memory cells. To do this the contents of the microwells are divided after the primary MLC, and the fractions analyzed separately.

B. Dilution of Microcultures

The extent to which the contents of individual wells can be divided before CTL activity is no longer detectable is determined by performing a ^{51}Cr release assay on serially diluted microcultures. After removal of the MLC supernatant, the cells in the microwells are resuspended in 100 μl of RPMI–10% FCS_Δ.

With a 50-μl Paintbrush dispenser serial twofold dilutions are made into the neighboring wells of the microtiter plate (provided they were left empty) or the wells of a fresh plate, each filled with 50 μl of RPMI–10% FCS$_\Delta$. Labeled target cells are added to each well, and the ^{51}Cr release assay carried out as described previously. It is important also to dilute the stimulator cell controls serially, since the spontaneous release values are often higher when fewer cells are present in the wells (Section V,A). The specific ^{51}Cr release at a given dilution is calculated with reference to the amount of ^{51}Cr released with the same dilution of stimulator cells alone.

C. Specificity Studies

The contents of individual wells can be divided and each part assayed with different target cells. The number of assays that can be performed with the contents of a well is limited by the smallest fraction of a positive well which allows detection of cytolytic activity, as determined above.

To perform an assay, for example, with two different targets, the contents of the wells are resuspended in 100 μl RPMI–10% FCS$_\Delta$. With a Paintbrush dispenser, 50 μl is removed from each microwell and placed in the same pattern on each of two new microtiter plates. The labeled target cells are then added to the plates, and the ^{51}Cr release assay carried out as described above.

Aliquots of the initial microcultures can also be assayed with the same target cells under different conditions, such as in the absence and presence of excess cold target inhibitors (Fischer Lindahl and Hausmann, 1980), antibodies (against different target cell determinants or in different concentrations) for specificity studies, or phytohemagglutinin (final concentration 10 μg/ml) to assay lytic activity regardless of specificity (Bevan and Cohn, 1975).

Assays of this type often involve more than 2000 samples. By replicating the pattern of the original microtiter plates containing the primary MLC in identical setups for the assay and later for the counting tubes, one obviates the necessity for labeling each well and facilitates subsequent comparison of the performance of individual microcultures under different conditions.

D. Comparison of Proliferative and Cytotoxic Activity

Proliferation of responding cells, as measured by the incorporation of thymidine, can be assessed in the same cultures to be tested for cytotoxic activity. Analysis of such data gives information on the relative frequencies of proliferating and cytotoxic cells. Ryser and MacDonald (1979) investigated the proliferative responses on the day of the ^{51}Cr release assay by removing a constant proportion of cell suspension from each microculture and incubating them for 18–24 hr in the presence of [³H]thymidine, while the rest of the culture was assayed for cytotoxic activity. Alternatively, proliferation and cytotoxicity can be measured with the same cells using [¹⁴C]thymidine rather than [³H]thymidine (Fischer Lindahl and Wilson, 1977b). Approximately 16–24 hr before the cytotoxicity assay, 0.1 μCi (in 25 μl) of [¹⁴C]thymidine is added to each culture. After this incubation, the microtiter plates are centrifuged at 500 g for 5 min and the supernatants removed. Excess (1000-fold) cold thymidine is added to each well in 50 μl of RPMI–10% FCS$_\Delta$ (assay medium), and the plates incubated for 1–2 hr (this ensures that free [¹⁴C]thymidine will not be taken up by the target cells). Target cells are then added, and the cytotoxic assay is carried out as described in Section III,E. After removal of the supernatants for ⁵¹Cr counting, the cell pellets are harvested on glass fiber filters, washed with distilled water, and air-dried. The incorporation of [¹⁴C]thymidine is assessed by liquid scintillation counting with the threshold settings adjusted such that minimum levels of ⁵¹Cr are detected.

E. Restimulation of Limiting Dilution Microcultures

Limiting dilution assays have also been used to study the relationship between CTL-P and memory cells in long-term MLC or to generate long-term clones of CTL (Teh et al., 1977; MacDonald et al., 1980). Briefly, after the primary MLC, the cultures are split; one part can be assayed for cytotoxic activity and the other part cultured further. The cultures can be maintained and expanded by restimulation with irradiated cells and the addition of TCGF (see Chapter 11, Vol. I, by von Boehmer), and samples can dition of TCGF, and samples can be removed when required for ⁵¹Cr release assays as described above.

F. Analysis of Data from Split Wells

The responder cell doses should be chosen such that there is a high probability of not having more than one CTL-P per well (Section VII). Before testing the split wells on different targets, it is necessary first to establish that wells divided and assayed on the same target cells in replicate cultures have comparable activity in each half-well.

For every microculture the ⁵¹Cr release values of each half-well are plotted as shown in Fig. 4, using only responder cell doses near or below the dose containing on the average one CTL-P per well. As in Fig. 4a, the wells are divided and both halves tested on the same target. The ⁵¹Cr release values for each half-well are comparable; however, a few cultures with very low activity score positive only in one half-well.

Figure 4b shows the results of an experiment with split wells assayed with two different targets with the same major histocompatibility complex

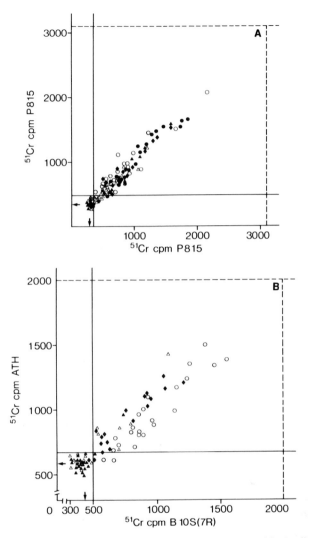

Fig. 4. Comparison of the cytotoxic activity of each half of the sensitized cell populations from single microwells split on the day of assay. (A) Groups of 24 wells containing 100 (solid triangles), 300 (open triangles), 500 (diamonds), 750 (open circles), or 850 (solid circles) normal C57BL/6 lymph node cells and 10^6 irradiated DBA/2 spleen cells. Both halves of the microwells were tested on ^{51}Cr-labeled P815 target cells. (B) Groups of 24 microwells containing 100 (solid triangles), 300 (open triangles), 500 (diamonds), or 750 (circles) normal A.CA (H-2^f) lymph node cells and 10^6 irradiated A.TH (H-2^{t2}) spleen cells. One half of each microwell was tested on ^{51}Cr-labeled A.TH Con A blasts, and the other half tested on ^{51}Cr-labeled B10.S(7R) target cells (H-2^{t2}). The solid lies represent the threshold values [mean spontaneous release (arrows) plus 2 SDs of the mean]. The dashed lines represent the mean maximum release of ^{51}Cr from each target.

(MHC) haplotype (H-2^{t2}) but with different non-MHC backgrounds. The counts obtained from each half-well are comparable; CTL which kill A.TH target cells also kill B10.S(7R) targets. Again a few cultures with low activity scored positive in one half only.

VII. LIMITATIONS OF THE ASSAY

The Poisson formula defines a probability distribution: in this case, the probability that a particular well contains CTL-P. An assay therefore is required which clearly distinguishes between a positive well (i.e., one containing CTL-P) and a negative well. One of the main problems in using the limiting dilution assay for the determination of CTL-P frequency is that there is no such distinction. The distribution of ^{51}Cr release values at any given responder cell dose is often continuous and shifts upward as the responder cell dose is increased (Fig. 2). In order to make the data amenable to analysis, it is necessary to decide on an arbitrary ^{51}Cr release value which defines a positive or negative culture. This value is generally chosen to exclude false positives from the calculation. Consequently, it may also exclude valid responses. Thus the CTL-P estimate is minimal.

If the culture conditions are optimal and the addition of growth-promoting factors sufficient, every CTL-P that responds should develop into a clone of roughly 1000 CTL, assuming a doubling time of 18 hr over the 8-day culture period. Since a lytic interaction takes between 5 and 30 min, and a CTL can accomplish several rounds of killing, every active CTL should kill several cell targets during the assay period, and near maximal ^{51}Cr release should be seen in every responding culture. However, although the lytic activity per responder cell is markedly higher in microcultures than in bulk cultures, it is still far from maximal, and the sensitivity of the ^{51}Cr release assay is still a critical factor. This problem is evident in the analysis of split wells (Fig. 4). If a culture has very low cytotoxic activity, one half-well may score positive and the other negative when assayed with the same target cells. This complicates interpretation of the same phenomenon occurring when two different targets are used.

If the data conform to single-hit kinetics, it is reasonable to assume that only a single component is limiting. However, this need not be the CTL-P. Furthermore, even if only the CTL-Ps are limiting, they need not be activated with maximal efficiency. If every specific CTL-P has the same probability of being stimulated and responding, single-hit kinetics and a straight-line plot will result, whether this probability is 1 or 100%. It is therefore necessary to work constantly to improve culture conditions and ensure maximal efficiency. Published data may serve as a guideline: If the frequency obtained in a given strain combination is lower than that found by others, the system as used is clearly deficient; if the frequencies are comparable, this should stimulate attempts to improve the system, since, for all the reasons discussed, the frequency is likely to be underestimated. Only loss of specificity would lead to an overestimate of the true frequency.

Finally, a word of caution is necessary concerning the use of limiting dilution for cloning. It must be remembered that responder cells are randomly distributed over the cultures, and even when there is *on the average* less than one precursor cell per well, some wells will contain more than one. From the general form of the Poisson distribution [Eq. (1)], the probability of having more than one CTL-P in a well can be calculated:

$$F_{>1} = 1 - F_0 - F_1 = 1 - (1 + \mu)e^{-\mu} \tag{5}$$

With an average of one CTL-P per well ($\mu = 1$), 26.4% of the *total* wells will contain more than one CTL-P; with an average of 0.1 CTL-P per well, $F_{>1}$ is 0.47%. The probability that a *positive* well will contain only one precursor, and thus that the CTLs belong to a single clone, is

$$F_1/(1 - F_0) = \mu e^{-\mu}/(1 - e^{-\mu}) \tag{6}$$

Thus we obtain 58.2% for $\mu = 1$, 77.07% for $\mu = 0.5$, and 95.8% for $\mu = 0.1$. It follows that only at very high dilutions of responder cell input, where less than 10% of all the wells are positive, will the probability that a positive culture is derived from a single precursor be above 95%.

ACKNOWLEDGMENT

We wish to thank Drs. H. R. MacDonald and M. B. Widmer for helpful advice and discussions.

REFERENCES

Bevan, M. J., and Cohn, M. (1975). *J. Immunol.* **114**, 559.
Fischer Lindahl, K., and Hausmann, B. (1980). *Eur. J. Immunol.* **10**, 289.
Fischer Lindahl, K., and Wilson, D. B. (1977a). *J. Exp. Med.* **145**, 500.
Fischer Lindahl, K., and Wilson, D. B. (1977b). *J. Exp. Med.* **145**, 508.
Gillis, S., and Smith, K. A. (1977). *Nature (London)* **268**, 154.
Iscove, N. N., and Melchers, F. (1978). *J. Exp. Med.* **147**, 923.
Lefkovits, I., and Waldmann, H. (1979). "Limiting Dilution Analysis of Cells in the Immune System." Cambridge Univ. Press, London and New York.
MacDonald, H. R., Cerottini, J.-C., Ryser, J.-E., Maryanski, J. L., Taswell, C., Widmer, M. B., and Brunner, K. T. (1980). *Immunol. Rev.* **51**, 93.

Miller, R. G. (1979). *In* "Regulation by T Cells" (D. G. Kilburn, J. G., Levy, and H.-S. Teh, eds.), p. 77. University of British Columbia, Department of Microbiology, Vancouver.

Miller, R. G., Teh, H.-S., Harley, E., and Phillips, R. A. (1977). *Immunol. Rev.* **35,** 38.

Piazza, A. (1979). *In* "Immunological Methods" (I. Lefkovits and B. Pernis, eds.) p. 419. Academic Press, New York.

Pilarski, L. M. (1977). *J. Exp. Med.* **145,** 709.

Ryser, J.-E., and MacDonald, H. R. (1979). *J. Immunol.* **122,** 1691.

Ryser, J.-E., Cerottini, J.-C., and Brunner, K. T. (1978). *J. Immunol.* **120,** 370.

Schilling, R. M., Phillips, R. A., and Miller, R. G. (1976). *J. Exp. Med.* **144,** 241.

Teh, H.-S., Phillips, R. A., and Miller, R. G. (1977) *J. Exp. Med.* **146,** 1280.

13

Induction of an Antibody Response in Cultures of Human Peripheral Blood Lymphocytes

Alma L. Luzzati

I. OBJECTIVE

The study of the complex mechanisms involved in the triggering, expression of function, and regulation of human B cells requires the successful establishment of methods for the induction and measurement of specific antibody responses in cultures of human peripheral blood lymphocytes (PBLs).

In spite of considerable effort it has been difficult to obtain with these cells reproducible antigen-induced and antigen-specific responses similar to those generated in the murine system of Mishell and Dutton. Only recently

IMMUNOLOGICAL METHODS, VOL. II

have a few laboratories reported some success in this area (Fauci and Ballieux, 1979).

In our laboratory we have established culture conditions under which a specific antibody response to heterologous erythrocytes can consistently be induced in human PBLs. Essential for this successful approach are (1) the removal of adhering inhibitory cells and (2) the provision of an inductive stimulus in addition to the antigen.

Here we describe in detail a method for specifically triggering an anti-sheep red blood cell (SRBC) response in the presence of Epstein–Barr (EB) virus as an additional stimulatory agent (Luzzati *et al.*, 1977, 1979).

II. PRINCIPLE OF THE METHOD

Blood is filtered through a column packed with synthetic wool, in order to remove adhering inhibitory cells (Luzzati and Lafleur, 1976), and then layered on a Ficoll–Urovison gradient. The cells harvested at the interface are cultured in plastic tissue culture wells in the presence of antigen (SRBCs) and EB virus.

The occurrence of a specific immune response is ascertained at different intervals by visualizing and enumerating the anti-SRBC plaque-forming cells (PFCs) with a modification of the gel hemolysis method.

III. MATERIALS

A. Synthetic Wool

A mixture of different synthetic fibers (polyester, polypropylene, acrylic), sold by a local dealer as cushion filling (No. 609.002, Coop, Basel, Switzerland), is used in our laboratory. The wool is soaked overnight in detergent (7 ×) and rinsed under running tap water for 24–48 hr and then in several changes of distilled water. The washed wool is dried, teased, and packed in weighed amounts into plastic syringes (see tabulation below) which are then autoclaved at 120°C for 30 min and dried.

Syringe	Wool (gm)	Blood (ml)[a]
10 ml	0.6	4
20 ml	1.2	8
50 ml	3.0	20

[a] The volume of blood that can be accommodated on a given amount of wool.

B. Ficoll–Urovison

Ficoll 400 (Pharmacia, Uppsala, Sweden), 46.20 gm
Urovison (Schering AG, Berlin, West Germany), 125 ml
Distilled water, 597 ml
The above ingredients are dissolved with stirring for 60 min at room temperature in the dark. The pH is brought to 7 with 0.1 N NaOH. If necessary, the density is adjusted to 1.077 with distilled water. The solution is autoclaved at 110°C for 20 min or sterilized by filtration through a 0.45-μm filter and then stored at 4°C in the dark.

C. Hanks' Balanced Salt Solution

Hanks' balanced salt solution (BSS) can be obtained from Microbiological Associates, Bethesda, Maryland (No. 10–508).

D. Culture Medium

Iscove's modified Dulbecco's medium (IMDM, a new medium formulation that can be obtained from Grand Island Biological Co., Grand Island, New York) supplemented with 8% human AB serum, 5 × 10⁻⁵ M β-mercaptoethanol, and 50 U/ml of streptomycin and penicillin) No. 17603 F, Microbiological Associates) is used.

The human serum is heat-inactivated and absorbed three times in the cold with 0.5 ml of packed erythrocytes per 10 ml of serum.

E. Antigen: Sheep Red Blood Cells

Sheep blood is collected in Alsever's solution (1 vol of blood in 1 vol of Alsever's solution) and allowed to age for at least 1 week before use.

The red cells are pelleted by centrifugation at 2500 rpm for 10 min and washed twice, care being taken to remove the buffy coat. The washing is usually performed in saline (0.15 M NaCl) when the erythrocytes are used as indicator cells, whereas it is performed in sterile Hanks' BSS when they are used as antigen *in vitro*.

F. Epstein–Barr Virus

Epstein–Barr virus is a moderate-risk oncogenic virus according to National Cancer Institute–National Institutes of Health standards. Therefore both the virus and the human and monkey transformed cells must be handled with caution. The use of ventilated safety cabinets (biohazard hoods) is mandatory.

The virus is prepared from the marmoset lymphoblastoid cell line B95–8.

The line is cultured at 37°C in RPMI 1640 medium (Grand Island Biological Co., Grand Island, New York) supplemented with 10% fetal calf serum (FCS) and 50 U/ml of streptomycin and penicillin in 1-liter plastic tissue culture bottles. The starting cell density is about 5×10^5 cells/ml.

After 7 days cells and debris are removed by low-speed centrifugation. The virus-containing supernatant is centrifuged at 100,000 g for 1 hr. Then 95% of the supernatant is sucked off, and the pelleted virus is resuspended in the remaining 5% (20 × stock). The 20× concentrated virus preparation is aliquoted in plastic culture tubes and stored at 4°C.

G. Eagle's Minimum Essential Medium

Eagle's minimum essential medium (MEM) can be obtained from Grand Island Biological Co., Grand Island, New York.

H. Agar for Enumeration of Plaque-Forming Cells

A 1% solution of agar (Bacto agar; Difco, Detroit, Michigan) in distilled water is diluted 1:1 with twice concentrated MEM (prewarmed at 43°C) and placed in a 43°C water bath. Shortly before use 0.15 ml of a 3% solution of DEAE–dextran (Pharmacia, Uppsala, Sweden) in 0.15 M NaCl is added to 10 ml of diluted agar.

I. Complement

Reconstituted lyophilized guinea pig complement (Behringwerke AG, Marburg/Lahn, West Germany) is absorbed twice in the cold with SRBCs (0.3 ml of packed SRBCs per 10 ml of complement). Absorbed complement is stored at −70°C.

IV. PROCEDURE

A. Preparing the Cells and Setting Up the Cultures

1. Blood from human donors is collected in heparin (50 U/ml).

2. Syringes packed with synthetic wool are accommodated on a rack specially designed to hold them in a vertical position. The syringe nozzle is sealed. The plunger is removed, and the wool is made compact by pushing it down with the aid of a pipette. Measured aliquots of blood are then distributed on top of the wool. The optimal ratio between amount of wool and volume of blood in a given syringe was given in Section III,A. With the aid of the plunger, the blood is forced into the wool until it reaches the far end, care being taken that it does not flow out of the wool. Even distribu-

tion of blood throughout the wool is achieved by tapping the syringe. The filled syringes are placed in a tray and put in a humidified CO_2 incubator at 37°C for 45 min. At the end of this period the blood is squeezed out of the syringes, and the wool is rinsed twice with warm Hanks' BSS, each time with a volume equal to one-half the initial volume of blood. Both the blood and the washing fluids are squeezed out of the wool by pushing the syringe plunger down as far as possible.

3. The wool-filtered blood diluted with the washing fluids is layered on the Ficoll–Urovison mixture (usually 30 ml of diluted blood on 15 ml of Ficoll in 50-ml conic glass tubes). Centrifugation is carried out at 20°C for 40 min with an interface force of 400 g. The cells at the interface are harvested, washed in Hanks' BSS, and suspended in tissue culture medium at a concentration of 8–9 × 10^6 cells/ml.

4. Antigen is added in the form of 0.05 ml of 1% SRBCs in Hanks' BSS per milliliter of cell suspension.

5. The cell suspension is distributed in 0.1-ml aliquots into the wells of Microtest II tissue culture plates (type 3040, Falcon Plastics).

6. Virus is added in the form of 25–50 μl of 20 × concentrated supernatant per well.

7. The cultures are incubated in a humidified 5% CO_2 incubator at 37°C without further treatment until assayed.

B. Assay of Plaque-Forming Cells

At the time of harvesting, the contents of five wells are pooled and the cells washed once in Hanks' BSS and resuspended in 0.25 ml of MEM.

The number of PFCs is assayed using a modification of the gel hemolysis method. Portions of 0.4 ml of the agar–DEAE–dextran mixture are distributed in 50 × 8 mm glass tubes and kept in a 43°C water bath. Twenty microliters of 20% SRBCs, 10–50 μl of the lymphoid cell suspension, and 50 μl of a 1:4 dilution of guinea pig complement are added to the tubes in rapid sequence. When high activity is expected, 10 μl of one or more dilutions of the lymphocyte suspension should be tested. The mixture is spread on glass microscope slides precoated with agar. After the agar has solidified, the slides are placed in a humidified box in a CO_2 incubator at 37°C. After 2.5 hr plaques can be enumerated with an automated colony counter by holding the slides under a magnifying lens in indirect light.

V. COMMENTS

The induction of a primary anti-SRBC response in cultured human PBLs is reproducible if a second appropriate stimulus, besides the antigen, is given to the cells. Very few if any failures are met with the system described here, which employs EB virus. The plaques obtained are of a size and quality comparable to those induced in mice and rabbits.

Maximum response is usually observed after 8–9 days of culture. The number of PFCs can then stay at almost a plateau level for several days or drop rapidly to a low value. In some instances a second peak can be seen on about day 13. Plaques are always of the direct type only.

Control cultures grown without antigen and/or without virus usually produce a very low number of plaques or no plaques at all. In some rare instances, cultures stimulated by EB virus may produce a sizable number of anti-SRBC plaques in the absence of the specific antigen. However, in this case the number of plaques is always smaller than that obtained with both stimuli and very rapidly drops to zero.

Although there is a great difference from donor to donor in the degree and the kinetics of the response, repeated experiments performed with samples of blood taken from the same donor give very consistent results. Thus the method can be used to evaluate an individual's capacity to mount an antibody response *in vitro*. Moreover it opens up possibilities for monitoring variations under clinical conditions (Luzzati *et al.*, 1979).

REFERENCES

Fauci, A. S., and Ballieux, R. E., eds. (1979). "Antibody Production in Man: In Vitro Synthesis and Clinical Implications." Academic Press, New York.
Luzzati, A. L., and Lafleur, L. (1976). *Eur. J. Immunol.* **6**, 125.
Luzzati, A. L., Taussig, M. J., Meo, T., and Pernis, B. (1976). *J. Exp. Med.* **144**, 573.
Luzzati, A. L., Hengartner, H., and Schreier, M. H. (1977). *Nature (London)* **269**, 419.
Luzzati, A. L., Heinzer, I., Hengartner, H., and Schreier, M. H. (1979). *Clin. Exp. Immunol.* **35**, 405.

(Fig. 1a and b). The tendon of the knee is then cut, so that the rectus femoris can be lifted. It is crucial to do this carefully, so that no muscle tissue remains on the upper side of the femur (Fig. 1c and d). Subsequently the femur is slightly lifted with surgical forceps, and the knee joint is cut (Fig. 1e). The femur is lifted again, and the muscles on the lower side are cut. Finally, the femur is elevated so that the joint capsule which keeps the head of the femur toward the ilium becomes stretched and can be cut (Fig. 1f).

Before isolating the bone marrow from the femur, the residual muscle

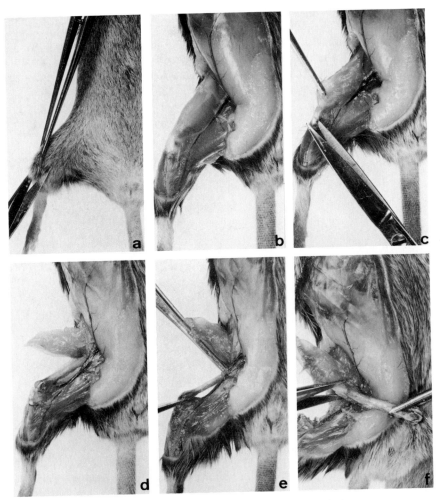

Fig. 1. Procedure for removing the femur of a mouse. For description see text.

tissue is removed with a tissue. The marrow can most easily be isolated after cutting the head of the femur and a small piece of the greater trochanter on the upper side, and a small piece of the condyle on the lower side. By means of a 2- or 5-ml syringe equipped with a 25G × 0.6 needle, a hole is pricked in both spongious ends of the femur. Then the marrow is collected by flushing the marrow cavity with 1 or 2 ml of a balanced salt solution (BSS) from the syringe (Fig. 2). Whether or not the marrow has been completely extracted from the femur can be judged from the color of the shaft. Bone marrow from long bones other than femurs can be similarly isolated by flushing the marrow cavity with BSS.

A single-cell suspension from the bone marrow can most easily be obtained by gently squeezing the latter through a nylon gauze filter with 100-μm openings (Stokvis and Smits Textielmij, Haarlem, The Netherlands). The nylon is stretched between two aluminium rings with a diameter of 3 cm. This setup is used in combination with a 50-ml glass beaker (Fig. 3).

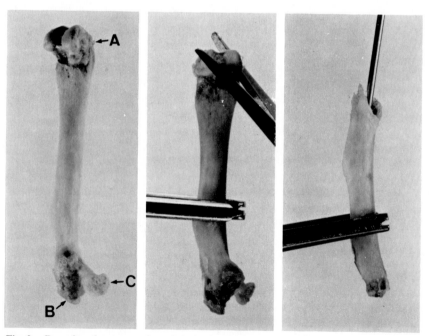

Fig. 2. Procedure for preparation of the bone marrow from a mouse femur. For description see text.

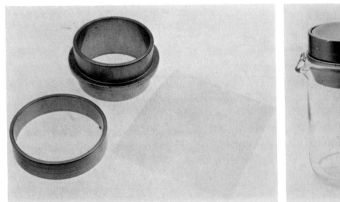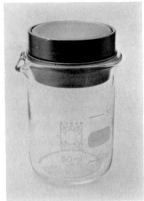

Fig. 3. Nylon gauze filter for preparation of single-cell suspensions.

B. Collection of Marrow from Flat Bones

Bone marrow from a flat bone is not easily isolated by flushing the marrow cavity. Therefore we prefer to break the bone in BSS with a mortar and pestle. When this is done carefully, the viability of the bone marrow cells is equal to that obtained after flushing long bones with BSS, i.e., over 90%. Large bone fragments can be removed by centrifuging for 30 sec at 125 g. Tiny bone fragments can be separated from the marrow by gently squeezing the supernatant through a nylon gauze filter with 100-μm or, if necessary, 30-μm openings.

III. DISTRIBUTION OF ANTIBODY-FORMING CELLS OVER VARIOUS BONE MARROW COMPARTMENTS

After mice are immunized the plaque-forming cell (PFC) activity is approximately the same in different bone marrow compartments. This is apparent from studies in which the PFC activity was determined in bone marrow cell suspensions obtained from femur, tibia, humerus, rib, and sternum. Such a comparative study was made during the primary response to *Escherichia coli* lipopolysaccharide (LPS) and the secondary resposne to sheep erythrocytes (SRBCs) (Table I). In view of the absence of significant differences between the PFC responses of marrow cells from these different compartments, the femoral marrow should be considered a reliable representative of the total bone marrow.

In similar studies on the distribution of surface Ig-positive (B) cells over various bone marrow compartments, equally high frequencies were found (Rozing *et al.*, 1978).

TABLE I

Comparison of Plaque-Forming Cell Activity in Various Compartments of Mouse Bone Marrow during the Primary Response to Lipopolysaccharide and the Secondary Response to Sheep Red Blood Cells[a,b]

Source of bone marrow cells	Anti-LPS PFCs	Anti-SRBC PFCs[c]		
		IgM	IgG	IgA
Femur	2492	820	4914	1568
Tibia	3415	1037	4648	1935
Humerus	2937	1640	4971	1882
Rib	2986	1667	5795	2137
Sternum	2960	n.d.	n.d.	n.d.

[a] From Benner and van Oudenaren, 1975, 1976.

[b] Female (C57BL × CBA) F_1 mice were either immunized by a single iv injection of 10 μg *E. coli* LPS or primed with 10^7 SRBCs iv and boosted with 4 × 10^8 SRBCs iv 4 months later. The PFC assay was performed 5 days after immunization with LPS and 7 days after the booster injection of SRBCs. The figures represent the number of PFCs per 10^7 viable nucleated cells.

[c] n.d., not determined.

IV. CALCULATION OF THE ANTIBODY-FORMING CELL ACTIVITY OF THE TOTAL BONE MARROW

Comparison of the PFC response of the bone marrow with that of the other lymphoid organs after immunization requires quantitation of the PFC response per whole organ. For spleen and lymph nodes this is easy to do, since the plaque assay can be performed with a sample from a cell suspension made from the whole organ. For bone marrow this is not feasible. In view of the comparable PFC activity in various bone marrow compartments (Table I), and in view of the fact that bone marrow cells can be easily isolated from femurs, we advocate determination of marrow PFC response in the femoral marrow, with subsequent calculation of the PFC response of the total bone marrow by using a conversion factor. This conversion factor can be deduced from the distribution of intravenously (iv) or intraperitoneally (ip) injected ^{59}Fe over the various parts of the skeleton. Three independent groups of investigators have performed such studies (Chervenick *et al.*, 1968; Schofield and Cole, 1968; Smith and Clayton, 1970). They found that of the total amount of ^{59}Fe which localized in the bone marrow, 5.9, 7, and 6%, respectively, was bound by the femoral marrow. The reciprocal value of the mean of these three percentages is 15.87. Thus the PFC response of the total bone marrow can be calculated to be 15.87 times the response of the bone marrow of a single femur. This calculation is based on the assumption that all bone marrow cells can be extracted from a femur. But sometimes it is difficult to remove all the visible (red) bone marrow from a femoral shaft. Consequently, the calculated bone marrow PFC response is too low. In order to reduce this factor we prefer to collect the marrow from both femurs of a mouse. Then we can use a conversion factor of 7.9.

V. KINETICS OF THE RESPONSE

Whether or not immunization of mice leads to antibody formation in the bone marrow is dependent on a number of factors (discussed in Section VI). Generally, secondary iv immunization with T-dependent antigens induces bone marrow antibody formation. The bone marrow PFC response has characteristic kinetics, independent of the type of T-dependent antigen and independent of the booster dose (Benner *et al.,* 1974). The response can be divided into two phases. The first phase, of about 1 week's duration, is characterized by a much higher number of PFCs in the spleen than in the marrow. During the second phase, on the other hand, the PFC response in the bone marrow is much higher than in all the other lymphoid organs combined (Benner *et al.,* 1974). This relatively high PFC activity in the bone marrow is found for IgM as well as IgG and IgA antibody production (Fig. 4).

VI. CRITICAL FACTORS

A. Primary versus Secondary-Type Responses

As stated in Section I, all initial studies in which the occurrence of antibody formation in mouse bone marrow was investigated revealed little or no PFC activity in this organ after immunization (reviewed in Benner and Haaijman, 1980). Almost all of these studies were limited in one aspect which proved to be crucial: Antibody formation in the bone marrow was assayed only during the primary response. Secondary immunization with a T-dependent antigen, however, induces antibody formation in the bone marrow. This result was found for heterologous erythrocytes (Fig. 4), protein antigen (Hill, 1976), and a variety of T-dependent hapten–carrier com-

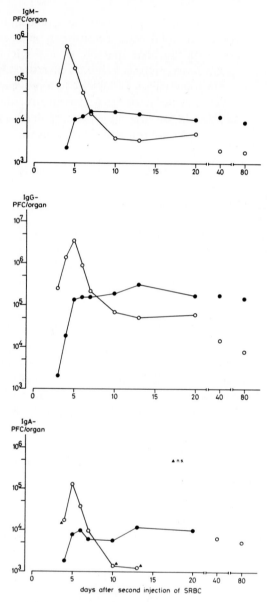

Fig. 4. Number of IgM, IgG, and IgA PFCs in (C57BL × CBA) F₁ mouse spleen (open circles) and bone marrow (solid circles) after two iv injections of SRBCs. The mice were primed with 10⁷ SRBCs and boosted with 4 × 10⁸ SRBCs 3 months later. A triangle indicates that the number of IgA PFCs above the number of IgM PFCs in the indirect plaque assay was not significant.

plexes (Koch *et al.,* 1981a) provided normal, thymus-bearing, mice were used. Secondary immunization of nude mice with SRBCs does not lead to significant antibody formation in the bone marrow.

Sometimes antibody formation occurs in the bone marrow after a single injection of a high dose of a T-dependent antigen. However, in such cases PFCs only occur in the marrow during the late phase of the primary response. We have shown that antibody formation in mouse bone marrow is dependent on the availability of memory B cells at the time of booster injection (Koch *et al.,* 1981a). Therefore the most likely explanation for bone marrow antibody formation during the late phase of the primary response is that in fact a secondary-type response is occurring. The generation of memory B cells during the first phase of the primary response and persistence of the injected antigen probably account for this phenomenon (see also Section VI,D).

B. Type of Antigen

Thus far, we did not observe exceptions to the rule that secondary iv or ip immunization of thymus-bearing mice with a T-dependent antigen dissolved in saline evokes the appearance of PFCs in the bone marrow. The kinetics of such bone marrow PFC responses has been described in Section V.

Although we have made only minimal investigations into whether antibody formation in the bone marrow also occurs after secondary immunization with T-independent antigens, we have studied the primary response to T-independent antigens. Intravenous immunization with a T-independent antigen such as pneumococcus, *E. coli* bacterium, α-1, 6-dextran, or 2, 4-dinitrophenyl (DNP)–Ficoll leads to a weak antigen-specific PFC response in the bone marrow and induces large numbers of PFCs in the spleen (Koch *et al.,* 1981b). However, immunization of mice with 10 μg *E. coli* LPS or 100 μg 1,3,5-trinitrophenyl (TNP)-LPS induces high PFC activity in the marrow. After abolishment of the mitogenic moiety of LPS, the lipid A component, by detoxification according to von Eschen and Rudbach (1976), the residual polysaccharide was no longer capable of inducing bone marrow antibody formation (Benner and Haaijman, 1980). The same result was found for the TNP-detoxified LPS complex. Thus antibody formation in the bone marrow after primary immunization with a T-independent antigen seems to require a second signal from a lipid A-like component. T cells are not required for the formation of bone marrow antibody to LPS and TNP-LPS. This can be deduced from the observation that BALB/c nude mice respond to an iv injection of LPS with bone marrow antibody formation. Although the kinetics of the response of nude mice is essentially the same as that of their euthymic littermates, the number of PFCs in the marrow of nude mice is generally 50–70% lower (Benner and van Oudenaren, 1979).

C. Route of Antigen Administration

Antibody formation is generally most prominent in the lymphoid organ draining the site of immunization. This rule also holds for antibody formation in bone marrow during the secondary response to T-dependent antigens. The highest bone marrow PFC responses are observed with iv or ip booster injections. At low booster doses a splenectomy just before the booster injection can almost completely prevent the bone marrow PFC response (Benner et al., 1977). Thereby the migration of antigen-activated memory B cells from the spleen into the bone marrow is prevented. These antigen-activated memory B cells, which normally migrate into the bone marrow during the first few days after the booster injection, account for the bone marrow PFC response (Koch et al., 1981a).

The decrease in the bone marrow PFC response resulting from a splenectomy can be overcome by using a high booster dose. This is illustrated in Table II for SRBCs as antigen. High iv booster doses of SRBCs probably stimulate the lymph nodes so that these organs can replace the spleen. Subcutaneous (sc) booster injections also lead to bone marrow antibody formation, both in nonsplenectomized and in splenectomized mice, but only with high antigen doses (Table II). Thus the antigen must be present in the peripheral lymphoid organs as well as in the bone marrow for PFCs to appear in the latter organ.

Whether or not secondary immunization with a T-dependent antigen will lead to bone marrow antibody formation is independent of the route of primary immunization; iv, ip, and sc priming are all effective. However, in the case of SRBCs as antigen, a 100-fold higher antigen dose is required for sc priming than for iv or ip priming in order to prepare for an equally high secondary bone marrow PFC response (Benner et al., 1974). The preparation for bone marrow antibody formation by iv priming with low or moderately high doses of SRBCs can be completely prevented by a prior splenectomy. A splenectomy before iv priming with a high dose of SRBCs is ineffective (Benner and van Oudenaren, 1975; Benner et al., 1977), probably as a result of the stimulation of lymph node tissue by the large amount of iv injected antigen.

TABLE II

Influence of the Route of Booster Immunization on the Extent of the Bone Marrow Plaque-Forming Cell Response[a]

Surgery	Booster dose of SRBCs	PFCs per bone marrow	
		IgM	IgG
Sham Sx	10^6, iv	8,830 (6,150–12,700)	45,760 (37,090–56,450)
Sx	10^6, iv	2,340 (1,570–3,990)	8,530 (7,380–9,860)
Sx	10^6, sc	860 (610–1,220)	8,340 (6,360–10,940)
Sham Sx	4×10^8, iv	29,510 (26,950–32,310)	255,400 (239,410–272,470)
Sham Sx	4×10^8, sc	8,480 (5,490–13,090)	91,030 (82,970–99,870)
Sx	4×10^8, iv	44,970 (33,110–61,060)	298,900 (232,920–383,590)
Sx	4×10^8, sc	21,820 (20,260–23,500)	96,760 (74,440–125,790)

[a] Female (C57BL × CBA) F_1 mice were primed with 10^7 SRBCs iv and boosted with either 10^6 or 4×10^8 SRBCs 3 months later. The mice were either splenectomized (Sx) or sham-splenectomized (sham Sx) 3 weeks before the booster immunization. The PFC assay was performed 7 days after the booster injection. Values shown are the geometric mean and 95% confidence limits.

D. Use of Adjuvants

The use of an adjuvant can interfere with bone marrow antibody formation. Adjuvants which induce excessive granulopoiesis within the bone marrow [e.g., complete Freund adjuvant (CFA) and high doses of LPS] abolish the ongoing Ig synthesis in this organ. This is apparent from the observation that several days after such a treatment the presence of Ig-synthesizing cells in the bone marrow can no longer be revealed with the protein A plaque assay. This excessive granulopoiesis can last for 1–4 weeks, depending on the dose and type of adjuvant used.

Secondary immunization of mice with heterologous erythrocytes or hapten–carrier complexes emulsified in CFA does not lead to antibody formation in the bone marrow during the first few weeks after the booster injection. This is merely due to the adjuvant, since injection of an equal amount of the same antigen in saline induces bone marrow antibody formation. Adjuvants which do not induce excessive granulopoiesis, such as alum, do not interfere with antibody formation in the marrow.

In our experience, the occurrence of excessive granulopoiesis, and thus the possibility of detecting antibody formation in the bone marrow, can usually be predicted from the color of the femoral shaft. Excessive granulopoiesis in the marrow is associated with a severe depression of erythropoiesis in this organ. Thus the femur is observed to be white instead of reddish.

Primary immunization with an antigen emulsified in adjuvant leads to prolonged antibody synthesis as compared to that observed after immunization with the antigen dissolved in saline. This can be concluded from comparison of the serum antibody titers of animals treated differently. However, the adjuvant also affects organ distribution of the antibody-producing PFCs. Several months after a single injection of antigen together with adjuvant, large numbers of PFCs occur in the bone marrow (Table III). The primary response becomes a secondary-type response, probably because of the slow release of antigen from the adjuvant-induced granuloma.

TABLE III

Influence of the Use of Adjuvant on the Number and Organ Distribution of Antibody-Forming Cells 3 Months after Primary Immunization with a Dinitrophenyl–Carrier Complex[a]

		PFCs per spleen		PFCs per bone marrow	
Antigen	Adjuvant	IgM	IgG[b]	IgM	IgG[b]
DNP-KLH	—	1,287 (1,005–1,647)	n.s.	< 500	3,790 (2,707–5,306)
DNP-KLH	Alum	3,815 (2,512–5,794)	n.s.	1,569 (581–4,238)	18,301 (8,200–40,845)
DNP-CGG	—	< 500	n.s.	< 500	n.s.
DNP-CGG	Alum	2,683 (1,010–7,125)	n.s.	865 (424–1,764)	23,924 (13,851–41,321)
DNP-CGG	CFA	2,639 (2,044–3,406)	n.s.	5872 (2,499–13,799)	84,692 (71,912–99,744)

[a] Female (C57BL × CBA) F_1 mice were immunized with 100 µg DNP10–chicken gamma globulin (DNP-CGG) or DNP200–keyhole limpet hemocyanin (DNP-KLH) ip 3 months previously. The DNP/carrier ratio is expressed as the number of DNP groups per protein molecule. The antigen was administered either dissolved in saline, precipitated on alum, or emulsified in CFA. Values shown are the geometric mean and 95% confidence limits.

[b] n.s., the number of IgG PFCs above the number of IgM PFCs in the indirect plaque assay was not significant.

E. Corticosteroid Level

The extent of the immune response is dependent upon the corticosteroid level (Garbielsen and Good, 1967). Generally, an increase in the corticosteroid level decreases the response, whereas a decrease in the corticosteroid level can increase the response (van Dijk *et al.,* 1976). In mice, corticosteroids have a differential effect upon antibody formation in spleen and bone marrow (Benner *et al.,* 1978; Benner and van Oudenaren, 1979). Daily injections of corticosteroid suppress the primary and secondary anti-SRBC IgM, IgG, and IgA PFC response in the spleen. Bone marrow IgM, IgG, and IgA PFCs were found to be rather resistant to corticosteroid-mediated suppression. These responses were not affected by daily doses of dexamethasone up to 4 mg/kg body weight. A daily dose of 16 mg/kg body weight decreased the bone marrow PFC response when the injections were started before the booster injection. When the corticosteroid injections were started 5 days after the booster injection, the dose of 16 mg/kg body weight did not suppress the bone marrow PFC response, in contrast to the splenic PFC response (Benner *et al.,* 1978).

The primary response to the thymus-independent antigen LPS is also affected by corticosteroid injection. In this case also, suppression of the splenic PFC response was proportional to the dose of corticosteroids administered. However, the anti-LPS bone marrow PFC response showed dose-dependent enhancement after daily corticosteroid injections. Thus antibody formation in mouse bone marrow, in contrast to antibody formation in mouse spleen, seems to be very resistant to corticosteroid-mediated suppression.

F. Age

Primary immunization of adult mice with LPS or TNP–LPS and secondary immunization with a T-dependent antigen lead, regardless of the age of the mice used, to antibody formation within the bone marrow. With aging, the day of peak PFC activity in the bone marrow occurs later, just as in the spleen. The extent of the bone marrow PFC response decreases somewhat with increasing age. This is especially true of the IgG PFC response (Blankwater, 1978).

Insight into the actual Ig-synthesizing activity of a mouse can be obtained by measuring the number of Ig-secreting cells or the number of C-Ig cells in various lymphoid organs. When this is done for mice of various ages, a clear age-related increase is found in the total number of C-Ig cells in all lymphoid organs. At 8 weeks of age a plateau is attained, which is maintained until death (Haaijman *et al.,* 1977). However, organ distribution of

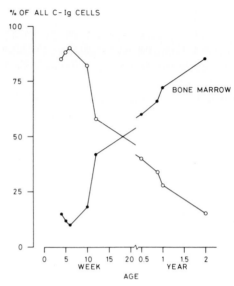

Fig. 5. Relative contribution of the bone marrow (solid circles) and the other (open circles) lymphoid organs (spleen, mesenteric lymph nodes, and Peyer's patches combined) to the total number of C-Ig cells in male CBA mice of various ages. From Haaijman *et al.*, 1977.

C-Ig cells changes considerably during aging. With time, C-Ig cells accumulate in the bone marrow (Fig. 5), and this holds for C-IgM cells as well as C-IgG and C-IgA cells (Haaijman *et al.*, 1977). The gradual increase in the importance of the bone marrow as a site of Ig synthesis throughout the life span probably reflects the gradual adaptation of individual mice to their antigenic environment. As an individual ages, the more often antigenic stimuli from the environment will have been experienced before, and thus more secondary-type responses will prevail. As outlined in Section VI,A, such secondary-type responses involve the bone marrow.

ACKNOWLEDGMENT

We sincerely thank Mr. T. M. van Os and Mr. J. G. H. Fengler for expert photography, and Mrs. Cary Meijerink and Rita Boucke for typing the manuscript.

REFERENCES

Askonas, B. A., and White, R. G. (1956). *Br. J. Exp. Pathol.* **37,** 61.
Benner, R., and Haaijman, J. J. (1980). *Dev. Comp. Immunol.* **4,** 591.
Benner, R., and van Oudenaren, A. (1975). *Cell Immunol.* **19,** 167.

Benner, R., and van Oudenaren, A. (1976). *Immunology* **30**, 49.

Benner, R., and van Oudenaren, A. (1979). *Cell. Immunol.* **48**, 267.

Benner, R., Meima, F., van der Meulen, G. M., and van Ewijk, W. (1974). *Immunology* **27**, 747.

Benner, R., van Oudenaren, A., and de Ruiter, H. (1977). *Cell. Immunol.* **34**, 125.

Benner, R., van Dongen, J. J., and van Oudenaren, A. (1978). *Cell. Immunol.* **41**, 52.

Benner, R., Rijnbeek, A.-M., Bernabé, R. R., Martinez-Alonso, C., and Coutinho, A. (1981). *Immunobiol.* (in press).

Blankwater, M.-J. (1978). Ph.D. Thesis, University of Utrecht, The Netherlands.

Chervenick, P. A., Boggs, D. R., Marsh, J. C., Cartwright, G. E., and Wintrobe, M. M. (1968). *Am. J. Physiol.* **215**, 353.

Gabrielsen, A. E., and Good, R. A. (1967). *Adv. Immunol.* **6**, 91.

Haaijman, J. J., Schuit, H. R. E., and Hijmans, W. (1977). *Immunology* **32**, 427.

Haaijman, J. J., Slingerland-Teunissen, J., Benner, R., and van Oudenaren, A. (1979). *Immunology* **26**, 271.

Hijmans, W. (1975). *In* "The Immunological Basis of Connective Tissue Disorders" (L. G. Silvestri, ed.), p. 203. North-Holland Publ., Amsterdam.

Hijmans, W., Schuit, H. R. E., and Hulsing-Hesselink, E. (1971). *Ann. N.Y. Acad. Sci.* **177**, 290.

Hill, S. W. (1976). *Immunology* **30**, 895.

Koch, G., Osmond, D. G., Julius, M. H., and Benner, R. (1981a). *J. Immunol.* (in press).

Koch, G., van Oudenaren, A., and Benner, R. (1981b). In preparation.

McMillan, R., Longmire, R. L., Yelenosky, R., Lang, J. E., Heath, V., and Craddock, C. G. (1972). *J. Immunol.* **109**, 1386.

Rozing, J., Brons, N. H. C., and Benner, R. (1978). *Immunology* **34**, 909.

Schofield, R., and Cole, L. (1968). *Br. J. Haematol.* **14**, 131.

Smith, L. H., and Clayton, M. L. (1970). *Exp. Hematol.* **20**, 82.

Turesson, I. (1976). *Acta Med. Scand.* **199**, 293.

van Dijk, H., Testerink, J., and Noordegraaf, E. (1976). *Cell Immunol.* **25**, 8.

von Eschen, K. B., and Rudbach, J. A. (1976). *J. Immunol.* **116**, 8.

15

Long-Term Culture and Cloning of Specific Helper T Cells

Max H. Schreier and Reet Tees

I. OBJECTIVE AND PRINCIPLE OF THE METHOD

The observations of Morgan *et al.* (1976) and Ruscetti *et al.* (1977) that supernatants of alloantigen or mitogen-stimulated lymphoid cells promote growth of T cells have resulted in a method for obtaining large numbers of apparently untransformed functionally defined T-cell populations. The growth-promoting activity of such conditioned media, termed T-cell growth factor (TCGF, Gillis *et al.*, 1978) or interleukin-2 (IL-2)[1], has been

---

[1] This revised name for TCGF was proposed at the Second International Lymphokine Workshop, Ermatingen, Switzerland, 1979. (Letter to the Editor, 1979.)

IMMUNOLOGICAL METHODS, VOL. II

used successfully in establishing and maintaining lines (Gillis and Smith, 1977) and clones of specific cytolytic T cells (reviewed by Smith, 1980). Similar attempts to maintain antigen-specific helper T cells in long-term TCGF-dependent proliferative culture (Schrier *et al.,* 1979; Watson, 1979; Schreier, 1979) have been successful, and clones of helper T cells specific for heterologous erythrocytes have been established (Schreier and Tees, 1980; Tees and Schreier, 1980).

In the initiation and maintenance of helper T-cell lines four phases can be distinguished: (1) *in vivo* induction of a sufficiently high fraction of helper T cells of a given specificity, (2) *in vitro* specific helper T-cell enrichment by selective antigen-induced clonal expansion, (3) TCGF-dependent, antigen- and adherent cell-independent proliferative culture, and (4) single-cell cloning and subcloning of helper T-cell lines.

This chapter describes the establishment and maintenance of lines and clones of helper T cells specific for sheep erythrocytes (SRCs) or horse erythrocytes (HRCs).

II. MATERIALS

A. Mice

Young adult female C57BL/6J mice have been most frequently used for the generation of *in vivo*-activated helper T cells. Congenic male or female C57BL/6J *nu/nu* mice (8–10 backcrosses) are used for testing the activity and specificity of *in vitro*-propagated helper T cells both *in vitro* and *in vivo*. Congenic mouse strains B10.A, B10.A (4R), and B10.A (5R) required for monitoring the depletion of alloreactive T cells during long-term *in vitro* culture and for H-2 restriction experiments have been obtained from OLAC, Ltd., Blackthorn, Bicester, Oxon, England. All mice must be specific-pathogen-free and are kept in isolators (three to five animals per cage).

For the generation of TCGF Lewis rats of either sex (170–220 gm) have been used. Occasionally used outbred strains yield comparable factor activity.

B. Salt Solutions, Media, and Medium Supplements

Earle's balanced salt solution (BSS) without $NaHCO_3$ contains, per 1000 ml glass-distilled water, 6.8 gm NaCl, 0.4 gm KCl, 0.14 gm $NaH_2 PO_4$ • H_2O, 0.2 gm $MgSO_4$ • $7H_2O$, 0.2 gm anhydrous $CaCl_2$, 1.0 gm $D(+)$-glucose, and 0.01 gm phenol red. The solution is sterilized by passing it through a 200-nm pore-filter and stored indefinitely at 4°C.

Ca^{2+}- and Mg^{2+}-free PBS used for detachment of adherent cells contains, per liter, 8.2 gm NaCl, 0.2 gm KCl, 2.88 gm Na$_2$HPO$_4$ • 12H$_2$O, 0.2 gm KH$_2$PO$_4$, 0.29 gm Na$_2$ EDTA • 2H$_2$O, and 1.5 ml 1% phenol red solution.

Iscove's medium (IMDM), an enriched modification of Dulbecco's modified Eagle's medium (Guilbert and Iscove, 1976; Iscove and Melchers, 1978), has recently become commercially available as tissue culture powder (No. 430,2200, Gibco). However, virtually all our experience has been with IMDM prepared by supplementing Dulbecco's modified Eagle's medium with additional amino acids and vitamins and adjusting it to optimal osmolarity according to the formula of these authors. When supplemented with a combination of albumin, transferrin, and lipids (Guilbert and Iscove, 1976; Iscove and Melchers, 1978; Iscove *et al.*, 1980) as serum replacement, we refer to the complete medium as IMDM-ATL.

IMDM-ATL is prepared from the following solutions:

1. Dulbecco's modified Eagle's medium, 2× (No. 430-2100, formerly H-21 Gibco): One package of powder (13.4 gm) is dissolved in 500 ml H$_2$O, and the solution filtered through a 0.45-μm filter and stored at 4°C.
2. NaHCO$_3$ solution, 5%: 5 gm NaHCO$_3$ is dissolved in 100 ml H$_2$O, and the solution sterile-filtered, and stored at 4°C.
3. HEPES buffer (No. 563, Gibco): 1 *M*, pH 7.3.
4. Amino acid mixture: 0.18 gm alanine, 0.156 gm asparagine, 0.216 gm aspartic acid, 0.54 gm glutamic acid, 0.288 gm proline, 0.792 gm sodium pyruvate, and 72 ml H$_2$O. These components are dissolved at approximately 40°C with repeated agitation, and 0.48 ml of a vitamin B$_{12}$–biotin solution (see below) is added. The sterile-filtered solution is stored in aliquots at −20°C.

The vitamin B$_{12}$–biotin solution consists of 0.005 gm vitamin B$_{12}$, 0.005 gm biotin, 20 ml H$_2$O, and 0.01 ml 1 *M* HCl. The solution is sterile-filtered and stored frozen in 1-ml aliquots.

5. Cystine: 0.7 gm cystine is dissolved in 100 ml 0.25 *M* HCl, and the solution is sterile-filtered and frozen in aliquots.
6. Selenium: 2.8 mg Na$_2$SeO$_3$ is dissolved in 100 ml H$_2$O, and the sterile solution is stored at 4°C.
7. 2-Mercaptoethanol (2-ME): 0.7 ml of 2-ME is dissolved in 100 ml BSS to give a 0.1 *M* sterile solution which can be stored for several months in a foil-covered bottle at 4°C.
8. Bovine serum albumin (BSA): In contrast to the original description the charcoal extraction and Amberlite treatment (Guilbert and Iscove, 1976; Iscove *et al.*, 1980) have been omitted; 20 gm pure BSA (Behringwerke, Marburg, West Germany) is dissolved in water, and the volume is adjusted to 100 ml. The sterile-filtered solution is stored at 4°C.

9. Transferrin iron (one-third saturated): 0.9 gm transferrin (human transferrin, Behringwerke, Marburg/Lahn, West Germany) is dissolved in 9.0 ml ($1 \times$) Dulbecco's bicarbonate-free medium buffered with HEPES, pH 7.3 (0.01 M); then 1.0 ml of a 7.9×10^{-3} M $FeCl_3$ solution (in 0.001 M HCl) is added; the sterile-filtered transferrin–iron solution is stored indefinitely at 4°C.

10. Soybean–lipid–cholesterol suspension: 0.24 gm soybean lipid (No. PH75, Nattermann, Cologne, West Germany) is spread on the bottom of a 200-ml glass beaker, and 0.138 gm cholesterol is evenly dispersed over this lecithin layer. Then 60 ml of a 1% BSA solution in 1 × Dulbecco's bicarbonate-free medium is placed in the beaker which is immersed in ice water and sonicated for 1 hr at maximum energy on a Measuring and Scientific Equipment sonicator. The 2-cm-diameter probe is placed close to the bottom of the beaker for the first 30 min and then raised to about 1 mm below the surface for the consecutive 30 min of sonication. The yellow suspension is filtered through a Whatman GF/A 4.7-cm glass-fiber filter placed over a Millipore Pyrex base mounted on a 200-ml suction flask and consecutively filtered through 1.2-μm and 0.45-μm Millipore membranes. It is stored for up to several months at 4°C.

IMDM-ATL is prepared by combining 82 ml 2× Dulbecco's modified Eagle's medium, 10.0 ml 5% $NaHCO_3$ solution, 5.0 ml HEPES buffer, 1.6 ml amino acid mixture, 0.8 ml cystine, 0.16 ml Na_2SeO_3, 0.1 ml 0.1 M 2-ME, 1.0 ml 20% BSA solution, 0.07 ml transferrin–iron, 5.0 ml lipids (soybean–lipid–cholesterol suspension), 2.0 ml penicillin–streptomycin (No. 514, Gibco), and 92.3 ml H_2O to a final volume of 200 ml. The complete medium is sterile-filtered (0.45 μm) and stored at 4°C for up to 4 weeks.

C. T-Cell Growth Factor

1. Preparation and Procedure

TCGF is prepared and partially purified as in published procedures (Shaw et al., 1978; Watson et al., 1979a,b; Schreier et al., 1980a) from concanavalin A (Con A)-induced rat spleen cell cultures.

Lewis rats are killed in CO_2 by placing five animals at a time for about 5 min in a 5000-ml glass beaker which contains a layer of dry ice below a layer of paper towels and is covered by a cork board. The spleens are aseptically removed and cut into small pieces with bent scissors over a stainless steel grid placed over a 6-cm tissue culture dish containing approximately 15 ml BSS. The cells are forced through the grid with the plunger of a 10-ml plastic syringe, transferred to Falcon No. 2070 50-ml tubes, filled up to 50 cm^3 with BSS, and spun for 10 min at 400 g. The washing is repeated, and the spleen cells are resuspended in IMDM and counted. They are then cultured in IMDM supplemented with BSA (0.25 mg/ml), antibiotics, 2-ME (5 × 10^{-5} M) and containing 5 μg Con A/ml. Then 250-ml cell suspensions (5 × 10^6 cells/ml) are cultured for about 40 hr in 174-cm^2 culture bottles (No. 1475, Nunclon Delta) in a horizontal position (250 ml per bottle) in a water-saturated atmosphere of 5% CO_2 in air at 37°C. The medium from about 20 bottles is decanted and freed of cells and cell debris by centrifugation in 250-ml screw-cap bottles in a Sorvall GSA rotor for 10 min at 9000 rpm (13,000 g). The supernatant is cooled to 4°C in an ice bath, and solid $(NH_4)_2SO_4$ (Ultrapure, No. 901946, Schwarzmann) is added slowly with stirring to 85% saturation (55.9 gm/100 ml). After 1 hr of stirring the precipitate is collected by centrifugation at 25,000 g. The precipitate is resuspended in HEPES-buffered water (0.02 M HEPES, pH 7.3) and dialyzed for 1 $\frac{1}{2}$ –2 hr against 2 liters of HEPES-buffered saline (0.01 M HEPES, pH 7.3) in a 2-liter graduated cylinder. The dialysis bag (dialysis membrane, 20 DM × 100 ft, Union Carbide, Chicago, Illinois) has been pretreated according to widely used procedures (McPhie, 1971) for removal of heavy-metal ions and sulfurous compounds. The tubing is cut into pieces of suitable length and boiled in two changes of 2 liters of 0.1 M Na$_2$CO$_3$ and 0.02 M sodium EDTA in an Erlenmeyer flask, followed by boiling in two to three changes of distilled water in which it is stored indefinitely.

During dialysis of the $(NH_4)_2SO_4$-precipitated Con A supernatant, a brownish heavy precipitate develops which is removed by centrifugation at 20,000 g. The clear supernatant (up to 30 ml) is applied to a 5 × 95 cm G-100 column equilibrated with HEPES-buffered saline (0.01 M HEPES, pH 7.3) and eluted at 1.2 ml/min. Then 12-ml fractions are collected. Rat TCGF-containing material elutes with an apparent molecular weight of 15,000–18,000. After use the column is washed with 30 ml of a 0.5 M α-methylmannoside solution.

A small aliquot of every second fraction is sterile-filtered (Millex disposable filter unit, SL GS 025 OS, Millipore SA, Molsheim, France) and tested for TCGF activity.

2. Assay

TCGF can be readily assayed and quantitated by using long-term cultured T-cell lines or clones of killer or helper T cells which are strictly dependent on TCGF for growth and survival (Gillis *et al.*, 1978; von Boehmer *et al.*, 1979). Then 10^3–10^4 cells are cultured in 0.2 ml IMDM-fetal bovine serum (FBS) or IMDM-ATL on Falcon II microtiter plates, and 1–5 μl of the column fractions is added to duplicate cultures. After 48–72 hr of culture [^{3}H]thymidine incorporation is determined.

If continuously growing TCGF-dependent T cells are not available, the elution profile of the G-100 column can be determined in cultures of mouse thymocytes (5–10 × 10⁵/ml) containing Con A (1–2 μg/ml) (costimulator activity, Paetkau et al., 1976). Both types of assays reveal identical profiles.

For routine use, the active fractions of the G-100 column are pooled, supplemented with BSA (0.5 mg/ml), and stored frozen at −70°C. Once thawed, they are kept at 4°C for up to 4 weeks.

D. Sheep and Horse Red Blood Cells

The antigenicity of individual SRCs or HRCs can vary among individuals and differ in its susceptibility to lysis. Therefore heterologous erythrocytes are obtained from the same selected donor which is bled at 1-to 2-week intervals over several years (50–100 ml/week). The blood is collected in an equal volume of Alsever's solution and can be stored for up to 4 months. Blood from a single bleeding is distributed in aliquots equivalent to 5 ml packed cells and washed three times in sterile BSS prior to use.

One milliliter of packed erythrocytes, the pellet obtained after centrifugation at 600–700 g, contains 2 × 10¹⁰ red blood cells. Fifty microliters of a 1% solution is regarded as equivalent to 10⁷ erythrocytes.

E. Counting of Viable Cells

The counting of viable cells in the presence of large numbers of dead cells is conveniently carried out with the fluorescein diacetate (FDA) method of Rotmann and Papermaster (1966). A 100× stock solution containing 0.5 mg FDA (No. 21575, Serva) in acetone is stored in an aluminum-covered bottle at −20°C. For cell counting 25 μl of a 100-fold dilution in PBS containing Ca^{2+} and Mg^{2+} is added together with 25 μl of a cell suspension to 0.2 ml Ca^{2+}- and MG^{2+}-free PBS. The viable brightly flourescing cells are counted in a Burker hemocytometer using a standard fluorescence microscope.

F. Incubation Boxes and Gas Mixture

To establish an atmosphere of 7% O_2, 10% CO_2, and 83% N_2 the culture bottles are gassed with this mixture, tightly capped, and placed in a 37°C incubator. Microtiter plates are placed in airtight incubation boxes, and the boxes are perfused for 5–10 min. We use small Lucite boxes which accommodate 12 microtiter plates. They are commercially available from Biotec, Schoenenbuch, Switzerland.

III. PROCEDURE

A. *In Vivo*-Activated Helper T Cells

Female C57BL/6J mice are lethally irradiated with 700–750 rads with an x-ray machine (Philips RT 305) by applying 100 rads/min at a distance of 25 cm. After irradiation the mice are injected intraperitoneally with 40 U USP heparin in a volume of 0.2 ml BSS (Liquemin Roche, Hoffmann-La Roche, Basel, Switzerland). Within a few hours the mice are injected intravenously with 0.5 ml of a cell suspension in BSS which contains 10^8 syngeneic thymocytes and 10^7 SRCs or HRCs per milliliter.

Seven days after reconstitution the mice are killed, and a cell suspension is prepared from their spleens. One mouse spleen yields on the average 3 × 10^6 viable cells, i.e., *in vivo*-activated helper T cells (Miller and Mitchell, 1967).

B. Antigen-Specific Stimulation and Propagation *in Vitro*

In vivo-activated helper T cells are cultured in Falcon No. 3013 tissue culture flasks containing, in 5 ml IMDM-ATL, 5 × 10^6 viable cells and 1.25 × 10^7 SRCs or HRCs. They are cultured in an atmosphere of 10% CO_2, 8% O_2, and 82% N_2 in an upright position in a 37°C incubator. Microscopic inspection reveals clusters of proliferating cells after several days of culture, the proliferation being strictly antigen-dependent. In the absence of antigen or in the presence of unrelated antigen no viable cells remain after 1 week of culture. At weekly intervals 3 ml of the supernatant is removed and spun at 400 g in Falcon No. 2095 screw-cap tubes. The spent medium is discarded, and the cells are resuspended in 3 ml fresh IMDM-ATL and added back to the culture from which they originated. Some of the cells can be removed for testing for specific helper activity (Section III,E). Every second week homologous antigen is added to the cultures (2.5 × 10^7 SRCs or HRCs per bottle). After 3–4 weeks of culture, when the cells cease to grow, x-irradiated (3300 R) congenic *nu/nu* spleen cells (5 × 10^6/5 ml culture) or normal syngeneic peritoneal macrophages (10^6/5 ml culture) are added to the cultures. Under these conditions cell growth is very slow, however, as judged by titration of specific helper activity, it is highly specific (Schreier *et al.,* 1980a).

C. T-Cell Growth Factor-Dependent Propagation of Helper T Cells

Adding Con A-induced partially purified TCGF (Section II,C) to the antigen-stimulated helper T cells after 2–12 weeks of culture leads to a vigorous proliferation of specific helper T cells. This proliferation is independent of antigen and adherent cells. Prior to the change to TCGF-supplemented IMDM-ATL, antigen and dead cells can be removed by spinning the long-term-cultured cells over a Urovison–Ficoll gradient (density 1.077) for 15 min at 700 g. The dose of TCGF required for maximal proliferation of T cells is determined by titrating the factor preparation against a line of killer or helper T cells or against an aliquot of long-term-cultured T cells (10^4 cells/0.2 ml culture).

The cells are subcultured into fresh TCGF-supplemented medium every 2–3 days. Cell growth is best when the cells are seeded at a density of at least 5×10^4 cells/ ml. After about 3 weeks of TCGF-induced growth the growth rate decreases significantly. An increasing number of small, round cells appear. Such cultures can be restimulated with homologous antigen and I-A-compatible irradiated syngeneic spleen cells (10^6/ml) or peritoneal macrophages (2×10^5/ml). After this restimulation addition of TCGF again induces vigorous cell growth. This requirement for restimulation with antigen differs widely among individual lines.

D. Cloning of Helper T Cells

Cloning is carried out under conditions of limiting dilution in Falcon II microtiter plates. On the average, each culture well contains, in a volume of 0.2 ml TCGF-supplemented medium (IMDM-ATL), one viable long-term-cultured T cell, 2×10^5 irradiated congenic *nu/nu* spleen cells, and 5×10^5 SRCs or HRCs, depending on the specificity of the helper T cells. For cloning we double the concentration of TCGF and add, in addition to albumin, transferrin, and lipids, 2% FBS or 1% mouse serum.

The microtiter plates are placed in incubation boxes, which contain open petri dishes with water for humidification, and perfused with the gas mixture. They are placed in a 37°C incubator or a warm room. The gas mixture is renewed at 4- to 6-day intervals.

After 12–15 days of culture without feeding the cultures are scored for cell growth, using an inverted microscope at low magnification. The cultures containing confluently growing T cells are transferred to a Costar well containing the same filler cells and medium supplements as used for the cloning procedure. After 4–5 days, 1 ml TCGF-supplemented IMDM-ATL is added per well and replaced at 3- to 5-day intervals. When the cells have grown to confluence, they are transferred to 5 ml TCGF-supplemented medium and further propagated as described in Section III,C.

For cloning (and subcloning) we establish at least 300 culture wells per long-term-cultured T-cell line. As judged from a great number of cloning experiments, cell growth is observed in 5–40% of the established culture wells. Cloning is best carried out when the cells are transferred from antigen- and adherent cell-dependent growth to TCGF-supplemented medium.

E. Testing for Specific Helper Activity

Specific helper activity of long-term culture T cells is monitored regularly at 2-week intervals. The test is carried out in Falcon II microtiter plates under the culture conditions described recently (Schreier, 1978).

Aliquots of a cell suspension (0.1 ml), containing, per milliliter IMDM-ATL, 2×10^6 anti-theta-treated or congenic *nu/nu* spleen cells together with 5×10^6 washed SRCs or HRCs are distributed into the wells of a microtiter plate. To this 0.1 ml, containing 2×10^5 T-cell-depleted spleen cells and 5×10^5 heterologous erythrocytes, another 0.1 ml IMDM-ATL is added which contains 10^1–10^5 helper T cells. Three to four replicate cultures are set up for each input of T cells. Maximal helper activity, as judged by the number of plaque-forming cells (PFCs) determined on day 5 after initiation of culture, is obtained with 10^5 to 2×10^5 *in vivo*-activated T cells or with about 10^3 long-term-cultured or cloned helper T cells (Schreier *et al.,* 1980a). In the absence of antigen or specific helper T cells no background PFCs arise under these culture conditions (Schreier, 1978, 1980).

The specificity of helper T cells is assessed by culturing the helper T cells in the presence of homologous and unrelated antigen. On day 5 the individual cultures are harvested, washed in BSS, and resuspended in a suitable volume. The number of PFCs directed against either antigen is enumerated with a modified plaque assay. 2×10^5 *nu/nu* spleen cells, containing about 50 B-cell precursor cells which recognize the antigen SRC, give rise to about 10^4 direct specific PFCs after 120 hr of culture.

F. *In Vivo* Reconstitution of Syngeneic *nu/nu* Mice

Specific helper T cells maintained *in vitro* for up to 2 years, reveal specific helper activity *in vivo* as they do *in vitro* (Tees and Schreier, 1980). Male or female congenic *nu/nu* mice are injected intravenously with 2–5×10^6 helper T cells together with 2×10^7 SRCs or HRCs. This injection is preceded by 30 min by an intraperitoneal injection of 40 U USP heparin (Liquemin Roche) in a 0.2-ml volume. Five to six days later the reconstituted mice are bled to determine the hemagglutination titer, and the number of specific PFCs per spleen is enumerated in a specific plaque assay.

G. Freezing and Thawing of Helper T Cells

Helper T cells can be readily frozen and thawed according to established procedures. Once a cell line or clone is established, the cells are spun down and the pellet is resuspended at 4°C in freezing medium (2–5 × 10⁶ cells/ml), i.e., IMDM-ATL, supplemented with 20% FBS and 10% DMSO (v/v). The freezing vials are wrapped in foam rubber or paper to ensure slow freezing and placed in a − 70°C freezer for about 1 day; then they are transferred to liquid nitrogen.

For thawing the cells are warmed up quickly to 4°C in a 37°C waterbath and transferred to 15 ml IMDM-ATL kept on ice. After centrifugation the pellet is resuspended in TCGF-supplemented IMDM-ATL and cultured as described.

IV. CRITICAL APPRAISAL

The establishment and maintenance of lines and clones of specific helper T cells are in line with the current concept of T-cell stimulation and proliferation. Mitogenic or antigenic stimulation of nonactivated, resting small T cells leads to the expression of a receptor for TCGF (Smith *et al.*, 1979; Coutinho *et al.*, 1979). The same stimulus leads to the production of TCGF, which requires both (Ly-1 +) T cells and I-A bearing accessory cells. The actual proliferation of T cells is promoted by TCGF which acts on all activated T cells displaying a receptor for this growth factor.

The initiation of a helper T-cell line requires a source of *in vivo*-immunized T cells containing a large fraction of specific helper T cells. This has been achieved by injecting the antigen into the base of the tail or into the footpad and using the draining lymph nodes as starting material (Schrier *et al.*, 1979; Julius and Augustin, 1979). For the antigens SRCs or HRCs *in vivo*-activated helper T cells, i.e., spleen cells of irradiated thymocyte reconstituted and immunized mice (Section III,A) are a potent source of helper T cells. The number of injected heterologous erythrocytes is critical. While 10⁶–10⁷ SRCs or HRCs induce a reproducibly large fraction of specific helper T cells, the injection of 0.2 ml of a 5–10% erythrocyte suspension (2–4 × 10⁸) induces low and greatly variable helper activity (Schreier, 1980).

Culture conditions are chosen such that nonspecific blast transformation of T cells by constituents of the medium (such as fetal calf serum) is avoided. Ideally, only T cells specific for the immunizing antigen should be in the blast stage and therefore susceptible to TCGF, which is generated in such cultures upon interaction of helper T cells, antigen, and adherent cells (Schreier *et al.*, 1980a).

While others have successfully used low concentrations of mouse serum (Schreier *et al.,* 1979), or selected human serum (Julius and Augustin, 1979), we have over the last 4 years employed a combination of albumin, transferrin, and lipids (Guilbert and Iscove, 1976; Iscove and Melchers, 1978) as a serum replacement to avoid nonspecific T-cell stimulation (Schreier 1978). Although we have obtained consistent results with various batches of these components over a long period of time, we have recently become aware of some batch-to-batch variation of these components, and similar observations have been brought to our attention by others. This may not be surprising for soybean lipids, which may contain variable amounts of the active components, such as linoleic acid (Iscove *et al.,* 1980; Schreier *et al.,* 1980a). Individual transferrin batches are titrated for maximal growth-promoting activity both on T-cell lines and in the *in vitro* helper assay. We have recently omitted the charcoal extraction of albumin as described by Guilbert and Iscove and Iscove *et al.* (1980) and have not as yet noticed a significant difference between treated and untreated material.

Large-scale production of TCGF has been a remarkably reproducible procedure in our hands. Some batch-to-batch variation of Con A has been observed, and individual batches should be titrated for maximal activity prior to large-scale factor production. The relative yield of TCGF activity from a column increases with high input of dialyzed, $(NH_4)_2SO_4$-precipitated material. We apply the material of at least 50, preferentially 100, rat spleens to a 2-liter column. Needless to say, the factor activity as prepared for routine use may contain numerous activities such as lymphocyte-activating factor (LAF, interleukin-1). However, this partially purified material is devoid of Con A and certain high-molecular-weight inhibitory components. The TCGF activity can be absorbed out with killer or helper T cells (Gillis and Smith, 1977; Schreier *et al.,* 1980a).

When evaluating the specificity of helper T cells *in vitro,* it is important to consider that the strict specificity of helper T cells can be masked by the *in vitro* "bystander effect." We use this term for the phenomenon in which helper T cells specific for either SRCs or HRCs can help induce an antibody response against both erythrocytes, provided both antigens are present in the culture at the same time (Schreier and Tees, 1980). For example, if SRC-specific helper T cells containing SRCs from previous antigenic stimulation are added to T-cell-depleted spleen cells and HRCs, they can aid in the induction of an anti-HRC response. If the residual SRCs are removed on a Ficoll gradient, the strict specificity of the helper T cells becomes evident. This consistent phenomenon reveals that the antigens required for T-cell induction and B-cell induction need not be the same.

A background of PFCs against unrelated antigens can also arise if the T-cell-depleted spleen cell population used in testing for helper activity contains a large fraction of B-cell blasts. These may be induced by mitogenic components of FBS in the culture or by anti-theta and complement treatment. The clonal expansion of B-cell blasts is due to the induction of growth factor(s), which is generated upon interaction of specific helper T cells, antigen, and I-A-compatible adherent cells (Schreier *et al.,* 1980a). This activity promotes antigen-independent and H-2 unrestricted proliferation of B-cell blasts but not of resting small B cells. It can be avoided by using nonstimulatory culture conditions, monoclonal anti-theta serum and a selected source of complement.

The establishment of lines and clones of helper T cells as described here has proved to be a remarkably reproducible procedure over the last several years. However, the present methodology will certainly require further improvements. The original interpretation that TCGF-supplemented medium promotes permanent growth of any T-cell blast may represent the exception rather than the rule. Although we hardly ever failed to establish a specific helper T-cell line in C57BL/6J mice and to maintain it for at least 5 or 6 months in continuous culture, some of these lines ceased to grow. The same holds for a significant fraction of the established clones at various periods of time after cloning. In several instances we have also observed that cells maintained in culture for up to 2 years lost their specific helper activity both *in vivo* and *in vitro*. In each case this loss of activity coincided with a rapid increase in growth rate. Active clones could be reestablished by subcloning or by reactivation of frozen stock.

It is obvious that this recent promising technology will greatly profit from further improvements in culture media and the definition of biologically active mediators required for survival and growth of T cells in culture.

ACKNOWLEDGMENT

We would like to thank Dr. N. N. Iscove for valuable advice on preparation of the culture medium.

REFERENCES

Coutinho, A., Larsson, E. L., Grönvick, K. O., and Andersson, J. (1979). *Eur. J. Immunol.* **9,** 587.
Gillis, S., and Smith, K. A. (1977). *Nature (London)* **268,** 154.
Gillis, S., Ferm, M. M., Ou, W., and Smith, K. A. (1978). *J. Immunol.* **120,** 2027.
Guilbert, L. J., and Iscove, N. N. (1976). *Nature (London)* **263,** 594.
Iscove, N. N., and Melchers, F. (1978). *J. Exp. Med.* **147,** 923.

Iscove, N. N., Guilbert, L. J., and Weyman, C. (1980). *Exp. Cell Res.* **126**, 121.

Julius, M. H., and Augustin, A. A. (1979). *Eur. J. Immunol.* **9**, 671.

Letter to the Editor (1979). *J. Immunol.* **123**, 2928.

McPhie, P. (1971). *In* "Methods in Enzymology (W. B. Jacoby, ed.), Vol. 22, p. 23. Academic Press, New York.

Miller, J. F. A. P., and Mitchell, G. F. (1967). *Nature (London)* **216**, 659.

Morgan, D. A., Ruscetti, F. W., and Gallo, R. C. (1976). *Science* **193**, 1007.

Paetkau, V., Mills, G., Gerhart, S., and Monticone, V. (1976). *J. Immunol.* **117**, 1320.

Rotmann, B., and Papermaster, B. W. (1966). *Proc. Natl. Acad. Sci. U.S.A.* **55**, 134.

Ruscetti, F. W., Morgan, D. A., and Gallo, R. C. (1977). *J. Immunol.* **119**, 131.

Schreier, M. H. (1978). *J. Exp. Med.* **148**, 1612.

Schreier, M. H. (1980). *In* "Lymphokine Reports 2" (E. Pick, ed.). Academic Press, New York, 31.

Schreier, M. H., and Tees, R. (1980). *Int. Arch. Allergy Appl. Immunol.* **61**, 227.

Schreier, M. H., Iscove, N. N., Tees, R., Aarden, L. A., and von Boehmer, H. (1980a). *Immunol. Rev.* **51**, 315.

Schreier, M. H., Andersson, J., Lernhardt, W., and Melchers, F. (1980b). *J. Exp. Med.* **151**, 194.

Schrier, R. D., Skidmore, B. J., Kurnick, J. T., Goldstine, S. N., and Chiller, J. M. (1979). *J. Immunol.* **123**, 2525.

Shaw, J., Monticone, V., and Paetkau, V. (1978). *J. Immunol.* **120**, 1967.

Smith, K. A. (1980). *Immunol. Rev.* **51**, 337.

Smith, K. A., Gillis, S., Baker, P. E., McKenzie, D., and Ruscetti, F. W. (1979). *Ann. N.Y. Acad. Sci.* **332**, 423.

Tees, R. and Schreier, M. H. (1980). *Nature (London)* **283**, 780.

von Boehmer, H., Hengartner, H., Nabholz, M., Lernhardt, W., Schreier, M. H., and Haas, W. (1979). *Eur. J. Immunol.* **9**, 592.

Watson J. D., Aarden, L. A., and Lefkovits, I. (1979a). *J. Immunol.* **122**, 209.

Watson, J.D., Gillis, S., Marbrook, J., Mochizuki, D., and Smith K. A. (1979b). *J. Exp. Med.* **150**, 849.

Watson, J. D. (1979). *J. Exp. Med.* **150**, 1510.

16

The Cloning of Alloreactive
T Cells

Hans Hengartner and C. Garrison Fathman

I. OBJECTIVE

Cytotoxic or proliferating antigen-specific murine T cells are generated following *in vivo* or *in vitro* immunization (Fathman and Hengartner, 1978; Hengartner and Fathman, 1980; von Boehmer *et al.*, 1979; for review, see *Immunol. Rev.* Vol. 51, 1980). The specificity of such cells may be retained in bulk tissue culture by repetitive restimulation with the appropriate antigens (Fathman *et al.*, 1977). The restimulated bulk cultures are enriched with antigen-specific responder cells but contain large numbers of cells which are nonspecifically costimulated during the immune response.

The following procedures provide a means of analyzing bulk cultures of

277

IMMUNOLOGICAL METHODS, VOL. II

T cells which specifically recognize histocompatibility antigens by the derivation of monoclonal proliferating T cells. These clones can be stimulated using either unique or shared mixed lymphocyte reaction (MLR) determinants expressed on spleen cell surfaces. Clones can be increased to large numbers of cells by repetitive stimulation which permits serological and biochemical analysis of such cells.

A slightly modified procedure is also applicable to the cloning of cytotoxic T lymphocytes (von Boehmer *et al.*, 1979) and soluble antigen-reactive murine T cells (Kimoto and Fathman, 1980).

II. PRINCIPLE

Lymph node cells of mice of strain A are stimulated *in vitro* using x-irradiated stimulator spleen cells of strain B6. After three to four restimulations, at 14-day intervals, the bulk cultures consist mainly of primed responder T cells (PRCs) which proliferate upon restimulation with spleen cells of strain B6. Alloreactive cytotoxic T cells, which are induced in primary mixed lymphocyte cultures (MLCs), are lost after three to five restimulations. Prior to soft agar cloning, such PRCs are restimulated for 24–48 hr in suspension and then distributed at various cell densities in soft agar. After 3–5 days, colonies of up to 30 cells can be picked, transferred, and restimulated in 0.2-ml cultures. The growing colonies can be expanded by restimulation every 10–14 days and increased to large numbers quite rapidly. Subcloning in soft agar or by limiting dilution allows the isolation of clones of alloreactive T cells.

III. MATERIALS

Complete medium: RPMI 1640 (Gibco Bio-Cult, Paisley, Scotland); penicillin–streptomycin, 100 U/ml; L-glutamine, 2 mmol/ml; β-mercaptoethanol, 5×10^{-5} M; 10% fetal calf serum (FCS), heat-inactivated, RPMI 1640 ($10\times$)

Freezing medium: complete medium containing 20% FCS plus 10% dimethylsulfoxide (DMSO), stored at 4°C after sterile filtration

Tritiated thymidine: (TRA.310, The Radiochemical Centre, Amersham, England), 1 mCi/ml in PBS diluted 25-fold in complete medium

Phosphate-buffered saline (PBS): 16 gm NaCl, 0.4 gm KCl, 2.3 gm $Na_2HPO_4 \cdot 2H_2O$, and 0.4 gm KH_2PO_4 in 1500 ml water plus 0.2 gm $MgCl_2 \cdot 6H_2O$ in 200 ml water plus 0.26 gm $CaCl_2 \cdot 2H_2O$ in 200 ml water

Balanced salt solution (BSS): 10 liters containing 0.1 gm phenol red, 1.4
gm CaCl$_2$ • 2H$_2$O, 80 gm NaCl, 4 gm KCl, 2 gm MgSO$_4$ • 7H$_2$O, 2 gm
MgCl$_2$ • 6H$_2$O, 0.6 gm KH$_2$PO$_4$, and 2.4 gm Na$_2$HPO$_4$ • 2H$_2$O

2.5% Bacto agar (Difco Laboratories, Detroit, Michigan) in triple-distilled water, autoclaved

Fluorescein diacetate (FDA) (Serva Feinchemica, Heidelberg, West
Germany), 5 mg/ml acetone kept at −20°C

Concanavalin A (Con A) (Pharmacia, Uppsala, Sweden), 5 μg/ml in
complete medium

Petri dishes, 10-cm diameter (No. 1001, Falcon, Becton-Dickinson,
Grenoble, France)

Costar trays (Nos. 3596 and 3524, Costar, Data Packaging Corp., Cambridge, Massachusetts)

Nalgene filters, 0.2 μm (Nalge Corp., Rochester, New York)

Animals: The responder lymph node cells are taken from 6- to 8-week-
old female A/J mice, and the stimulator spleen cells from 6- to
12-week-old female C57BL/6 or (C57BL/6 × A/J) F$_1$ animals. Rat
spleen cells as a source of T-cell growth factor (TCGF, also termed in-
terleukin 2 or IL-2) are from 6- to 12-week-old albino or Lewis rats of
either sex.

IV. PROCEDURES

A. Preparation of Responder T Cells

Responder T cells may be aseptically collected from the cervical, ax-
illary, mesenteric, and inguinal lymph nodes. The nodes are placed in a
petri dish (No. 1007, Falcon) with 4 ml BSS and minced with scissors. The
suspension is squeezed through a steel net mesh (width approximately 0.5
mm), using a 2-ml syringe piston, and flushed with cold BSS.

The cells are then transferred to a plastic tube (No. 2059, Falcon) and
resuspended by repetitive gentle pipetting in a total of 12 ml BSS. Larger
cell aggregates and connective tissue residues are allowed to sediment for 5
min. The single-cell suspension in the supernatant is washed twice by centrifugation for 10 min at 170 g at 4°C.

B. Preparation of Stimulator Spleen Cells

Aseptically removed spleens are placed in 10-cm-diameter bacteriological-type petri dishes (No. 1001, Falcon) containing 10 ml of BSS.
The cells are teased from the capsule with forceps and gentle flushing with

BSS using a 10-ml syringe and a No. 21 needle. After gentle resuspension by repetitive pipetting using a 10-ml plastic pipette, they are finally transferred to a 50-ml plastic tube. After 5 min, during which cell aggregates and debris sediment, the supernatant is transferred to a new tube and washed three times by centrifugation at 170 g for 10 min at 4°C. The cells are then resuspended in normal medium at a density of 5 × 10^7 ml in 50-ml plastic tubes. They should be kept on ice until X-irradiated with 3300 R from a regular x-ray machine or a cesium source.

C. Counting of Viable Cells

In order to count the viable cells directly in MLR mixtures, which contain large numbers of dead cells and debris, we use the FDA method rather than the indirect trypan blue exclusion technique (Rotman and Papermaster, 1966). A solution of 5 mg/ml FDA in acetone is kept at −20°C. The solution is diluted 100 times with PBS and then can be used as a 10 × stock solution for the viability assay; it must be prepared fresh daily and kept on ice.

One part of the 10× stock solution is added to 9 parts of cell suspension. After 1–5 min at room temperature, viable cells fluoresce brightly when observed under a fluorescent light microscope using appropriate excitation and barrier filters.

D. Primary Mixed Lymphocyte Cultures

Lymph node responder cells (40 × 10^6) are cultured with 80 × 10^6 x-irradiated (3300 R) stimulator spleen cells in 15 ml complete culture medium in 75-cm^2 tissue culture bottles (No. 3024, Falcon) in an upright position. The bottles are incubated in a 37°C incubator with a water-saturated atmosphere of 5.5% CO_2 in air. The culture can be left for 10–14 days without changing the medium.

E. Secondary Mixed Lymphocyte Cultures

Ten to fourteen days after initiation of the primary MLC, cells are centrifuged, washed once with BSS, and counted by the FDA method. At this point, most of the stimulator cells are dead, and the culture consists mostly of viable T cells. These cells (2 × 10^6), called PRCs, are resuspended in 15 ml normal medium together with 50 × 10^6 stimulator spleen cells in 45 ml normal medium in the same tissue culture flask in a horizontal position. The restimulation of PRCs can be repeated every 10–14 days for months.

F. Proliferation Assay

In principle PRCs or cloned alloreactive T cells are cocultured with syngeneic and allogeneic stimulator spleen cells. The stimulatory effect is measured by tritiated thymidine uptake after different periods of stimulation (2, 3, and 4 days).

Ten to fourteen days following the last stimulation, 1×10^4 to 5×10^4 PRCs are cocultured with 1×10^6 x-irradiated (3300 R) stimulator spleen cells in 0.2 ml of complete medium on tissue culture plates with flat-bottom wells (No. 3596, Costar). Proliferation is assayed 48 or 72 hr after initiation of the MLC by adding 0.05 ml of complete medium containing 2 μCi of tritiated thymidine (2 Ci/mmol, TRA.310, The Radiochemical Centre, Amersham, England). After 16 hr, the cells are harvested by a semiautomatic cell harvester onto glass-fiber filters (GF/A, 13 $\times$ 19.5 cm, Whatman, Ferriers, France) and rinsed with distilled water.

The filters are dried on a hot plate and transferred to vials containing 5 ml scintillation fluid (Instafluor II, Packard) which are then counted in a liquid scintillation photospectrometer.

Each MLC is prepared in duplicate or triplicate. The results are then expressed as the mean counts per minute of replicate samples. The alloreactivity can be expressed as difference or as the ratio between the mean values derived from allogeneic and syngeneic combination of the MLCs.

G. Cloning and Subcloning of Alloreactive T Cells

At any time following four restimulations by irradiated stimulator spleen cells, PRCs are more than 95% Thy-1-positive and do not exhibit any alloreactive cytotoxic activity. For cloning, $2-3 \times 10^6$ resting PRCs are collected 10–14 days after the last stimulation and transferred to 15 ml fresh culture medium containing 5×10^7 x-irradiated allogeneic stimulator cells. Twenty-four hours after initiation of the MLR, cells are centrifuged at 170 g for 10 min at 4°C and diluted to various concentrations for cloning on soft agar in petri dishes 10 cm in diameter (No. 1001 Falcon). The bottom layer consists of 10 ml 0.5% Bacto agar (Difco Laboratories, Detroit, Michigan) prepared as follows. First, 30 ml of 2.5% Bacto agar in water is dissolved in boiling water and kept in a 45°C water bath. Then 117 ml prewarmed complete medium and 3 ml 10 $\times$ RPMI are added, and the solution kept at 45°C. After pouring without air bubbles, the agar layer is allowed to solidify for 15 min at room temperature. The bottom layer can contain 5×10^6 x-irradiated (3000 R) spleen cells which increase the cloning efficiency. In the meantime, the stimulated PRCs are counted by the FDA method and distributed into 1 ml complete medium in 5-ml plastic tubes in a 37°C water bath without being separated from the stimulator cells. We usually spread 1×10^6, 0.5×10^6, 0.25×10^6, and 0.1×10^6 PRCs per petri dish. Then 2 ml of 0.5% agar in a 5-ml plastic pipette is added to the 1-ml aliquot of PRCs, thoroughly mixed by pipetting twice, and immediately evenly distributed by dropping onto the bottom agar layer. The plates are kept for 10 min at room temperature and then incubated on a horizontal plate holder at 37°C in a water-saturated atmosphere containing 5% CO_2. After 4–6 days of incubation, colonies of up to 20–40 cells start to appear. Under an inverted microscope these colonies can be picked with Pasteur pipettes drawn out to fine capillaries. The proliferating cells are transferred to 0.2 ml complete medium containing 10^6 x-irradiated stimulator spleen cells on Costar microtiter plates (No. 3596). Proliferating cultures can be scored very easily by microscopic inspection. With a Pasteur pipette, 0.2-ml proliferating cultures are transferred directly to 2 ml complete medium containing 10×10^6 x-irradiated stimulator spleen cells. After 10–14 days, these cultures contain $0.5–1.5 \times 10^6$ cells which can be further increased in 5-ml cultures in 25-cm² tissue culture bottles in an upright position or in 15- or 45-ml cultures in upright or horizontal 75-cm² tissue culture bottles. They contain starting cell densities of $6–8 \times 10^4$ cloned proliferating T cells and 3×10^6 x-irradiated stimulator spleen cells.

These colonies can be subcloned by following the procedure outlined above, with the difference that the 10 ml 0.5% Bacto agar feeder layer must contain supernatant from rat Con A-activated spleen cells as a source of TCGF. In this case the 0.5% Bacto agar feeder layer consists of 30 ml of 2.5% dissolved Bacto agar in water, 87 ml of complete medium, 30 ml of supernatant from Con A-activated rat spleen cells, and 3 ml of $10 \times$ RPMI. No colony formation is observed in the absence of Con A supernatant. All the subsequent steps are carried out as described above.

Cloning by limiting dilution is carried out by plating 33 cells in 10 ml from a soft agar colony onto 98-well flat-bottomed microtiter plates (No. 3396, Costar) each well containing 1×10^6 x-irradiated (3300 R) stimulator cells and 10% Con A supernatant in 100 μl. The cultures are maintained as above, and growth is observed by microscopic inspection. No fresh medium need be added during culture. Growing clones can be increased by transferral to Costar plates (No. 3524) containing 1×10^7 irradiated (3300 R) stimulator cells in the absence of Con A supernatant.

H. Concanavalin A Supernatant

Supernatant of Con A-activated lymphocytes is produced by culturing 5 $\times 10^6$ spleen cells from 6- to 12-week-old albino or Lewis rats of either sex at a density of 5×10^6 cells/ml complete medium in the presence of 5 μg/ml Con A in 175-cm^2 tissue culture bottles (No. 3028, Falcon) at 250 ml/bottle. Forty-eight hours after initiation of the cultures, the supernatant is recovered by centrifugation at 1000 g for 10 min. Sterile-filtered aliquots kept at $-20°$C retain their TCGF activity for months.

I. Freezing and Thawing of Alloreactive T Cells

Cloned or long-term-cultured alloreactive T cells can be frozen. Ten to fourteen days following the last stimulation 3×10^6 alloreactive T cells are restimulated by 6×10^7 x-irradiated spleen cells in 15 ml complete medium. Twenty-four hours after initiation of the culture, the cells are centrifuged at 170 g for 10 min at 4°C and the pellet resuspended in 1 ml of freezing medium which contains complete medium, 20% FCS, and 10% DMSO. All cell manipulations in freezing medium are done at 4°C on ice. The cells are frozen in plastic vials by placing them in a $-75°$C deep freezer overnight in a styrofoam box. Freezing occurs at a rate of about 1°C/min. The following morning, the cells are removed from the freezer and stored in liquid nitrogen.

The cells can be thawed in a 37°C water bath. As soon as the last ice crystal disappears, the cell suspension is diluted 10 times by adding complete medium at 4°C. After centrifugation, the cells are resuspended in 15 ml complete medium containing 6×10^7 x-irradiated stimulator spleen cells.

V. CRITICAL APPRAISAL

Soft agar cloning has been carried out with long-term A/J anti-C57BL/6 and A/J anti-(C57G./6 $\times$ A/J) F_1 MLR cultures. The cell densities in soft agar must be rather high in order to obtain colony formation. The chances of not picking real clones after the first cloning are high, which makes subcloning absolutely necessary. As mentioned in Section IV, subcloning is only possible when a supernatant of Con A-activated spleen cells is present in the 0.5% agar feeder layer or by limiting dilution in the presence of a 5% Con A supernatant. When Con A supernatant is used in the following 0.2- and 2-ml cultures, the proliferating T-cell clones lose their specificity pattern. Thus, if Con A supernatant is used following subcloning, originally H-2 haplotype-specific responding T cells may be nonspecifically stimulated by any third party stimulator cells even in the absence of Con A supernatant. For this reason supernatant of Con A-activated spleen cells is omitted in cultures following the soft agar cloning or limiting dilution step.

The selection of FCS is rather critical. The mitogenic effect on spleen cells must be minimal (low background in a syngeneic MLC system), and the FCS must support a high MLR in an allogeneic system.

The cloning of cytotoxic T cells can be carried out by following a similar protocol. Specific cytotoxic T cells are induced *in vitro* in a primary MLC and kept in culture in complete medium containing 10% supernatant of Con A-activated spleen cells (Gillis and Smith, 1977; von Boehmer *et al.*, 1979). The cytotoxic T cells are then cloned after 2–3 weeks adaptation on soft agar or by the limiting dilution technique in 0.2-ml cultures in the presence of irradiated peritoneal macrophages.

REFERENCES

Fathman, C. G., and Hengartner, H. (1978). *Nature* (*London*) **272**, 617.

Fathman, C. G., Collavo, D., Davies, S., and Nabholz, M. (1977). *J. Immunol.* **118**, 1232.

Gillis, S., and Smith, K. A. (1977). *Nature* (*London*) **268**, 154.

Hengartner, H., and Fathman, C. G. (1980). *Immunogenetics* **10**, 175.

Immunol. Reviews Vol. 51, 1980.

Kimoto, M., and Fathman, C. G. (1980). *J. Exp. Med.* (in press).

Nabholz, M., and Miggiano, V. (1977). *In* "B and T cells in Immune Recognition" (F. Loor and G. E. Roelants, eds.), p. 261. Wiley, New York.

Rotman, B., and Papermaster, B. W. (1966). *Proc. Natl. Acad. Sci. U.S.A.* **55**, 134.

von Boehmer, H., Hengartner, H., Nabholz, M. Lernhardt, W., Schreier, M. H., and Haas, W. (1979). *Eur. J. Immunol.* **9**, 952.

17

The Technique of Hybridoma Production

Georges Köhler

I. INTRODUCTION

Conventional antisera have several disadvantages: The titers are low, the antibodies are heterogeneous even when specific for a single determinant, the supply is limited, and it is impossible to reproduce a combination of specific antibodies in a new animal.

IMMUNOLOGICAL METHODS, VOL. II
Copyright © 1981 by Academic Press, Inc.
ISBN 0-12-442702-2

The lymphocyte fusion technique provides a tool for overcoming these limitations. In short, spleen cells of mice, previously immunized with antigen, are fused to a myeloma line which grows in tissue culture. Hybrid lines are obtained which combine parental traits, tumoral growth, and specific antibody production (Köhler and Milstein, 1975).

In the past, cell fusion has mainly been used to study gene linkage and gene regulation. For both purposes, cells from distant species and of different ontogenetic origin were fused. Function rescue fusion (e.g., rescuing antibody production), however, works best if the tumor and normal cells are ontogenetically and phylogenetically matched (Shulman and Köhler, 1979).

Experiments are considered good if they yield over 100 hybrids, about 50% secreting new immunoglobulins (Ig's) of the IgM and IgG class and about 1–10% being specific for the immunogen injected into the donor mice. The frequency of specific hybridomas is over 10 times higher than expected from the number of antigen-specific B lymphocytes in the spleen. It is thought that a preferential fusion with the 1% dividing cells of the spleen occurs in which recently stimulated B lymphocytes represent a sizable fraction.

It is this unexpected bonus which has made the hybridoma technique so popular in such a short time. For reviews, see Melchers *et al.* (1978), Shulman and Köhler (1979), Raschke (1980), Milstein *et al.* (1980), McMichael and Bastin (1980), Goding (1980), and Kennett *et al.* (1980). Although the principle of the technique has not changed much, it has been simplified enormously by the use of polyethylene glycol (PEG) as fusing agent instead of Sendai virus.

Many different protocols for the generation of hybridoma lines exist. An attempt to sort out the many variables during the fusion process has been made by Stephen Fazekas of this institute (Fazekas de St. Groth and Scheidegger, 1980), and some of his suggestions are incorporated in the protocol presented here.

The production of monoclonal antibodies, however, depends not only on the generation of a large number of hybridoma lines but also on a basic knowledge of how to maintain tissue culture lines, how to test antibody specificity, and how to keep cell lines and purify monoclonal antibodies. This chapter therefore includes some basic accessory protocols aimed at enabling a beginner in the tissue culture field to grow and test hybridomas. Where possible, commercially available reagents are used.

From the beginning (immunizing an animal) to the end (harvesting monoclonal antibodies) 3–4 months' time will be required on a full-time basis.

II. PREFUSION STEPS

A. Basic Equipment

Our tissue culture room has a surface of 3×3.5 m, is under higher air pressure than the adjacent room, and is air-conditioned, which is essential for small rooms (but not if the equipment is installed in a corner of a large room). In an area this size one person can easily operate, but two persons would result in overcrowding. The heavy equipment listed below should be arranged so that most of it can be reached from a sitting position: vertical or horizontal sterile laminar-flow hood, $37°C$ wet incubator CO_2, $37°C$ dry incubator, small $+4°C$ refrigerator, small $-20°C$ freezer, inverted microscope, sink with water supply, suction line connected to a flask containing Hycolin disinfectant, gas flame in hood, supply of 10% CO_2, 7% O_2, and 83% N_2 gas mixture, and $37°C$ and $45°C$ water baths.

Outside the culture room, a low-speed centrifuge, liquid nitrogen containers, and a $-70°C$ freezer are needed.

B. Choice of Animal

The choice of animal depends mainly on the availability of appropriate tissue culture lines for fusion. So far only rat and mouse myeloma lines are available. Cross-species fusions work for mouse myeloma and rat lymphocytes but not very efficiently for mouse myeloma and rabbit or human lymphocytes (Melchers *et al.*, 1978). At the Fourth International Congress of Immunology in Paris, a rabbit line TRSC-1.8 was presented by A. B. Schreiber and his colleagues. This line produced intracellular IgG and gave rise to few hybrids, but only one was found to contain an additional heavy chain. Since no Ig secretion was obtained, this line is not yet optimal for monoclonal antibody production. Olsson and Kaplan reported the isolation of a human myeloma line (U–266AR$_1$) suitable for fusion, which seems to have properties similar to those of the mouse lines (Olsson and Kaplan, 1980). Although this line will enormously boost human monoclonal antibody production, especially with respect to the therapeutic implications, human beings are not very useful experimental systems. Thus, we are left with the mouse and the rat. At the moment the mouse seems to be the best choice, because myeloma lines exist which have lost their own Ig production (the rat line still expresses light chains) and all IgG classes of the mouse (but not the rat) bind to protein A of *Staphylococcus aureus,* which facilitates purification of Ig's (Section V,C).

All the myeloma lines are derived from the BALB/c strain of mice.

Hybridomas obtained with BALB/c lymphocytes will grow as tumors in this strain when injected intraperitoneally (ip), thus generating high-titered ascitic fluid. Since the immune response against a given antigen may not be optimal in the BALB/c strain, another strain of mice (e.g. C57BL/6) should also be used. We use female mice (which are easier to handle) 8–12 weeks old (Bomholtgård, Ry, Denmark).

C. Immunization

For soluble antigens inject 100 μg protein precipitated in alum and mixed with 2×10^9 killed *Bordatella pertussis* organisms ip. Boost with 10 μg antigen in saline. Remove spleens 3 days later. For cellular antigens inject 2×10^7 cells ip, repeat 2–3 weeks later, boost after 3 weeks with the same dose, and remove spleens 3 days later. In general, animals should have 3 weeks rest before the last boost. This boost should be given ip or intravenously (iv) so that the antigen reaches the spleen. Dependence on only one spleen should be avoided; either three spleens should be pooled or three separate fusions made. If the major response appears to occur in the lymph nodes, fusion with lymph node cells will work equally well. One shouldn't, however, expect miracles; a mouse with no serum antibody against a given antigen will generate work but not specific hybridomas. *In vitro* antigen stimulation of primed spleen cells or transfer of primed spleen cells together with antigen into irradiated host mice may help to produce extra enrichment of the B cells of interest (Luben and Mohler, 1980; Eshhar *et al.*, 1980).

D. Choice of Myeloma Cells

In the early days myeloma cells secreting Ig were used: X63-Ag8 (IgG$_1$, $\varkappa$) and MPC-11 (IgG$_{2b}$, $\varkappa$). Variants of these lines were selected to contain only light chains and finally no chains at all.

All the lines listed in Table I have worked in several laboratories. But cell lines change, and sometimes the fusion frequency drops or antibody synthesis is unstable in the hybridoma lines generated. Therefore it is best not to rely on one line. At least three different lines (perhaps some nonproducers) should be obtained, and the first fusions(s) made with all of them. The one which gives the most satisfying results should be selected, and a large stock frozen for use. These cells grow in Dulbecco's modified Eagle's medium (DMEM) or equally well in RPMI medium supplemented with 10% fetal calf serum (FCS). Optimal growth is obtained at concentrations between 10^4 and 5×10^5 cells/ml. Cells in the logarithmic growth phase should be used for fusion.

TABLE I

Myeloma Cell Lines

Cell line	≠ chrom.	Ig	Derived from	Ref.
X68-Ag8	65	$\gamma_{1,}{}^{\varkappa}$	MOPC-21	Köhler and Milstein (1975)
NSI-Ag4/1	65	Intracellular $\varkappa$	X63	Köhler et al. (1976)
X63-Ag8.6.5.3	58	None	X63-Ag8	Kearney et al. (1979)
Sp2/0-Ag14	72	None	X63-Ag8 × BALB/c	Shulman et al. (1978)
FO	72	None	Clone of Sp2/O-Ag14	Fazekas de St. Groth and Scheidegger (1980)
S194/5.XXO.BU.1		None	BALB/c	Trowbridge (1978)
MPC11-45.6, TG 1.7	62	$\gamma_{2b,}{}^{\varkappa}$	BALB/c	Margulies et al. (1976)
210.RCY3.,Ag 1.2.3.	39	$\varkappa$	Lou rat	Galfré et al. (1979)

III. PREPARATION OF MEDIUM CONSTITUENTS, MEDIA, AND CELL SUSPENSIONS

A. Preparation of 100 × Stock Solutions of Hypoxanthine, Aminopterin, and Thymidine

Hypoxanthine, MW 136.1 [6-hydroxypurine (No. 26040, Serva, or No. H-93771, Sigma)]: For a 10^{-2} M solution in H_2O, 136.1 mg is dissolved in 100 ml distilled water and heated to 45°–50°C for 1 hr to dissolve.

Aminopterin, MW 440 [4-aminofolic acid, 4-aminopteroylglutamic acid (No. A-2255, Sigma)]: For a 4×10^{-5} M solution, 1.76 mg aminopterin is added to about 90 ml of distilled water. Then 0.5 ml 1 N NaOH is added to dissolve. After the volume is adjusted to 100 ml the solution is neutralized by adding 0.5 ml N HCl.

Thymidine, MW242.2 (No. T-9250, Sigma): For a 1.6×10^{-3} M solution, 1, 1 N HCl 37.8 mg is readily soluble in 100 ml H_2O.

It is convenient to dissolve hypoxanthine and thymidine together in 100 ml H_2O at 45°–50°C. This leaves two 100× stock solutions, hypoxanthine–thymidine and aminopterin. The solutions are sterile-filtered and stored frozen at -20°C in 100 ml aliquots. Aminopterin must be protected from light.

B. Preparation of Media

Complete DMEM is prepared from the following constituents: 450 ml DMEM tissue culture medium, 1× [No. 320-1965, Gibco, or No. 12-332-54 (1-001M), Flow]; 5 ml 100 mM sodium pyruvate (No. 629, Gibco); 5 ml penicillin-streptomycin solution, 10,000 U/ml (No. 514, Gibco); 5 ml 200 mM L-glutamine (No. 514, Gibco); 50 ml FCS (No. 629, Gibco); and 250 μl 2-mercaptoethanol from a 0.1 M stock solution.

This complete medium can be stored at 4°C for up to 6 weeks. Media made with 10 × DMEM or powder are equally good, but workers just starting tissue culture work may prefer not to depend on their own water supply. Horse serum is cheaper than FCS and can be used with equally good results but may interfere with antigen testing and antibody purification from supernatants because of its Ig content.

Hypoxanthine-aminopterin-thymidine (HAT) medium and hypoxanthine-thymidine (HT) medium are prepared by adding 5 ml of the respective 100× stock solutions of aminopterin and hypoxanthine-thymidine to 500 ml complete medium.

GKN buffer [a glucose (G), potassium (K), and sodium (Na)-containing buffer] consists of 8 gm NaCl, 0.4 gm KCl, 1.77 gm $Na_2HPO_4 \cdot 2H_2O$, 0.69 gm $NaH_2PO_4 \cdot H_2O$, 2 gm glucose, and 0.01 gm phenol red in 100 ml H_2O, pH 7.2, which are mixed and then autoclaved.

C. Preparation of a Polyethylene Glycol Solution

Ten grams of PEG, MW 4000 (No. 9729, Merck, for gas chromatography) is melted and sterilized by autoclaving. It is cooled to 50°C (at which temperature it is still liquid) and combined with 10 ml of warm GKN buffer. The resulting 50% PEG solution (w/v) can be stored in 1-ml aliquots at room temperature for several weeks.

D. Preparation of Cell Suspensions

1. Mouse Spleen Cells

Mice are killed by neck dislocation, and their spleens are removed aseptically and transferred to a bacteriological-type plastic petri dish containing 10 ml GKN. The cells are teased from the capsule with a spatula. Clumps of cells are further dispersed by pipetting up and down with a 10-ml plastic pipette. The suspension is transferred to a 15-ml polycarbonate tube where the clumps are allowed to settle for 2-3 min. The cell suspension is decanted into another tube and centrifuged for 15 min at 170 g at 4°C. The cells are resuspended and washed again in GKN. An aliquot of the cells is counted

(20 μl plus 1 ml trypan blue solution) (0.1% w/v in phosphate-buffered saline (PBS). Cell suspensions with a viability above 75% can be used for fusion.

2. Mouse Peritoneal Macrophages

Normal peritoneal cells are collected and washed under conditions selected to avoid cell clumping and adherence. They are obtained from normal mice by flushing the peritoneal cavity with about 4 ml of 0.34 M sterile-filtered sucrose. The pooled fluids are centrifuged for 10 min at 2000 rpm at 4°C in 50-ml Falcon No. 2070 tubes. The pellet is resuspended in culture medium at the required cell density. A normal mouse yields about 3×10^6 cells. No attempt should be made to increase the number of macrophages by irritating the mice, for example, with thioglycollate. Activated macrophages will destroy the hybrids. Spleen cells at 2×10^5 cells/ml can replace the peritoneal cells and are easier to obtain. The advantage of peritoneal cells is that the plates look tidier; they eat the debris, but occasionally also the hybrids (about every fiftieth fusion). The source of macrophages is not critical [mouse, rat, and guinea pig have been tried (Fazekas de St. Groth and Scheidegger, 1980)].

IV. CELL FUSION WITH POLYETHYLENE GLYCOL

Figure 1 gives an overview of the technique. First, 10^8 mouse spleen cells and 5×10^7 8-azaguanine-resistant myeloma cells (X63-Ag8,6.5.3;FO; SP2/0-Ag14), washed once in GKN buffer, are combined in a 50-ml conical tube (No. 2070, Falcon). The tube is filled with GKN buffer and spun for 10 min at 170–200 g at room temperature.

The supernatant is carefully withdrawn. A total of 0.5 ml 50% PEG solution is added dropwise to the pellet with agitation over a period of 1 min. During this operation the tube is kept at room temperature. After 90 sec 10 ml of serum-free DMEM is added slowly (initially dropwise) over a period of 5 min to dilute out the PEG. The mixture is left for 10 min and then diluted into 500 ml of complete HAT medium containing either 10^8 spleen cells or 2.5×10^7 peritoneal cells as feeder cells. One-milliliter aliquots are distributed into 480 wells of Costar trays (Costar Tissue Culture Cluster 24, No. 3524, Costar, Cambridge, Massachusetts). The feeder cells can be seeded into HAT medium the day before fusion. The trays are kept in a fully humidified incubator at 37°C in an atmosphere of 5% CO_2 in air.

After 3 days, and twice a week thereafter, 1 ml medium is removed using a Pasteur pipette fitted to suction pumps and replaced with HAT medium. If possible, the Pasteur pipette should be changed for each culture.

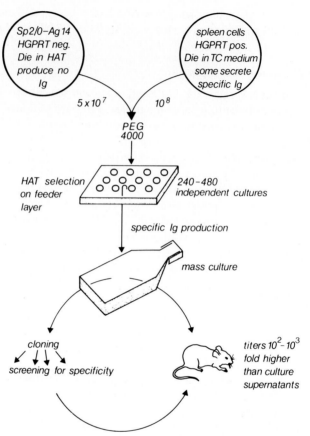

Fig. 1. The generation of hybridoma lines. HGPRT, Hypoxanthine-guanine phosphoribosyltranferase; HAT, addition of hypoxanthine, aminopterin, and thymidine to tissue culture (TC) medium.

After 7–10 days the wells are scored for hybrids, and supernatants of growing hybrids (at least 10% of the bottom should be covered) are removed and tested for specific antibody. After a culture of potential interest has been identified, the cells are detached from the bottom of the well by sucking the medium up and down in a Pasteur pipette. The original well is fed with HAT medium. The detached cells are diluted in four twofold steps into 2-ml Costar wells containing 1 ml of HT medium. If the cells grow without difficulty, they should be transferred to 75-cm^2 Falcon bottles (20 ml of DMEM-HT, 5 ml of cells). The bottles are gassed with 10% CO_2–air, closed so that they are airtight, and placed in a dry incubator at 37°C (to avoid risk of infection). Several aliquots of about 5 × 10^6 cells are frozen. The cells are cloned as early as possible in soft agar or immediately under limiting dilution conditions (Köhler, 1979; Lefkovits, 1979). Feeder cells (e.g., 5 × 10⁴ peritoneal cells/ml) are advised when growth problems of the hybridoma cells are noticed. If hybrid lines repeatedly fail to generate, it is possible that the parental lines are contaminated with mycoplasmas. Procedures for detecting mycoplasmas are described in Russel *et al.* (1975) and McGarrity *et al.* (1979).

V. PRODUCTS OF FUSION

A. Test of Antibody Specificity

The most commonly used test system with the broadest application range is solid-phase enzyme immunoassay (EIA). The principle of this assay is based on the observation that protein sticks tightly to certain plastics, e.g., polyvinyl chloride. Once the plastic is saturated with protein, no new attachment occurs. If the antigen is not a protein, it might be covalently attached to protein. Membrane antigens can be tested by attaching cells to plastic wells (Stocker and Heusser, 1979).

Usually the antigen is fixed to the plastic, and then incubation with hybridoma supernatants containing antibody follows. The antibody is then detected by using a rabbit anti-mouse Ig antiserum to which an enzyme has been covalently linked. The enzymatic activity is revealed by incubation with a substrate, giving rise to a colored product. The intensity of the color can be measured using a Titertek Multiscan (Flow, Scotland) to obtain semiquantitative results. Since quantitation [which is better achieved with radioimmunoassay (RIA)] is not required in the first screening for supernatant activity, EIA is quicker (the results are read by eye) without being less sensitive than RIA. The assay system should be tested using a conventional mouse antiserum against the antigen *before* hybridization is started; growing hybridomas do not allow time to be invested in assay modifications.

1. Materials

Polystyrene or polyvinyl chloride 96-well microtiter plates (Falcon)
Rabbit anti-mouse Ig covalently linked to alkaline phosphatase
    [self-made according to Kearney *et al.* (1979), a firm advertising it is
    Monoclonal Ab Inc., 719 Colorado Ave., Palo Alto, California]
Substrate: *p*-nitrophenyl phosphate (Merck, Darmstadt, West Germany)

2. Buffers

Saline: 0.15 *M* NaCl, 0.05% Tween 20, 0.02% NaN₃.
Blocking buffer: saline containing 10 m*M* phosphate, pH 7.2, and 1%
    bovine serum albumin (BSA).

Enzyme buffer: 0.05 M Tris–HCl, pH 8.0, 1 mM MgCl$_2$, 0.04% NaN$_3$, 5% BSA.

Substrate buffer: 10% diethanolamine in H$_2$O, 0.25 M MgCl$_2$, pH 9.8, adjusted with HCl; 60 mg of p-nitrophenyl phosphate is added per 100 ml substrate buffer which is made fresh each time.

3. Procedure

a. Coat plastic with antigen by pipetting 0.1 ml of about a 10μg/ml solution in PBS into the microtiter wells. Leave at least 2 hr at room temperature or overnight at 4°C.

The antigen preparation does not have to be pure; even in highly impure solutions antigen might bind. Remove antigen solution by flicking it out.

b. Block unreacted sites with 0.2 ml of blocking buffer for 2 hr at room temperature. Wash twice with saline.

c. Add 0.1 ml test solution (hybridoma supernatant) and incubate for 2 hr at room temperature. Wash three times with saline.

d. Add 0.2 ml of an appropriate dilution (around 50 mg protein) of enzyme-linked rabbit antimouse Ig. (Leave for 2 hr at room temperature.) Wash three times with saline.

e. Add 0.2 ml freshly prepared substrate mixture. Leave for 10–30 min or longer. Positive wells are indicated by the development of a yellow color. Stop the reaction by adding 50 μl 3 M NaOH.

Each assay includes negative (medium only; plastic is coated with unrelated antigen) and positive controls (conventional mouse antiserum at various concentrations).

a. If no color develops, check the test system by coating some wells with mouse Ig.

b. If color develops in all wells, check washing; attached cells may have some intrinsic enzymatic activity.

c. If color develops in all except negative controls, it may be the result of residual spleen cell activity (this happens if the test is performed too early with too few media changes). If all wells are indeed positive, multiple clones per well are present.

d. If later tests become negative for certain wells, the specific clone has been overgrown by an unrelated clone or has stopped Ig production probably as a result of chromosome loss. Early cloning might help maintain the clone.

e. If the test is positive for some wells even when unrelated antigen is used, it may be due to unusual "stickiness" of this particular Ig (often IgM). The contents of these wells cannot be further analyzed unless, in addition to antigen binding, other biological activities of the Ig are measured, e.g., lytic activity of IgM.

The EIA can only be a first screening in order to eliminate negative cultures. An inexperienced investigator is well advised not to keep too many cultures going.

a. Positive supernatants should if possible be checked with a different technique (immunofluorescence, a biological test, precipitation).

b. The EIA might not be the best test for the antigen in the first place; antigens which are easily attached to sheep erythrocytes may benefit from easy immunological tests (agglutination, lysis) performed with erythrocytes.

B. Storage of Antibodies

In order to make a high-titered supernatant, leave a culture so that cells overgrow and start to die. Such a supernatant usually contains 1–10 μg/ml IgM and 10–50 μl/ml IgG antibodies. Add 0.1% NaN_3 to prevent bacterial growth and store at $-20°C$. These supernatants will still be active after 2 yr of storage. If too many supernatants accumulate in the freezer, there are ways to alleviate the problem. Administer ip injections of 5×10^6 cells, washed in PBS, to mice. Beware of using mice which match the hybridoma antigens; e.g., if a BALB/c myeloma was fused with C57Bl/6 lymphocytes, the hybridoma should be injected into (BALB/c $\times$ C57Bl/6) F_1 mice. Hybridomas obtained with F_1 lymphocytes other than BALB/c cannot be grown in mice. So far, tumor growth has always been observed in over 50% of the injected animals, often in ascitic form. We usually kill a mouse with a well-developed ascites by bleeding it out and mixing its blood with the ascitic fluid. This enhances the clotting of the ascitic fluid which otherwise often clots after storage. Tumor cells can be spun out of the ascitic fluid and reinjected into new hosts or regrown in tissue culture. The fluid obtained contains between 1 and 10 mg antibody/ml, IgM generally giving lower, and IgG higher, concentration. The fluid should be aliquoted and stored frozen at $-70°C$. A disadvantage of ascitic fluid is contamination of the monoclonal antibody with normal mouse Ig.

C. Purification of Antibodies

1. Immunoglobulin G Antibodies

a. Materials

All mouse IgG antibodies (only one rat IgG) bind to protein A–Sepharose (Pharmacia) at pH 8.2. The bound IgG's elute at pH values between 6 and 3, which is characteristic of their subclass (Ey *et al.*, 1978). To simplify the procedure only three buffers are made (all solutions should contain 0.1% NaN_3 to prevent bacterial growth): buffer A:1 M Tris–HCl, pH 8.2; buffer B: 0.05 M Tris–HCl, pH 8.2, 0.15 M NaCl; buffer C: 0.05 M sodium citrate–citrate, pH 3.5, 0.15 M NaCl.

b. Procedure

  i. To 100 ml culture supernatant add 5 ml buffer A.

  ii. At room temperature, pass the supernatant slowly over a column containing 1 ml protein A–Sepharose swollen and washed in buffer B.

  iii. Wash column with 10 ml of buffer B.

  iv. Elute with 4 ml of buffer C into 2 ml of buffer A to raise the pH.

  v. Dialyze eluate against buffer B.

  vi. Recover column by washing with 10 ml of buffer B (the column can be used many times).

2. Immunoglobulin M Antibodies

a. Materials

  Immunoglobulin M antibodies can be partially purified from culture supernatants by 45% $(NH_4)_2SO_4$ precipitation and concanavalin A (Con A) affinity chromatography. The following buffers are made: buffer D: 0.05 M Tris–HCl, pH 7.4, 0.5 M NaCl, 10^{-4} M $CaCl_2$, 10^{-4} M $MgCl_2$, 10^{-4} M $MnCl_2$, 0.1% azide; buffer E: same as buffer D but containing 0.1 M α-methylglucoside.

b. Procedure

  i. To 100 ml of cold culture supernatant add slowly, with stirring, 28 gm of $(NH_4)_2SO_4$.

  ii. Leave overnight at 4°C.

  iii. Collect precipitate by centrifugation at 10,000 g for 20 min.

  iv. Wash precipitate with 45% $(NH_4)_2SO_4$ and recentrifuge.

  v. Solubilize pellet in 100 ml buffer D.

  vi. Pass slowly over 20 ml Con A–Sepharose (Pharmacia).

  vii. Wash with buffer D (check that OD_{280} drops to baseline).

  viii. Elute with 160 ml of buffer E (collect 10-ml fractions), measure OD_{280}, and pool fractions.

  ix. Concentrate over XM300 Amicon filters.

  x. Dialyze again with buffer B (Section V,C,a).

  xi. Restore Con A column by passing 60 ml of buffer D. (The column can be used many times.)

  This procedure also copurifies some FCS components, so preparing culture supernatants with the lowest possible FCS concentrations (between 1 and 5%) is advantageous.

D. Ouchterlony Test for Immunoglobulin Class and Subclass

  The easiest way to determine class and subclass specificity is an Ouchterlony analysis. For this the supernatants should be concentrated about 10-fold.

1. To 1 ml of supernatant add 1 ml of a saturated $(NH_4)_2SO_4$ solution. After 1 hr in the cold centrifuge at 10,000 g for 10 min, take up the pellet in 0.1 ml of water.
2. Use class- plus subclass-specific rabbit anti-mouse μ, α, $\gamma_{1,2a,2b,3}$ and χ, antisera (Litton Bionetics, Kentington, Maryland).
3. Place about (No. H401, Meloy, Springfield, Virginia) 20 μl of concentrated culture supernatant in the center of an Ouchterlony plate and arrange 20 μl of specific antisera around it. Use 20 μl normal mouse serum diluted 1:5 as a control for antisera activity.

It is advisable to countercheck serological determinants by, for example, sodium dodecyl sulfate polyacrylamide gel electrophoresis (SDS–PAGE) of radiolabeled supernatants. This separates μ, ϵ, α, and γ and may reveal γ_{2b} as a double band running slightly slower than the other γ subclasses (Köhler *et al.*, 1978). Functional properties can also be used [lytic activity of IgM, IgG_{2a}, and IgG_{2b}, or protein A or Con A binding (IgG versus IgM)].

VI. FREEZING AND THAWING OF HYBRIDOMA CELLS

A. Freezing of Cells

To 180 ml culture medium containing 20% serum, add 20 ml of dimethyl sulfoxide (DMSO, No. 802912, Merck, Hohenbrunn, West Germany). Do not try to filter-sterilize or autoclave the pure DMSO, because the filters are destroyed by DMSO and the DMSO is destroyed by autoclaving. The DMSO is so toxic that it should be sterile by itself, however, the freezing medium can be filter-sterilized. Always keep medium at 4°C.

Centrifuge down (170 g) about 5×10^6 cells (keep cold) and add 1 ml of *cold* freezing medium to the pellet. Transfer the freezing mixture to sterile 2-ml screw-cap vials. Avoid wetting the top. Close the vials so that they are airtight. Place the vials in a rack in a styrofoam box having a lid with walls about 1-cm thick. Keep the closed box at $-70°C$ for 1 day and then transfer the vials to liquid nitrogen.

B. Thawing of Cells

Take the vials out of the liquid nitrogen and thaw them quickly in a 37°C water bath. As soon as the medium is liquified, remove the cells with a Pasteur pipette and transfer them to a 50-ml tube containing *cold* growth medium. Pellet (170 g) the cells and wash them again with 50 ml *cold* medium. Grow the viable cells (as judged by trypan blue) at different dilutions. This is necessary because the trypan blue count often does not reflect the large fraction of cells which might die after a 1-day culture period.

ACKNOWLEDGMENT

Many of the protocols given in this chapter are based on a manual written for two EMBO courses on hybridoma techniques, held in Basel 1978 and 1980. The EMBO manual was written by Members of the Basel Institute for Immunology (M. Schreier, H. Hengartner, C. Berek, L. Forni, and M. Trucco) and by members of the Roche Project for Applied Immunology (T. Staehelin, J. Stocker, and B. Takacs). I want to thank them for their help in writing the manual and for their generosity in letting me use their protocols for this chapter.

REFERENCES

Eshhar, Z., Ofarim, M., and Waks, T. (1980). *J. Immunol.* **124**, 775.

Ey, P. L., Prowse, S. J., and Jenkin, C. R. (1978). *Immunochemistry* **15**, 429.

Fazekas de St. Groth, S., and Scheidegger, D. (1980). *J. Immunol. Methods* **32**, 297.

Galfré, G., Milstein, C., and Wright, B. (1979). *Nature (London)* **277**, 131.

Goding, J. W. (1980). *J. Immunol. Meth.* **39**, 285.

Kearney, J. F., Radbruch, A., Liesegang, B., and Rajewsky, K. (1979). *J. Immunol.* **123**, 1548.

Kennett, R. H., McKearn, T. J., and Bechtol, K. B. (eds.) (1980). "Monoclonal Antibodies." Plenum Press, New York.

Köhler, G. (1979). *In* "Immunol. Methods" (I. Lefkovits and B. Pernis, eds.), p. 397. Academic Press, New York.

Köhler, G., and Milstein, C. (1975). *Nature (London)* **56**, 495.

Köhler, G., Howe, S. C., and Milstein, C. (1976). *Eur. J. Immunol.* **6**, 292.

Köhler, G., Hengartner, H., and Shulman, M. J. (1978). *Eur. J. Immunol.* **8**, 82.

Lefkovits, I. (1979). *In* "Immunological Methods" (I. Lefkovits and B. Pernis, eds.), p. 355. Academic Press, New York.

Luben, R. A., and Mohler, M. A. (1980). *Mol. Immunol.* **17**, 635.

McGarrity, G. J., Vanaman, V., and Sarama, J. (1979). *Exp. Cell Res.* **121**, 159.

McMicheal, H. J., and Bastin, J. M. (1980). "Immunology Today." Elsevier/North Holland Biomedical Press, Amsterdam.

Margulies, P. H., Kuehl, W. M., and Scharff, M. D. (1976). *Cell* **8**, 405.

Melchers, F., Potler, M., and Warner, L. (eds.) (1978). "Current Topics in Microbiology and Immunology," Volume 81.

Milstein, C., Clark, M. R., Galfré, G., and Cuello, A. C. (1980). In "Immunology 80" (M. Fougereau and J. Dansset, eds.), p. 17. Academic Press, New York.

Olsson, L., and Kaplan, H. S. (1980). *Proc. Natl. Acad. Sci.* **77**, 5429.

Raschke, W. (1980). *Biochim. Biophys. Acta* **605**, 113.

Russel, W. C., Newman, C., and Williams, D. M. (1975). *Nature (London)* **253**, 461.

Shulman, M., and Köhler, G. (1979). *In* "Cells of Immunoglobulin Synthesis" (B. Pernis and H. Vogel, eds.), p. 275. Academic Press, New York.

Shulman, M., Wilde, D., and Köhler, G. (1978). *Nature (London)* **276**, 269.

Stocker, J. W., and Heusser, C. H. (1979). *J. Immunol. Methods* **26**, 87.

Trowbridge, I. S. (1978). *J. Exp. Med.* **148**, 313.

18

Enzyme Immunoassay for the Detection of Hybridoma Products

John W. Stocker, Fabio Malavasi,
and Massimo Trucco

I. INTRODUCTION

Enzyme immunoassays (EIAs) have found widespread application since their introduction (Engvall and Perlmann, 1971) and offer several advantages over radioimmunoassay (RIA). Enzyme-coupled reagents are generally stable during prolonged storage, thus eliminating the need for repeated labeling with isotopes which undergo decay. The use of enzyme-coupled reagents avoids the dangers and special precautions involved in working with radioactive isotopes. In addition, the change in the color of a substrate can be seen by the eye, thus circumventing the requirement for expensive equipment for measuring radioactivity.

Thus EIAs have been found to be ideally suited for screening for monoclonal antibody production in tissue culture (Fig. 1 shows a general

IMMUNOLOGICAL METHODS, VOL. II

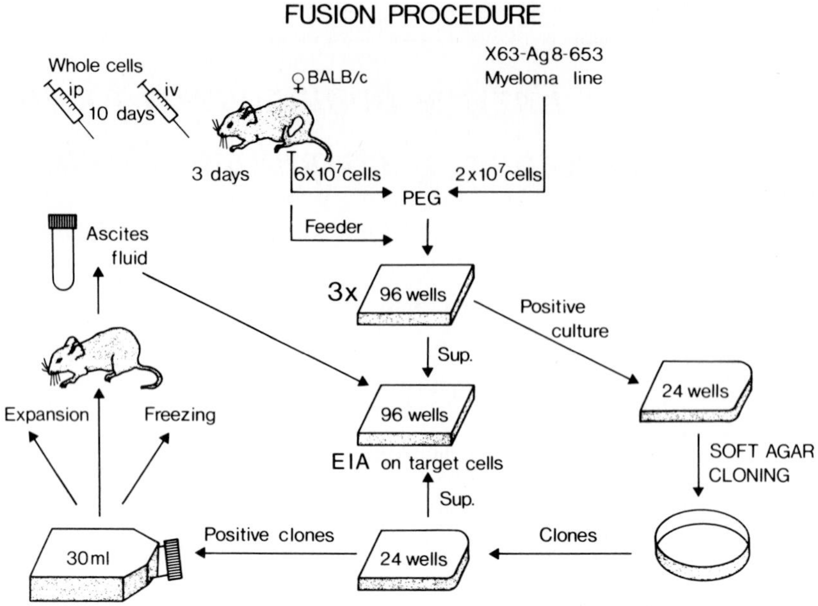

FUSION PROCEDURE

Fig. 1. Schematic description of the fusion procedure stressing three steps in which EIA is used to detect antibody binding: screening of primary cultures, screening of clones, and determination of the titer of an ascites fluid.

plan). In this application, antigen is immobilized on a plastic surface, and supernatant medium from the hybridoma culture is added. The binding of monoclonal antibodies to the antigen layer is detected in a second step by incubation with an enzyme-coupled anti-immunoglobulin (anti-Ig) having specificity for the monoclonal reagent. In this chapter, the application of this method in the detection of mouse hybridoma products will be described, and here the second step involves incubation with enzyme-coupled rabbit anti-mouse IgG.

Where the monoclonal antibody is directed against a soluble protein antigen, use has been made of nonspecific adsorption of proteins to a plastic surface to allow antigen immobilization (Catt and Tregear, 1967). This property has found application in the screening of monoclonal antibodies to soluble antigens by RIA and is equally suitable for EIA.

For antibodies against cell surface antigens, the screening assay has usually been performed using fresh or fixed cells in suspension and has required time-consuming centrifugation steps. A method has been recently described (Stocker and Heusser, 1979) for immobilizing cells on a plastic surface where the cell layer can be used as a solid-phase target for immunoassay procedures. The application of this principle in EIA for cell surface antigens will be described in this chapter.

The presence of intrinsic enzyme activity within and on the surface of cells can sometimes be a problem in EIA, where it results in a high background. This problem is not overcome by fixation of the cells and is best solved by choosing an enzyme not present on the cell surface. Alkaline phosphatase has been found to be a suitable enzyme for assays involving cell targets, and its use will be described here.

II. MATERIALS

A. Rabbit Anti-Mouse Immunoglobulin G

1. Immunization Schedule

Rabbits are injected intramuscularly (im) every second week with 200–500 μg of mouse IgG (Nordic Immunological Laboratories) in Freund's complete adjuvant (1 vol of adjuvant plus 1 vol of Ig in saline solution). After 3 months, sera from the injected rabbits are tested on Ouchterlony plates against mouse IgG.

2. Affinity Purification

Affinity purification is achieved by eluting the rabbit anti-mouse Ig's from mouse IgG coupled to Sepharose 4B (Jaton *et al.*, 1979).

3. Enzyme Labeling

Rabbit anti-mouse Ig is coupled with alkaline phosphatase using the general method of Kearney *et al.* (1979). Alkaline phosphatase (400 μl) (Boehringer, 5 mg/ml, 2000 U) is centrifuged for 10 min at 12,000 g in a Fisher centrifuge at 4°C. The supernatant is discarded, and the pellet resuspended in 50 μl 0.15 M phosphate-buffered saline (PBS), pH 7.2. The suspension is then transferred to a collodion bag (Sartorius GmbH, Göttingen, West Germany) and dialyzed against PBS. Then 100 μl affinity-purified rabbit anti-mouse IgG (5 mg/ml) is added, and the final volume adjusted to 200 μl with PBS. The mixture is then transferred to a plastic tube, and the volume brought to 500 μl with PBS. To 500 μl of antibody–enzyme mixture is added 4 μl of 25% glutaraldehyde solution, followed by incubation for 2 hr at room temperature. The volume is adjusted to 2 ml with PBS, and the solution dialyzed against PBS overnight at 4°C. The dialyzed material is diluted to 5 ml using Tris buffer [0.5 M Tris, 0.001 M MgCl$_2$,

0.04% NaN$_3$, 5% bovine serum albumin (BSA)]. The enzyme-linked antibody solution can be kept for at least 1 yr at 4°C.

4. Testing of the Conjugate

Cells of a human lymphoblastoid line are immobilized in microtiter wells (see below), and a solution of mouse monoclonal antibody known to bind to the line is added. The EIA is performed (Section III,A,1) using dilutions of the enzyme-linked antibody, and an optimal dilution is determined. This usually corresponds to about 1:500.

B. Monoclonal Antibodies

Fifty microliters of supernatant containing antibodies from a confluent hybrid cell culture is generally enough to give a strongly positive reaction against 2×10^5 target cells. From a single well of a microtiter tray into which the fusion mixture has been seeded (Fig. 1), 150 μl of supernatant is easily obtained. This allows three replicates to be set up for each hybrid culture. The antibodies used in the examples were either previously described monoclonal antibodies against HLA structures (Trucco *et al.,* 1979) or monoclonal antibodies directed against hepatitis B antigen (HBs) obtained using the general fusion procedure shown in Fig. 1.

C. Target Cells

Two methods allow the attachment of cells to the surface of wells on polyvinyl chloride (PVC) microtiter plates (No. 1–220–25, Cooke, Alexandria, Virginia) where the cell layer can be used as a solid-phase target for immunoassay procedures (Stocker and Heusser, 1979). Small cells, such as erythrocytes, splenocytes, thymocytes, and bacteria, can be immobilized by centrifugation followed by glutaraldehyde fixation, which results in a firm attachment of the cells to the PVC surface. Larger cells, such as human lymphoblasts, mouse myelomas, and human melanoma cells, require prior loading of the plastic surface with a protein which binds the cells. This "anchor" protein can be an antibody or lectin capable of binding to the cell target. Cells are centrifuged onto the coated plastic surface and can be used directly as targets or fixed with glutaraldehyde to provide increased stability of the cell layer during washing procedures. Furthermore, fixation permits storage of the assay plates.

D. Other Reagents

1. Substrate

For alkaline phosphatase, *p*-nitrophenyl phosphate dissolved in diethanolamine buffer is a suitable substrate. *p*-Nitrophenyl phosphate (20 mg) (No. 6850, Merck) is dissolved in 50 ml of diethanolamine buffer [48 ml of diethanolamine (No. 803116, Merck) and 24.5 mg of $MgCl_2$ (No. 5833, Merck) are added to 400 ml of H_2O; the solution is brought to pH 9.8 using HCl and adjusted to a final volume of 500 ml with water]. The substrate must be prepared immediately before use, while the diethanolamine buffer can be kept at room temperature in a brown glass bottle. In the presence of the enzyme, the colorless *p*-nitrophenyl phosphate is split to phosphate and *p*-nitrophenol, which is yellow. The reaction can be assessed visually or by using a photometer reading at 405.

2. Phytohemagglutinin P

Phytohemagglutinin P (PHA-P) is obtained from Difco Laboratories, Detroit, Michigan.

3. Egg White Buffer

Four to six hen's eggs are broken into a beaker, the yolk being retained in the eggshell. The egg white is stirred for about 1 hr in 500 ml PBS with 0.1% NaN_3. The suspension is then centrifuged at 10,000 g for 15 min to remove debris, and the A_{280} of the solution is measured in a spectrophotometer and adjusted to 14 by the addition of PBS.

E. Vertical Light Path Photometer

The Titertek Multiskan (Flow Laboratories) is a vertical light path photometer able to give rapid assessment of a color reaction in the wells of microtiter plates. It prints out the value of the absorbance to three decimal places. The printout identifies the vertical column by number, followed by the absorbance readings for wells in horizontal rows A to H of the microtiter trays. The instrument can also work with a preselected absorbance range which is divided into 10 equal parts represented by the numbers 0 to 9. These numbers are printed out in an 8 × 12 matrix corresponding to the layout of a microtiter tray (see example in Fig. 3).

III. ENZYME IMMUNOASSAY

A. Immobilized Cells

Cells from tissue culture are conveniently immobilized by centrifugation onto an anchor protein layer adsorbed to the plastic. In the example described here (Fig. 3) cells from two human lymphoblastoid cell lines are attached to microtiter plates using the lectin PHA-P, followed by glutaraldehyde fixation. When immobilizing small cells (Section II,C), the anchor protein layer can be omitted.

Binding of Hybridoma Products to Human Lymphoblastoid Cell Lines

1. To each well of the assay plate, 50 μl PHA-P and 20 μg/ml in PBS are added. Coating is accomplished by leaving the plate at room temperature overnight or by incubation for 1 hr at 37°C. Free lectin is removed by shaking over a sink and washing the plate three times in PBS.

2. The cells are harvested from the culture bottle, washed three times in PBS, and resuspended to 4×10^6/ml. Fifty microliters of cell suspension is added to each lectin-coated well.

3. The plate is centrifuged at 50–100 g for 1 min and then gently immersed in a beaker containing freshly prepared 0.25% glutaraldehyde solution in PBS. The plate must be immersed carefully to avoid disturbance of the cell layer and the trapping of air in the wells.

4. After fixation for 5–7 min, the plate is shaken over a sink to remove glutaraldehyde. It is then washed by three cycles of immersion in PBS, and the washing solution being shaken out each time.

5. The wells are then filled with egg white buffer (EWB) and kept for 30 min at room temperature to saturate protein-binding sites on the plastic and glycoprotein-binding sites of the lectin. It should be noted that a BSA solution meets the first but not the second requirement and is unsuitable for this assay.

6. Fifty microliters of monoclonal antibody solution (culture supernatant or ascites fluid diluted with EWB) is added to each well and kept at 4°C for at least 90 min (see Fig. 2). This incubation can extend overnight if the plate is kept in a moist chamber.

7. The plates are washed three times with PBS, and then 50 μl of appropriately diluted (Section II,A,4) enzyme-labeled anti-mouse Ig in EWB is added. The plates are kept at 4°C for 90 min.

8. After washing three times with PBS, 200 μl substrate solution is added to each well (Section II,D,1). Approximately 30 min later the colorless solution turns bright yellow in the wells where antibodies have bound to the

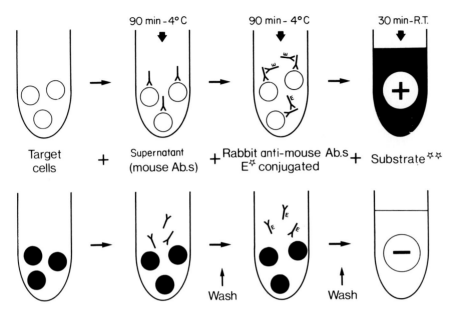

☆E = Alkaline phosphatase
☆☆p-nitrophenylphosphate in diethanolamine buffer

Fig. 2. The principle of the EIA (Enzyme Immune Assay) method. (+), positive reaction; (−), negative reaction; R. T., room temperature.

cells, and the reaction can be assessed by eye or by using a vertical light path photometer (Fig. 3 and Section II,E). The reaction can be stopped by adding 3 M NaOH at 25–50 μl per well. The plate must be kept in the dark before reading.

Example A. Cells from two different human lines were attached to microtiter wells using PHA-P. Daudi is a Burkitt lymphoma line which, because of the deletion of chromosome 15, lacks β_2 microglobulin and consequently also lacks HLA,A, B, and C antigens at the cell surface but still expresses HLA, D determinants. WT 18 is an Epstein–Barr virus-transformed cell line from an HLA homozygous donor. Both cell lines were tested against supernatants from different monoclonal hybrid cultures with known specificities against HLA structures.

As shown in Fig. 3, Daudi cells only bind antibodies directed against HLA-DR antigens, while WT 18 binds antibodies to β_2 microglobulin, non-polymorphic HLA,$\overline{ABC}$ and HLA, $\overline{DR}$ structures. The antibody recognizing the polymorphic specificity HLA, DRw 3 + 5 + 6 binds to Daudi, which bears this antigen, but not to WT 18, which carries HLA,DRw2.

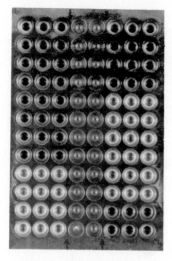

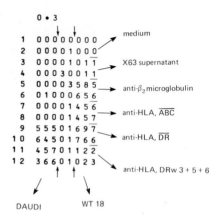

```
        0 • 3
           ↓   ↓
   1   0 0 0 0 0 0 0 0         medium
   2   0 0 0 0 1 0 0 0
   3   0 0 0 0 1 0 1 1         X63 supernatant
   4   0 0 0 3 0 0 1 1
   5   0 0 0 0 3 5 8 5         anti-β₂microglobulin
   6   0 1 0 0 0 6 5 6
   7   0 0 0 0 1 4 5 6
   8   0 0 0 0 1 4 5 7         anti-HLA, ABC
   9   5 5 5 0 1 6 9 7
  1 0  6 4 5 0 1 7 6 6         anti-HLA, DR
  1 1  4 5 7 0 1 1 2 2
  1 2  3 6 6 0 1 0 2 3
                              anti-HLA, DRw 3 + 5 + 6
       ↙      ↑   ↑      ↘
     DAUDI        WT 18
```

Fig. 3. Binding of various monoclonal antibodies specific for HLA-related structures to two lymphoblastoid lines. Hybridoma supernatants were reacted with immobilized cells of the DAUDI and WT 18 lines. The results of the EIA are shown in a photograph of the assay plate and on a printout from the vertical light path photometer. In the photograph the lightest wells represent a positive reaction, which is seen in the actual test as a yellow color. In the printout, the light absorbance is scored on a scale of 0 to 9, where 0 is a negative reaction. Rows 1 and 2 are controls containing cells with tissue culture medium. Rows 3 and 4 show reactions with supernatant from the X63 myeloma line, rows 5 and 6 with anti-β_2 microglobulin, rows 7 and 8 with anti-HLA, $\overline{ABC}$, rows 9 and 10 with anti-HLA, $\overline{DR}$, and rows 11 and 12 with anti-HLA, DRw $3 + 5 + 6$. Odd-numbered rows received 50 μl of supernatant and even-numbered rows received 25 μl.

B. Use of Soluble Antigen

Antigen dissolved in PBS is kept on a microtiter plate to allow nonspecific adsorption to the plastic and then used for solid-phase EIA. An example is given here of the use of the system to detect monoclonal antibodies to HBs in supernatant fluid from individual clones in a mixed population of antibody-producing and non-antibody-producing cells.

1. The protein antigen is diluted with PBS to a concentration of 1–5 μg/ml. Fifty microliters is added to each well, leaving some uncoated wells to serve as negative controls for nonspecific binding of reagents to the plastic (first column of the tray in Fig. 4).

2. The plate is kept for at least 2 hr at room temperature. Plates can be stored for weeks at this stage if 0.1% NaN$_3$ is added to the PBS and the

93	107	98	200	110	175	140	1280	225	2130	195	111
-	-	-	-	-	-	-	+	-	+	-	-
101	131	178	120	210	150	4510	170	130	180	215	5950
-	-	-	-	-	-	++	-	-	-	-	+++
131	156	137	175	200	275	162	280	155	235	225	
-	-	-	-	-	-	-	-	-	-	-	
107	138	191	120	170	215	3620	145	210	180	165	
-	-	-	-	-	-	++	-	-	-	-	
115	101	109	180	215	175	211	210	250	165	225	
-	-	-	-	-	-	-	-	-	-	-	
121	167	143	155	145	205	131	205	260	235	220	
-	-	-	-	-	-	-	-	-	-	-	
98	198	193	190	225	260	120	5040	220	165	5790	
-	-	-	-	-	-	-	+++	-	-	+++	
104	171	170	150	235	275	3400	210	160	155	6420	
-	-	-	-	-	-	++	-	-	-	+++	

Fig. 4. Comparison between EIA and RIA in screening supernatants from clones producing anti-HBs antibodies. Supernatants were tested in parallel for binding to HBs using EIA and RIA as described in Example B (see text). In each case one square represents assays with a single culture supernatant. The numbers are counts per minute of ^{125}I-rabbit anti-mouse Ig bound in the RIA. The symbols + and − refer to the score given in the EIA, where − is a negative reading and + to + + + are a measure of the strength of the positive color reaction. The first column, used as a blank, is a control without protein antigen; the second is a negative control where medium alone was used; the other squares are all individual clones tested for the production of anti-HBs monoclonal antibodies.

plates are stored in a moist chamber at 4°C or room temperature.

3. The wells are completely filled with a solution of 1% BSA in PBS to block the remaining sides on the plastic for nonspecific absorption. The EWB described above can also be used for this purpose and results in a lower background in EIA, especially where IgM monoclonal antibodies are to be detected. The plate is kept at room temperature for at least 30 min, followed by removal of the protein solution by flicking it into a sink. The wells are then filled with 100 μl (2 drops) of PBS, and the plates covered and stored at 4°C for weeks or months until use. Before use, the plates are rinsed again with PBS.

4. The EIA is then performed exactly as described in Section III,A, steps 6–8.

Example B. A cell population containing a mixture of hybridoma cells producing anti-HBs antibodies and non-antibody-producing cells was cloned by limiting dilution. Supernatant medium from the individual cultures was tested in an EIA and in a RIA against the HBs adsorbed to microtiter wells.

The supernatants were collected when cell growth had reached 10–20% confluence, in this case on day 8 following cloning. Figure 4 shows a direct comparison between the two assay methods. Note the complete agreement between the results obtained in the two systems.

IV. CONCLUSION

Enzyme immunoassay provides a safe, reliable, convenient screening test for the detection of monoclonal antibodies. It can be used to demonstrate antibodies in tissue culture supernatants and in ascites fluid from hybridoma-bearing mice. The test can be used for soluble antigens adsorbed to plastic or on immobilized cell layers where cell surface antigens are to be studied.

REFERENCES

Catt, K., and Tregear, G. W. (1967). *Science* **158**, 1570.
Engvall, E., and Perlmann, P. (1971). *Immunochemistry* **8**, 871.
Jaton, J.-C., Brandt, D. Ch., and Vassalli, P. (1979). "Immunological Methods" (I. Lefkovits and B. Pernis, eds.), p. 54. Academic Press, New York.
Kearney, J. F., Radbruch, A., Liesegang, B., and Rajewsky, K. (1979). *J. Immunol.* **123**, 1548.
Stocker, J. W., and Heusser, C. H. (1979). *J. Immunol. Meth.* **26**, 87.
Trucco, M. M., Garotta, G., Stocker, J. W., and Ceppellini, R. (1979). *Immunol. Rev.* **47**, 219.

Index

309